PRAISE FOR

Motherhood is a journey.
Mommy MDs are your guides.

It is fascinating to find the real experiences of physician moms interposed with solid data about healthy pregnancy and delivery. *The Mommy MD Guide to Pregnancy and Birth* is an enjoyable and enlightening book that will "hold hands" with women through their pregnancies.

—*Joanna M. Cain, MD, Chace/Joukowsky Professor and chair, assistant dean of women's health at the Warren Alpert Medical School of Brown University, and obstetrician and gynecologist-in-chief at Women & Infants Hospital, both in Providence, RI*

The Mommy MD Guide to Your Baby's First Year is fun, easy to read, and informative. I love that the advice from physicians is practical and based on experience, in addition to medical expertise. Since it is a series of vignettes, it's easy to read and pick up in between other activities, which is ideal for busy people like me and new moms. Best thing: I plan to use the tips I learned with our baby-to-be! It helped me feel some relief to know other physicians, who are supposed to be experts and who are in similar shoes as I soon may be, felt as nervous to become a mom as I am!

—*Jennifer Arnold, MD, a neonatologist and the medical director of the Pediatric Simulation Center at Texas Children's Hospital and an assistant professor at Baylor College of Medicine, both in Houston, and the star of TLC's* The Little Couple

I found a quiet corner in the living room and flipped open this new guide, *The Mommy MD Guide to Pregnancy and Birth*, about a topic I last experienced 10 years ago. The more I read, the more I kept thinking to myself, "I wish this book had been *around* 10 years ago." I would have devoured every word if I'd read it 20 years ago, as I plodded through my very first experience with the baffling world of pregnancy. This book really is different from every other pregnancy book I've read.

I loved the premise of advice coming from doctor moms. When our third child was born, we took him to our pediatrician to discuss his endless fussing. We got very different advice with that visit (I feel your pain!) than we had four years earlier, when we'd brought in our second child with the same problem (Just relax. You're making him stressed.) The difference? In that window of time, our pediatrician had married and had two little ones of his own. Suddenly, all of his advice had changed. There's something very comforting about knowing the person giving the advice has actually been in the trenches themselves.

The Mommy MD Guide to Pregnancy and Birth has advice from 60 doctors who are moms. Aside from the great medical advice, I was drawn to the anecdotal feeling of this book. As I read, I felt like I was sitting in the living room with these women as they shared their personal stories. I'm a person who loves to hear a good birth story, and I was really drawn to the personal nature of the advice. Instead of feeling like it was coming from a textbook, the advice feels like it's coming from a girlfriend who's just navigated the road herself. But it went beyond "just" a girlfriend's guide, because it was a girlfriend's guide times 60.

I highly recommend *The Mommy MD Guide to Pregnancy and Birth*. I have a feeling many dads wouldn't mind reading it either since it's not long chapters of information, but short snippets of advice, gathered in a very logical way.

I enjoyed the website that's hosted by the coauthors and look forward to the series this team is working on, covering the other stages of parenting, from newborn sleep issues to elementary school struggles. It's a great idea that was truly done right.

—*Judy Berna, a mom of four and a writer for GeekMom.com*

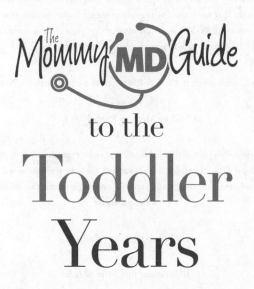

The Mommy MD Guide

to the

Toddler Years

Tips That 62 Doctors Who Are Also
Mothers Use During Their Children's Toddler Years

By Rallie McAllister, MD, MPH
and Jennifer Bright Reich

MOMOSA PUBLISHING

649.122
Mac

10/12
B+T

This book is intended as a reference volume only, not as a medical manual.
The information given here is designed to help you make informed decisions about
your child's health. It is not intended as a substitute for any treatment that may have been
prescribed by your child's doctor. If you suspect that your child has a medical problem,
we urge you to seek competent medical help.

Internet addresses given in this book were accurate at the time it went to press.

Printed in Hong Kong

Illustrations by Carrie Wendel

Book design by Leanne Coppola

Library of Congress Control Number 2012943917

ISBN 978–0–9844804–4–9

2 4 6 8 10 9 7 5 3 1 paperback

The Mommy MD Guides

Motherhood is a journey.
Mommy MDs are your guides.

MommyMDGuides.com

Contents

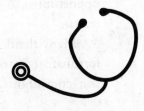

Acknowledgments

The books in the Mommy MD Guides series are proof positive that if we dream big, work hard, and believe in ourselves, we can accomplish anything we feel passionate about. If we're lucky enough to have the help and support of friends and family while we're at it, the process is a whole lot easier, and a lot more fun.

I feel incredibly blessed to have Jennifer as a friend, coauthor, and business partner. Although it's roughly 600 miles from my desk to hers, she's as close to me as a sister. Jennifer and I are both passionate about helping moms carry out one of the most important jobs in the world—raising healthy, happy children. We couldn't do this without the help of our awesome team at the Mommy MD Guides or the incredible physicians who generously shared the stories of their lives. I'm grateful to each of them.

I'm also grateful to my family—Robin, Oakley, Gatlin, Chad, Lindsey, Bella, and Cam—and very thankful for all the love and laughter we share.

—*Rallie McAllister, MD, MPH*

⌇⌇

First and foremost, thank you from the bottom of my heart to Rallie. Publishing our third Mommy MD Guide is a dream come true! Every day that I get to work with her on this amazing adventure is a gift. I will always be grateful to her!

Thank you to the dozens of smart, kind doctors who shared their stories and their wisdom with us for this book. Talking with them was both an honor and a delight, and I'm so happy for the opportunity to share their experiences and wisdom with our readers.

Many thanks also to the Mommy MD Guides team. I'm so fortunate to work with such a talented group: editor Amy Kovalski, consultant Jennifer Goldsmith, writer Marie Suszynski, factchecker Linda Hager, designer Leanne Coppola, layout designer Susan Eugster, illustrator Carrie Wendel, indexer Nanette Bendyna, executive assistant Crystal Smith, photographer Samantha Yob, and Magnum Offset Printing sales manager Alice Fan.

I am very grateful for the talented people at the Cadence Group, especially Amy Collins, Nicole Riley, and Bethany Brown, for helping us to achieve our goals of getting our books into more stores.

I am very grateful to Drew Frantzen, our logo designer, who has helped to establish the very tone and style of our brand.

Thank you to my mentors and friends who have shared their wisdom and advice: Susan Berg, Elly Phillips, Anne Egan, Chris Krogermeier, Joey Green, Tim Foster, Maggie Agentis-Ryan, and Buddy Lesavoy.

Most of all, thank you to my family— Mike, Tyler, and Austin Reich and John R. Bright, Mary L. Bright, Robyn Swatsburg, and Judy Beck—for all of your support, encouragement, and love and for making my life so rich, rewarding—and fun.

—*Jennifer Bright Reich*

Introduction

Looking back, our children's toddler years feel a bit like a blur. They don't call them the "terrible twos" and say "three is the new terrible twos" for nothing. Toddlers are challenging in many ways. They're learning and growing at an incredible rate, and at the same time, they're pushing and stretching against boundaries, in every direction. Toddlers are like pint-sized teenagers.

To create this book, we spoke with 62 Mommy MD Guides—doctors who are also mothers. Some of these Mommy MD Guides have children who are all grown up with toddlers of their own. They're Grammy MD Guides! Combined, these doctors have centuries of experience as physicians, and they have 142 children and 10 grandchildren.

These smart, funny, fascinating women opened their hearts and lives to us. They shared their challenges with picky eating, tantrums, and night terrors. They also talked with us about their joy as their toddlers celebrated birthdays and holidays, learned to use the potty, and enjoyed playdates, shopping trips, and vacations. These Mommy MD Guides generously shared the wisdom and tips that they learned to make it through their children's toddler years.

Because doctors so often see the things that can go wrong, they try to do everything as right as they can for their own health and for that of their families. Physicians are a healthier group than the whole. Even though women physicians sometimes will just suffer with things that affect them alone, caring for their children is different. Mommy MD Guides combine all of their experience and training as physicians with their wisdom and knowledge as moms to skillfully care for their toddlers.

The more than 900 tips and stories in this book are presented in the Mommy MD Guides' own words, and each tip is clearly attributed to the doctor who lived it. Most of these stories contain kernels of advice. This is what doctors who are also mothers did to make it through their children's toddler years. Other stories in this book are just that—true stories. The implied advice is: I made it through this pesky problem, and you can too!

Even though this book is filled with advice from a select group—all Mommy MD Guides—you'll find that they hold vastly differing opinions. Parenting is filled with issues that people feel very strongly about. When should children give up their bottles? Should you spank, or not? When should you move your toddler into a big-kid bed? We've presented many different viewpoints—but not with the intent to confuse or to offer conflicting advice. Instead, these diverse voices are presented so that you can choose what's best for you and your family.

As you read this book, keep in mind that every toddler is different, and in fact every mom is different. Children change and grow at different rates. We encourage you to use the index at the end of this book as a resource, in addition to reading topic by topic.

Welcome to the Mommy MD Guides! Best wishes for your family's health and happiness!

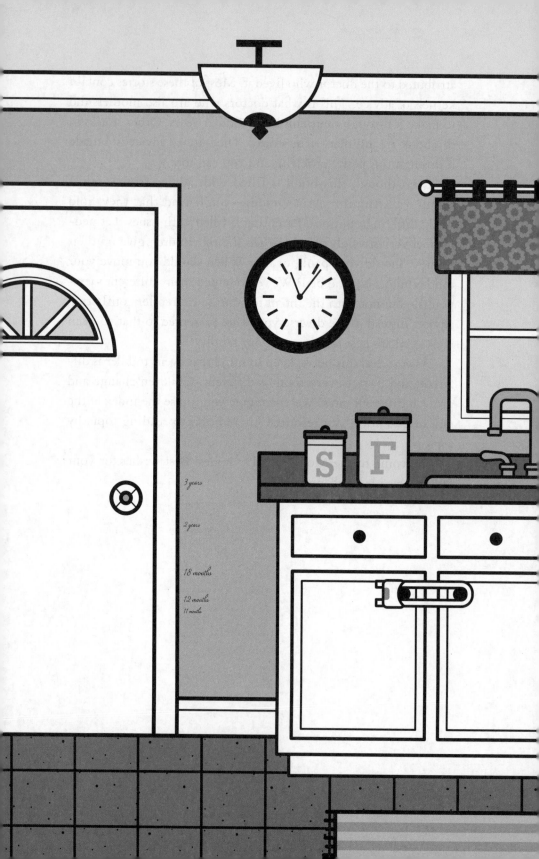

3 years

2 years

18 months

12 months
11 months

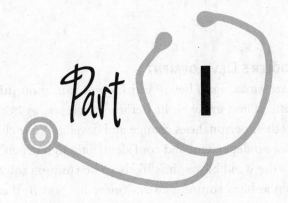

Part I

GROWTH AND DEVELOPMENT

Chapter 1
Watching Your Toddler Grow

YOUR TODDLER'S DEVELOPMENT

Toddlers are amazing: They're quirky and fun, inquisitive and spontaneous. They grow right before your eyes, as both their bodies and their personalities change and develop. Your child will become more independent and confident, although depending on which way the wind blows, he's likely to be running toward you just as often as he is running away. You're his port in the storm, and when all of the changes in his toddler world become too much, he'll cling to you for support. There's nowhere else he'd rather be.

TAKING CARE OF YOU

Your toddler will likely gain as many as 10 pounds from his first birthday to his third. You're probably hoping *not* to do the same! The fact that your child is gaining independence presents a great opportunity to take some time for yourself—to get into better shape than ever before. Why not join a gym such as Curves, take a fitness class like Zumba, or simply invite a neighbor or a friend to join you on regular walks? You're worth it!

JUSTIFICATION FOR A CELEBRATION

Your toddler is growing and developing so rapidly that there are many reasons to celebrate. During the transformative toddler years, your child's walk will break into a run. He'll kick his first ball. He'll walk up steps, and later he'll learn to walk back down again. He'll be able to pick up small items with the greatest of ease. In a few short years, your child's vocabulary will go from zero words to more than 300. Someday soon, your toddler will say these wonderful words: *I love you too, Mommy.* And you'll hear them in your heart forever.

Growing

As your baby turned one year old, you probably noticed his growth slowing. He might not be outgrowing his clothes as quickly as he did as an infant. Toddlers grow an average of 2½ inches each year, and they gain between three and five pounds each year.

You'll likely see an amazing transformation in your child's body as he grows from a baby—with a relatively large head and short legs and arms—to a toddler—with his head, arms, and legs in better proportion.

During the toddler years, you'll notice that your child's head growth also slows. The average toddler's head grows ¾ inch in his second year, but then it grows only ¾ to 1¼ inches in the next 10 years. Your child's pediatrician will probably stop measuring his head circumference after his two-year well-child visit.

Don't be surprised if you catch yourself looking at your toddler's face, searching for the baby face that was there just a few months ago! Your child's face will change in his toddler years. His lower jaw will become more pronounced, and his upper jaw will widen to make room for his permanent teeth. Your toddler's face will actually become larger, and his features will become more chiseled. The toddler years are a wonderful time of growth and change!

I found that one of the most amazing and rewarding parts of my kids' toddler years was how important I was to them. At this time in your child's life, you are the center of his universe. Toddlers really listen to and watch everything that you say and do. That's both a huge responsibility and an enormous privilege. This continues as a child grows, but at no time is it more important as in those first few years.

—*Ayala Laufer-Cahana, MD, a mom of 16- and 14-year-old sons and a 12-year-old daughter, a pediatrician, and the founder of Herbal Water Inc., in Wynnewood, PA*

∽◦◦

All through my girls' childhoods, they went to regular well-child doctor visits. The nurses carefully measured their weights and heights. After we got home, I marked their heights on charts that we hung on a wall in each of their rooms. My kids loved watching their heights change and how they compared with each other. I would always reinforce them by saying things like, "You're growing a healthy body" and "You've done such a good job eating your vegetables!"

—*Cathy Marshall, MD, a mom of 28-, 14-, and 11-year-old daughters and a pediatrician in private practice, in Encino, CA*

∽◦◦

When I take my sons to their well-child visits, the doctors always check their growth by taking their weight and height measurements and plotting them on a standard growth chart. They also write down the information in a small book I bring with me to each appointment so I can keep track too.

—*Deborah Kulick, MD, a mom of two-year-old and eight-month-old sons, a child and adolescent psychiatrist at the Everett Teen Health Center, and an instructor in psychiatry at Harvard Medical School and the Cambridge Health Alliance, in Boston, MA*

∽◦◦

My daughter has been growing well. In fact, she's in the 95th percentile for height. I do have to monitor her weight carefully, though. She's always been tiny. I have a bathroom scale at home, and every so often, I have her stand on it.

"Look! You're getting big and strong," I say.

—*Tanya Douglas Holland, MD, a mom of a two-year-old daughter, a women's health advocate, and a consultant in medical affairs to a pharmaceutical company, in Atlanta, GA*

My twins were small as toddlers, especially my daughter, who hovered around the 5th percentile. I wasn't too concerned because she was keeping to her own growth curve, which means she was growing at a steady rate, even if she was always in the 5th percentile. Some kids are just smaller than others. I'm not a huge person, and neither is my husband.

For a while, my daughter did drop off the growth chart altogether. I started giving her some PediaSure to drink each day to boost her calorie intake. Soon after that, my daughter was back on the chart again.

—*Ann Contrucci, MD, a mom of 13-year-old boy-girl twins who works as a pediatric emergency physician, in Atlanta, GA*

❧

My older son has always been small, and he continues to skim the bottom of the last percentile on the growth curve. I've tracked his growth very carefully, but I try not to worry about it. Someone has to be at the bottom of the percentiles after all! I'm Indian and small, and my husband isn't tall either, so I know my son comes by his size naturally.

I know my son isn't going to be a basketball player, or a football player for that matter. But he is following his own growth curve, and I take comfort in that.

—*Leena Shrivastava Dev, MD, a mom of 15- and 11-year-old sons, a general pediatrician, and an advocate for child safety, in Philadelphia, PA*

❧

My son eats like a horse, but he has always been a skinny kid. As my son became a toddler, he was growing but not filling out. At times he was in the 75th percentile for height, but not even on the growth chart for weight. Because he was meeting his milestones and had been breastfed, I tried not to obsess too much about the growth charts.

My son isn't a big meal eater, so I offer him lots of healthy snacks throughout the day. Now he's finally starting to get a little tummy.

—*Lennox McNeary, MD, a mom of a three-year-old son, a specialist in physical medicine and rehabilitation at Carilion Clinic, and a cofounder of the Mommy Doctors Bakery (makers of Milkin' Cookies), in Roanoke, VA*

My younger son was really small when he was born. He was barely on the growth chart.

During my son's first year, he was in the 3rd percentile. I tried not to worry about it too much because he was growing and developing normally.

When I took my son to his two-year well-child visit, he measured at the 25th percentile. I was very excited about that! It's helpful for parents to know that around two years of age, there is a bigger range of "normal" size, so the growth chart is more forgiving.

—*Rebecca Reamy, MD, a mom of seven- and two-year-old sons and a pediatrician in emergency medicine at Children's Healthcare of Atlanta, in Georgia*

Rallie's Tip

I worried about plenty of things when my boys were toddlers, but fortunately their rate of growth wasn't one of them. My husband and I are both tall, and my boys were all rather long at birth. I was happy to let our pediatrician track my boys' growth on their medical charts at his office, and he always let me know that they were following their growth curves nicely.

That doesn't mean that I didn't have fun tracking their growth unofficially at home. We had a door in our mudroom that served as our makeshift growth chart, and from the time my boys were old enough to walk, I would stand them next to that door and mark their height with the date I measured them. I had planned to do this a couple of times a year, but my boys enjoyed doing it so much that I usually ended up doing it a couple of times a month. They loved seeing those little lines move up the door so they could tell how much they had grown!

By the time my sons were old enough to hold crayons or pencils, they started scribbling their "names" on the door beside the line I had drawn right above their heads. When the boys had their cousins or their friends over to visit, we'd measure them as well, and we'd ask them to write their names on the door. Sometimes, we'd write a little note on the door if one of our sons had accomplished something impressive that week, such as "Oakley ate broccoli!" "Chad did a cartwheel!" or "Gatlin shared his fire truck with his brother!" With each passing year, the marks and the writing on the mudroom door inched upward.

When we moved into a new house, I couldn't bear the thought of leaving that door behind, and I finally talked my husband into taking it with us. Now it's in the basement of our new house. My sons are all over six feet tall now, and occasionally I can still talk them into letting me mark their height and write a few comments on the old mudroom door. While we're at it, we always take a minute to see how tall they were when they were toddlers, and then preschoolers and preteens, and we read some of the notes beside their names. It's a wonderful trip down memory lane for all of us, and that door has become one of my most treasured possessions.

When to Call Your Doctor

In general, the rate at which your child grows is more important than his specific measurements. Some toddlers are small and might grow at a slower rate compared to their friends, but they should reach the approximate height of their parents by the time they're adults.

A growth delay, however, can coincide with developmental delays and might signal a problem such as a chronic disease, an endocrine disorder, infection, poor nutrition, or emotional problems.

Talk with your pediatrician if you're concerned about your child's growth, particularly if he shows any of the following symptoms of failure to thrive.

- Your child's height, weight, and head circumference don't fall within the standards on growth charts.
- Your child's measurements fall below the 3rd percentile on growth charts or 20 percent below what's ideal for his height and weight.
- Your child's progress on the growth curve has slowed or stopped.

Walking, Running, and Gross Motor Skills

If your child hasn't started walking yet, he probably will before he's 16 months old. But your child won't be striding confidently for a little while. There's a good reason they're called toddlers: The first few months, walking is more like toddling, with legs wide apart, toes pointed outward, and arms at shoulder level for balance. Rather than smoothly walking forward, your toddler's motion will be more lurching from side to side. After about six months of walking practice, toddlers get the hang of it. By their second birthdays, most toddlers can walk without assistance, stand tentatively on tippy toes, carry toys while walking, pull a wagon or toy behind them—and then they begin to run.

As your toddler's walk transforms into a run, he'll develop his muscles and shed his baby fat. Almost before your eyes, your baby will grow into a toddler, with a more angular face and a better defined jawline.

Toddlers are quick studies. They learn lots of skills, including kicking a ball, walking up and down steps, and walking sideways and backwards. By age three, most toddlers walk with an easy heel-toe motion. They can usually ride a tricycle, play catch, and bend forward to pick something up—without toppling over.

~

I didn't really worry about my daughter meeting developmental milestones. I knew overall that she was growing and developing just fine. Actually, I was often surprised when my daughter would suddenly do something new, such as climb up the stairs or speak in a sentence, before I even expected that she could. She was constantly surprising me.

—*Dina Strachan, MD, a mom of a six-year-old daughter, a dermatologist and director of Aglow Dermatology, and an assistant clinical professor in the department of dermatology at New York University, in New York City*

~

All of my kids started walking at different ages. Three of my children are triplets, so that's really a great example of how every child develops differently. I just let my kids be, and I didn't stress about it. As long as children are developing within the normal range, you're good.

—*Sadaf T. Bhutta, MD, a mom of a six-year-old daughter and four-year-old triplets and an assistant professor and the fellowship director of pediatric radiology at the University of Arkansas for Medical Sciences and Arkansas Children's Hospital, both in Little Rock*

When my girls were toddlers, we played outside a lot. I wanted them to have plenty of opportunities to develop their motor skills running and playing. Our family loved to play Follow the Leader, Head of the Train, and Tag.

One thing that I found helped my toddlers develop motor skills was walking on curbs. Kids love to do this, as long as you provide close supervision—at arm's length in case you need to catch them! It can help toddlers improve their strength and balance.

—*Cathy Marshall, MD*

Giving a baby tummy time is a good way to help a child's development early on, but once a child is crawling and cruising, I'm not sure how much a parent can speed it up besides not holding their children back too much. Just let them learn and grow. Because I practice emergency medicine, I was never too worried about letting our kids climb. Falls from heights less than four feet are unlikely to cause any serious injury to toddlers, and learning to climb and fall is a natural part of maturing.

—*Amy Baxter, MD, a mom of 14- and 12-year-old sons and a 9-year-old daughter; the CEO of Buzzy4Shots.com; and the director of emergency research, Scottish Rite, of the Children's Healthcare of Atlanta, in Georgia*

My husband calls the toddler years the all-legs-and-no-brains years. He's an emergency physician, so he really knows what he's talking about. Toddlers can get around, and they crave independence, but they don't have a lot of judgment or impulse control to govern it.

As moms, our instinct is to try to protect our kids from everything. But I believe that we have to allow our kids to climb one rung higher than we're comfortable with. Moms' comfort zones are generally pretty small!

—*Deborah Gilboa, MD, a mom of nine-, seven-, five-, and three-year-old sons, a parenting speaker whose advice is found at AskDoctorG.com, and a family physician with Squirrel Hill Health Center, in Pittsburgh, PA*

∽◦∾

A wonderful incentive for my younger son to develop and learn new skills is trying to keep up with his older brother. I think that's why my younger son is very advanced in his motor skills. At the age of two, he can climb out of his crib, walk up and down stairs, and throw a ball.

One fascinating thing I'm noticing is that I think my younger son is left-handed. If that's the case, he'll be the first lefty in our family! I noticed it when he was learning to throw a ball and also as he learns to write. He almost always does these things with his left hand. It's amazing how this causes you to rethink things. Do I need to buy left-handed scissors? A left-handed desk?

My husband is an athlete, and he's a bit dismayed because being

When to Call Your Doctor

From the time you learned you were pregnant, you probably began looking forward to watching your child take his first steps. But putting one foot in front of the other doesn't always happen when parents expect. Some babies start walking before their first birthday, while others don't walk until they're almost two.

Walking can be an anxiety-ridden milestone for parents of children who are still on their hands and knees when their peers are on two feet. In general, most babies are able to stand and walk while holding onto furniture at age one, and most can walk alone by 18 months.

The National Center on Birth Defects and Developmental Disabilities recommends calling your doctor if your child can't walk at 18 months or doesn't walk steadily at age two.

left-handed can be a disadvantage in some sports. But not for baseball pitchers! For them, being a lefty is an advantage. Maybe my son will be a great baseball pitcher someday!

—*Rebecca Reamy, MD*

⌒◯⌒

During the toddler years, it's important to keep an eye on your child's developing skills. This is the time when some children start to "fall off the curve." If a toddler isn't hitting milestones, it's important to get help. Early intervention is very powerful, and I encourage parents to check in with their pediatricians if they have any concerns about their toddlers' development.

My older daughter had speech, occupational, and physical therapy when she was young. These interventions are critical, and the earlier they start the better.

—*Eva Ritvo, MD, a mom of 21- and 16-year-old daughters, a psychiatrist, and a coauthor of* The Beauty Prescription, *in Miami Beach, FL*

Talking

Your one-year-old understands a great deal more than you might think, and before you know it, he will start to answer you back. This is a special time, as many children "coin" their own words for the things that they love. You're likely able to crack the code and understand what your child says far better than other people can. It's common for beginning talkers to omit or change certain sounds. For example, a child might substitute sounds that he *can* say, like d and b, for sounds that he can't say. Or he might drop off the last parts of words, saying things like "ba" instead of "ball."

Usually by the time children are 1½ years old, they can say a few active words such as "go" and some directionals, such as "up." Your child might ask simple questions by raising his voice at the end of a word, such as "Out?" to go outside to play, probably accompanied by corresponding hand gestures! Typically, by the time children are two years old, they're able to say approximately 50 words. They can often speak in simple sentences, such as "Go out."

When your child is two years old, he will likely graduate from speaking in two-word sentences to using sentences with as many as six words. Many two-year-olds start to use pronouns, and they quickly understand the concept of "mine." Most two-year-olds can follow the storyline of a book—and even remember it. Also at this time, toddlers can follow two- or even three-part directions, such as "Go to the living room and bring me your stuffed lion." More people probably understand your toddler's speech now, but it's still common for about half of your child's sounds to be mispronounced. For example, a child might say "wabbit" instead of "rabbit." This endearing phase is fleeting. Enjoy it while it lasts!

Toddlers are quick learners, and by age three, your child probably has a vocabulary of more than 300 words. Many toddlers are little chatterboxes, practicing and improving their speech. They're often inquisitive, bombarding you with rapid-fire questions. Your child might even start to tell you stories at this age. What a wonderful window into what he's thinking about!

❧

When my daughters were toddlers, I really tried to approach them from their developmental level.

I spoke to my toddlers in very concrete language that they were more easily able to understand. For example, when we went out to eat in a restaurant, I would tell my daughters to sit in their seats and use their inside voices inside the restaurant, rather than telling them something more abstract like, "Be good girls."
—*Cathy Marshall, MD*

❧

At one year old, my daughter is really starting to talk. My husband jokes that she's loud, like her grandma! She's also very funny.

My daughter says "MaMa" and "DaDa," and random words here and there. One of my favorite things about this age is the words that she's created for the things that she loves. For example, she has a stuffed giraffe that she calls "Buh-Wa," which I think is her interpretation of "giraffe." I will miss this stage once she's able to say all of her words correctly.

—*Jennifer Bacani McKenney, MD, a mom of a one-year-old daughter and a family physician, in Fredonia, KS*

When my older daughter was five years old, she had brain surgery. My mother came to help out. My mother is a very bright woman, and she's also more patient than I am. She sat with my younger daughter, who was only eight months old, and taught her to say "duck," so she was very verbal, very early.

I never treated my daughters like they were babies, so I never "baby talked" to them. I considered my daughters to be people in small packages, not babies or toddlers. I always felt that I could talk to them, reason with them, and explain things to them. I spoke to my toddlers the way I'd speak to anybody! I know that might seem odd, but they were both very bright and verbal from early ages.

—*Eva Ritvo, MD*

I think most parents focus like a laser beam on their first child, carefully watching every stage of development. When my oldest child was around two years old and not talking fluently, my husband and I were concerned. We had a big medical evaluation done, and it all turned out to be perfectly normal.

Parents often get all twisted up into a pretzel about development concerns, but most of the time it's just fine. I think the key is not to compare your child with other kids.

—*Victoria McEvoy, MD, a mom who raised four children; a grandmom of six-, four-, and two-year-old grandsons; an assistant professor of pediatrics at Harvard Medical School; the medical director and chief of pediatrics at Mass General West Medical Group; and the author of* 24/7 Baby Doctor, *in Boston, MA*

One of the hardest things about toddlers is that they want to be independent and do things by themselves, but they can't communicate that yet. I found the best way to help my toddlers was to be patient and try to communicate with them on their level by giving them choices and using a lot of pointing to supplement their words.

Another thing that helps is to keep in mind that your toddler will be talking soon, and then he'll be talking nonstop.

—*Kristie McNealy, MD, a mom of nine- and six-year-old daughters and four-year-old and 22-month-old sons and a blogger at KristieMcNealy.com, in Denver, CO*

Before my son was able to communicate really well, he got very frustrated when my husband and I didn't understand what he was trying to say. My son would bang his head on the floor or walls. It made me nervous because I know that while head banging can be a normal phase of development, it can also be a harbinger of more serious concerns.

I mentioned the head banging to my son's pediatrician, who felt it was a normal phase. Now that my son is able to communicate better, he doesn't bang h.s head anymore. If the behavior had continued, I certainly would have brought it up to my pediatrician again.

—*Deborah Kulick, MD*

During my kids' toddler years, the lack of verbal skills typical for this age presented a challenge. I tried to focus on helping them develop their language skills. When my toddlers tried unsuccessfully to communicate something to me, I would make eye contact, clearly verbalize what I thought they wanted or needed, and repeat a single word.

For example, if my son was throwing a fit because he wanted a snack, I'd say, "Please, snack, please." When he expressed anything with good vibes, I'd say, "Yes, you may have a snack, please and thank you. Good work using your words, please, snack. Johnny said please snack, good work."

We parents must remember to be patient with toddlers because they understand so much more than they are able to communicate. We must also remember to be consistent in encouraging verbal communication, and of course to have patience during the learning process. Don't forget to show appreciation for any genuine attempt from your toddler.

—*Hana R. Solomon, MD, a mom who raised four children, a grandmom of three, a board-certified pediatrician, the president of BeWell Health, LLC, and the author of* Clearing the Air One Nose at a Time: Caring for Your Personal Filter, *in Columbia, MO*

I noticed pretty early on that my son wasn't as verbal as my daughter had been as a toddler. At the time, I kept thinking, *He's such a good, quiet baby!* I wasn't really worried about it.

When I took my son to his two-year-old well-child visit, the pediatrician told me that he hadn't hit a milestone and that we should look into it. I didn't take it very seriously. But I did follow through on the evaluation. It took about six months to go through the proper steps to have my son's speech evaluated, but we did then find out that something was wrong.

I encourage parents that if their child's pediatrician suggests checking into something, do so right away. If I had ignored our doctor's suggestion and hadn't pursued it, we would have been behind the eight ball when my son started school. If you check into it, and everything comes back normal, that's great! But if there's a problem, it's better to get help sooner rather than later.

My son received speech therapy until first grade, and now he's all caught up with his peers.

—Ann V. Arthur, MD, a mom of a 10-year-old daughter and an 8-year-old son, a pediatric ophthalmologist in private

Mommy MD Guides-Recommended Product
Signing Time

"When my kids were babies, I started to teach them sign language," says Jennifer Hanes, DO, a mom of a six-year-old daughter and a three-year-old son, an emergency physician, a certified forensic physician, and the founder of Empowered Medicine, PLLC, in Austin, TX. "Most people stop using sign language when their kids begin to talk. I found that continuing to sign has tremendous benefits for toddlers— and beyond. For example, when my kids were toddlers and we were at a park, if one of them was misbehaving, I could sign to them to stop, rather than calling them out in front of their friends. Also, my kids were sometimes able to sign things before they were quite able to say them. This helped eliminate frustration and prevent tantrums.

"I think that knowing sign language also helped my kids learn to read. Sign language is very logical, and it helped them to learn their letter sounds and how to spell. For example, some words, such as *park*, are finger-spelled. So to sign *park*, you actually sign the letters P, A, R, K. My son could spell 'park' at a very early age.

"Sign language is very easy to learn. I love the series Signing Time. The children learn signs, and they also learn how to use them together in a sentence. The series is filled with great lessons from spelling practice to how to set the table properly.

"One day when my daughter was five years old, she was signing with a deaf girl at the playground. The little girl's mom was very touched, and I was so proud!"

You can buy Signing Time volume 1 for $19.99 at **SIGNINGTIME.COM**.

practice at Park Slope Eye Care Associates, and a blogger at
WaterWineTravel.com, in New York City

∽◦

My oldest three children were all late talkers. When my oldest daughter was 18 months old, she spoke only a couple of words. She wasn't really putting any words together into sentences yet. That was concerning.

I talked with my daughter's pediatrician about it at her two-year checkup. She connected us with Early Intervention, which is a support system for children with developmental disabilities or delays and their families, and my daughter received speech therapy for about a year. The therapist came to our home once a week, for about a half hour each visit.

I learned a lot of very helpful things by watching the therapist, and I was better able to help my younger daughter and sons to learn to talk. For example, we'd play games that involved naming things, and any time I could name an item, I did. Sometimes parents put off talking with their pediatricians about speech delays. But I think it never hurts to at least call and have an evaluation done.

—*Kristie McNealy, MD*

∽◦

As a pediatrician, I'm very well aware of the window of language acquisition. If you don't take advantage of this time, it's lost forever. Newborns will pay attention to any speech, but by about six months, they start to really only focus on people speaking the language they hear most at home.

When my husband and I were looking for day care for our older daughter, we chose a woman who spoke Spanish. We instructed her to speak Spanish with the girls. I also really wanted our daughters to learn Chinese, and I played Chinese CDs for them. My older daughter now takes Chinese classes. I think teaching your children to speak a foreign language is an incredible gift.

—*Kate Tulenko, MD, MPH, a mom of four- and one-year-old girls, the author of* Insourced: How Importing Jobs Impacts the Healthcare Crisis Here and Abroad, *and a pediatrician and global health specialist with IntraHealth, in Washington, DC*

Fostering Hand-Eye Coordination

It's incredible to think that as your one-year-old is working to master walking and then running, he's also improving his fine motor skills and hand-eye coordination. At one year old, most babies have a hard time picking up small objects. But by 1½ years, most children can pick up tiny objects between their thumbs and forefingers—and get them into their mouths, of course.

By age two, most children are able to hold a pencil properly and create their first art masterpieces—well, scribbles anyway. At two, your child can probably color with sweeping vertical, and then circular, marks. It's in the second year that most children start to use one hand more frequently than the other. Soon you'll have the answer to the question: Is he right- or left-handed? By age three, a child can probably trace an object like a cookie cutter, draw a circle, and scribble very well.

Most two-year-olds can pick up a container and turn it over to pour out the contents, though don't expect your child to run for the dustpan and broom and sweep up the mess. At two, most children can stack four blocks into a tower—only to knock them right over again. Soon your child will be able to stack six or more blocks with ease.

Your two-year-old's attention span is lengthening. He might now be able to sit long enough to hear a whole storybook, and he can probably even turn the pages for you. He's starting to show many signs of independence, such as pulling off his shoes and unzipping his coat's zipper. By three, he can probably unbutton things as well.

At three years old, most toddlers can turn rotating handles. (Time to step up those babyproofing efforts!) Toddlers enjoy imitating the people they love by learning how to use tools, such as scissors and even flashlights, screwdrivers, and gardening shovels. "I'm a big kid now!"

⌒⌒

My daughter and I do a lot of things together to help improve her hand-eye coordination. She loves to color, and she enjoys doing arts and crafts. We also have a ball that we throw back and forth or kick.

—*Tanya Douglas Holland, MD*

∽◌

When my girls were babies, I found some soft block toys with black and white designs, and I would use them to have the girls track and reach. As they got older, we would play catch or tag together to improve their coordination.

—*Marra S. Francis, MD, a mom of eight-, seven-, and five-year-old daughters and a gynecologist, in San Antonio, TX*

∽◌

When my sons were toddlers, I did a lot to improve their hand-eye coordination. One fun thing I did was throw a ball to my sons in the family room while I was in the kitchen making dinner. I'd throw the

When to Call Your Doctor

Toddlers and preschoolers tend to be a little clumsy because they have a high center of gravity. Their legs don't develop in proportion to their upper bodies until they're around age six. Their center of gravity then becomes more like an adult's, giving them better balance. At the same time, toddlers' fine motor skills are still developing, which helps them with tasks such as tearing paper and cutting with scissors.

But it's important to pay attention to your child's hand-eye coordination. Preschool-age children who have learning disabilities tend to have a hard time coloring with crayons, writing with a pencil, using scissors, controlling zippers, fastening snaps, and learning to tie shoes.

Don't delay calling your doctor if you have concerns about your child's coordination. Although none of these problems necessarily means your child has a learning disability, it could be a red flag that should be looked into.

ball, and then I'd have 30 seconds to chop or stir! And quite often they would busy themselves for a minute or two and give me more time to get something done in the kitchen!

—*Leena Shrivastava Dev, MD*

I loved giving my sons Thomas the Tank Engine wooden trains with magnetic ends to play with. Because of the polarity of the magnets, the trains have to be pointing in the right direction to connect. Also, putting the trains on the track required my sons to carefully place the wheels in the grooves of the track. Playing with those trains was fun for my sons, and it also fostered good hand-eye coordination.

—*Jill Wireman, MD, a mom of 16- and 13-year-old sons and a pediatrician in private practice at Johnson City Pediatrics, in Tennessee*

The game technology we have today is very helpful for teaching kids hand-eye coordination and fine motor skills. My two-year-old son was playing Angry Birds by himself the other day! I believe computer games help kids learn numbers and letters too.

You have to be careful what you give kids, though. Over the holidays, we got a live Christmas tree. When we took the tree down a few weeks later, we found the old iPod Touch I let my younger son play with floating in the tree water. The lesson is to keep an eye on the two-year-old when he is playing with an expensive "toy" like that!

—*Rebecca Reamy, MD*

I have bad handwriting, and today all of my children have trouble with their handwriting and other fine motor skills. In retrospect, if I knew then what I know now, I might have done more activities with my toddlers to develop their fine motor skills. For example, I could have had them dry the silverware and pick up small items to strengthen the fine muscles in their hands and develop better dexterity.

But until you see what your kids are going to be good at, and not so good at, it's hard to know where to intervene.

—*Amy Baxter, MD*

RALLIE'S TIP

Hand-eye coordination is something that I was anxious for my kids to master early on so that they could start feeding and entertaining themselves without relying completely on me. I imagined that it would also come in handy for picking up their toys and putting them away, but that didn't exactly materialize.

One unexpected outcome of improved hand-eye coordination is that once your toddler can spot the object of his desire and effectively grasp it in his little hand, he can also put it into his little mouth, and if the object is small enough, it could present a choking hazard. Or if the object is toxic, it could present a poisoning hazard.

I encouraged my toddlers to develop their hand-eye coordination through play. We made games of picking up blocks and putting them one by one into a box while we counted each one. We had a toy workbench with wooden pegs, and all of my boys enjoyed hammering away at those pegs. My husband was convinced that each of our sons would be drafted by the NBA at any moment, so he bought a four-foot plastic basketball net, and he spent a lot of hours encouraging the boys to shoot hoops.

We also bought the boys a game called Whac-a-Mole, and that did wonders for their hand-eye coordination. The game features plastic moles that pop up from their burrows, and the challenge is to whack the poor moles with a plastic hammer before they disappear back into their burrows. My boys loved that game, and fortunately it didn't cause any of them to become violent later in life.

I think one of the best things moms can do to help their children develop better hand-eye coordination is to allow toddlers to do some things for themselves, even when it's not the easiest or most expedient way to do things. Of course we can zip and button our children's jeans and coats in two seconds flat, but it's important to allow toddlers to practice these skills, even if it takes an extra five minutes. Allowing toddlers to practice and perfect these skills and praising them for their efforts helps them develop better hand-eye coordination, and it also gives them greater self-confidence and pride in their accomplishments.

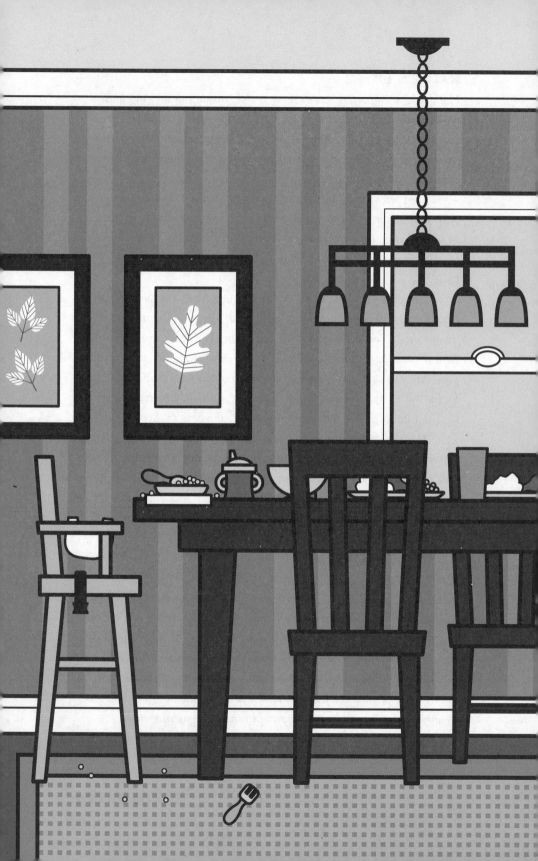

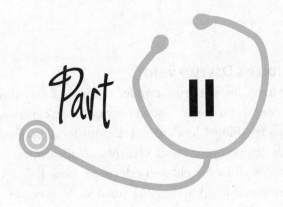

Part II

FOOD AND NUTRITION

Chapter 2

Introducing Finger Foods

YOUR TODDLER'S DEVELOPMENT

You might have already begun introducing finger foods to your toddler a few months ago. But it's a good bet you have plenty of nutritious foods still to try. Finger foods are perfect for toddlers. First, eating finger foods supports your toddler's growing independence; she can eat finger foods all by herself! Second, finger foods help toddlers to develop their pincer grasp, as they pick small foods up between thumb and forefinger. Plus, nutritious finger foods such as Cheerios, peas, cooked pasta, and pieces of cheese help your toddler to develop a taste for whole, healthy foods. And they're fun to eat to boot!

TAKING CARE OF YOU

What a joy it is to share your favorite foods with your toddler! Why not discover some new favorites together? Every nutritious food offers a different combination of vitamins and minerals. That's why eating a varied diet is so important. An apple a day might keep the doctor away, but an apple, and a pear, and a mango, and a nectarine, and a kumquat are even better. Take a trip to a farmers' market or a grocery store with a large produce section and pick out a few fruits and vegetables you've never tried. You might find a new favorite!

JUSTIFICATION FOR A CELEBRATION

When your toddler uses a spoon, and then a fork, for the first time, that's a wonderful reason to celebrate!

Trying New Foods

You want your toddler to try new, nutritious foods. That's a great idea, except that practically everything about being a toddler goes against her wanting to try new foods! First, a toddler's growth has slowed, so she needs to eat fewer calories. Second, toddlers are on the go, and they don't want to sit still long enough to eat anything, let alone something they're not sure they'll love. And third, toddlers tend to glom on to the same foods, wanting them over and over and over again. Why try a new food (broccoli) when you know that mac 'n cheese is super great?

Fortunately, this is one of many areas in life where persistence pays off. Experts say that it can take 10—or more—times of offering a food to a toddler before she'll eat it. Keep trying, and maybe someday she'll like it!

❧

In the toddler years, my sons have enjoyed eating finger foods because it gives them the independence they crave.

My sons love fruits such as cantaloupe and apple slices, crackers, and peanut butter and jelly sandwiches cut into small squares.

—*Bola Oyeyipo-Ajumobi, MD, a mom of four- and one-year-old sons, a family physician in private practice, and the owner of SlimyBookWorm.com, in Highland, CA*

❧

Even at this age, Cheerios are still an ideal finger food. They're inexpensive and nutritious—at least not as sugary or salty as some of the other food choices out there. When my sons were toddlers, I'd put a few Cheerios on their high chair tray and let them practice picking them up one by one. Cheerios are a great snack, and eating them helps toddlers to develop their hand-eye coordination and pincer grasp too. I did have to be careful, though, because if I gave them too many all at once, they would disappear either on the ground or too many in the mouth!

—*Leena Shrivastava Dev, MD, a mom of 15- and 11-year-old sons, a general pediatrician, and an advocate for child safety, in Philadelphia, PA*

Sometimes an "old" food in a "new" setting can create a totally different response. My son was a very picky eater. When he was about four years old, my mother took him for a grandparent-grandchild camp. In the afternoon, the only option for a snack was apples. Prior to this, my son wouldn't touch an apple. But at that camp, with apples being the only option, my son decided that he liked apples, and he's eaten them ever since.

—*Dana S. Simpler, MD, a mom of 25- and 20-year-old girls and a 23-year-old son and a specialist in internal medicine in private practice, in Baltimore, MD*

Kids like food because it tastes good. I use sauces, and I present veggies and ice cream in the same way: All foods are good! We had some fun with sweet red beets. When I told my daughter they'd turn her pee pink, she was pretty excited. Of course, this backfired with asparagus, which can make pee smell pretty funny.

It was helpful for us to always be pleasant at mealtimes, and offer the foods I want to cook and eat for the next 18 years, and never to push her to eat something she didn't want!

—*Katja Rowell, MD, a mom of a six-year-old daughter, a family practice physician, and a childhood feeding specialist with TheFeedingDoctor.com, in St. Paul, MN*

Trying new foods is a way of life with my toddler, but maybe not in the way one might imagine. My older son is a great eater, but he's constantly changing what he likes to eat. One week, for example, my son loves grapes, so I buy a big bunch of them. The next week, he dislikes grapes, but now he loves blueberries. I like to buy my son new foods so that he can experiment, try new things, and see what he likes—this week anyway.

—*Deborah Kulick, MD, a mom of two-year-old and eight-month-old sons, a child and adolescent psychiatrist at the Everett Teen Health Center, and an instructor in psychiatry at Harvard Medical School and the Cambridge Health Alliance, in Boston, MA*

I introduced my toddlers to new foods by eating them myself and saying, "Yummy! This is good." Then I'd ask, "Do you like it?" More often than not, my toddlers were at least willing to give this yummy new food a try. If they refused, I would try again. Each meal presented a new opportunity.

I never forced my kids to try new foods, and I never ever made threats regarding food. Food is for sustenance, not a reward nor a punishment.

—*Hana R. Solomon, MD, a mom who raised four children, a grandmom of three, a board-certified pediatrician, the president of BeWell Health, LLC, and the author of* Clearing the Air One Nose at a Time: Caring for Your Personal Filter, *in Columbia, MO*

My younger son is a fantastic eater. He eats a very wide range of foods. The other day, we went to a restaurant, and he ordered spicy Asian noodles! He's not just a chicken-nuggets-and-French-fries kid. He loves broccoli, and fresh tomatoes are his favorite food. If we're in a restaurant, and someone else has tomatoes on their plate, my son will reach over and snatch them!

I believe that my son is such a great eater because rather than following a traditional way of introducing new foods one at a time, I gave my son what we ate, cut into finger-food-size pieces. This strategy is called baby-lead weaning. One of my son's first foods was refried beans. He ate them then, and they are still one of his favorite foods.

—*Rebecca Reamy, MD, a mom of seven- and two-year-old sons and a pediatrician in emergency medicine at Children's Healthcare of Atlanta, in Georgia*

My daughter eats everything. She's a great eater! I know that a lot of kids don't like "slimy" foods, such as certain fruits. So I introduced them to my daughter pretty early so that she would get accustomed to them. I would cut slimy fruits, such as peaches, into small pieces and set them on her high chair tray. My daughter would study the food for a bit and then pick it up and give it a try.

Another trick I used was mixing together foods I knew she liked, such as pasta, with foods that might be new, such as peas. This way, when my daughter picked up a piece of pasta, she'd often get a pea along with it.

—*Shilpa Amin-Shah, MD, a mom of a two-year-old son and a one-year-old daughter and an emergency physician at Emergency Medical Associates, in Livingston, NJ*

From the day my kids started to eat table food, I exposed them to a broad variety of foods. My goal wasn't just for them to like a particular food, but rather for them not to be afraid or hesitant to try new things.

To break the ice when putting something new in front of them, I used a technique my husband and I called "culinary comparisons." For example, when we gave our kids falafel for the first time, I told them it was an "Egyptian hamburger," so it was not something completely new to them. In other words, my kids were very familiar with hamburgers, and falafel is shaped like hamburgers (even though it is made of chickpeas), so the Egyptian part was just a little added twist! This technique worked nine times out of 10!

—*Mona Gohara, MD, a mom of five- and three-year-old sons, a dermatologist in private practice, an assistant clinical professor in the department of dermatology at Yale University, and a cofounder of K&J Sunprotective Clothing, in Danbury, CT*

I'm a vegetarian, and when my daughter was a toddler and in preschool, she was very proud to be a vegetarian too. One of her preschool teachers was also a vegetarian, and the school made sure that my daughter and this teacher had extra-special foods for snacks. Pretty soon, all of the other kids in her class wanted to be vegetarians too!

Once my daughter got to pre-K, though, there weren't any other vegetarians in her class. One day my daughter came home from school and announced, "Mommy, I want meat!" It was like she felt I had been holding out on her, that there's this stuff called meat, and it's really good, and she wanted it!

Eating vegetarian was my choice, and I always felt that if my daughter didn't want to make that choice, that was fine. Today she eats all different types of meat, even very unusual things for children, such as duck pâté and salmon. She's very adventurous.

—*Dina Strachan, MD, a mom of a six-year-old daughter, a dermatologist and director of Aglow Dermatology, and an assistant clinical professor in the department of dermatology at New York University, in New York City*

The toddler years are a critical time in which tastes develop. Training your toddler's palate to prefer healthy foods is giving her the gift of lifelong healthy eating.

Kids are not born with a "kids' palate." Around the world, kids eat all sorts of different things—spicy foods, even bitter foods. Yet, in the United States, we often think that kids will eat only bland food, or worse yet sweet foods that are packaged to be fun and entertaining.

I think that during the toddler years, there should be a gradual weaning from breast milk to family meals. In my home, our meals were focused on fruits and vegetables. We ate very little added sugar and processed foods.

Generally, my husband and I simply mashed up the foods we were eating for our toddlers. Even if we were out with our kids, we'd take along a banana or pear and mash it. If you have to give your toddler packaged foods, choose ones that contain only the ingredients you have on hand and would cook with in your own kitchen.

—*Ayala Laufer-Cahana, MD, a mom of 16- and 14-year-old sons and a 12-year-old daughter, a pediatrician, and the founder of Herbal Water Inc., in Wynnewood, PA*

When my son was a year old, he took forever to eat. It would take him 15 minutes to chew a piece of chicken. I called him "the poucher" because he'd pouch the chewed food inside his cheeks sometimes for up to an hour.

I finally realized that I just needed to cook the food much longer and make it more tender. That way, half of the work was already done for him! Now I know to tell parents of beginning eaters to make sure to cut the food into very small pieces and make sure it is tender enough for toddlers who have no molars to masticate their food! Toddlers don't get all of their teeth until the year between their second and third birthdays, so it makes sense that it takes much longer for them to eat.

—*Cheryl Wu, MD, a mom of a four-year-old son, a pediatrician at LaGuardia Place Pediatrics in New York City, and a pediatric emergency physician at the Joseph M. Sanzari Children's Hospital of Hackensack University Medical Center, in New Jersey*

RALLIE'S TIP

When my boys were toddlers and I wanted to get them to try new foods, it helped if I encouraged them to play with their food. For instance, I'd put some yogurt or applesauce on the tray of their high chairs and show them how to swirl it around with their hands. One-year-olds naturally put their hands in their mouths, and when my sons tasted applesauce or yogurt on their fingers, they got the idea that they could feed themselves!

I also found it helpful to stop spooning food into my sons' mouths, and instead I encouraged them to feed themselves. I sat with them and kept them company and encouraged them, but I forced myself to sit still and refrain from helping them put the food into their mouths.

Choosing Organic Foods

The USDA estimated that in January 2012, it cost $1,067.30 a month to feed a family of four. That assumes you're making everything at home, yourself. Nothing is handed to you from a drive-thru window or delivered to you in a pizza box. No doubt about it, food represents a large percentage of any family's budget. Parents, wanting the best for their children, make the best choices that they can.

When food costs as much as it does, can you afford to choose organic foods, which generally cost even more than conventionally grown foods? More and more stores offer a choice of organically grown food. In fact, every food category now has an organic alternative. Many experts previously thought some crops—such as cotton—couldn't be grown organically, but farmers proved them wrong.

But what does "organic" mean? Organic foods are produced without genetically engineered seeds or crops, sewage sludge (Ick.), pesticides, herbicides, and fungicides. Organically raised animals are fed organically grown feed, are not given antibiotics or growth hormones, and are given fresh air and access to the great outdoors.

Organic farming offers many benefits, both to people and to our planet. A 2009 report from the President's Cancer Panel found that kids are at greater risk than adults of cancer from pesticides and other environmental toxins. What's more, organic farming doesn't release pesticides into the environment, which can harm wildlife. It also helps to preserve biodiversity and maintain fertile soil.

In addition to not causing harm, organic foods might offer more benefits. Some studies have found higher levels of nutrients in some varieties of organic foods. For example, a study conducted in England found that organic milk contained 67 percent more vitamins and antioxidants than conventional milk.

If you're standing at the grocery store comparing the price of organically grown food with conventionally grown—literally comparing apples to apples—you'll notice a price difference. Sometimes it's a very significant one. There are many reasons why. Farmers pay more for organically grown feed. Plus it costs a lot more to weed a field by hand than to spray it with herbicides. Also, conventional farmers can grow crops on every inch of farmland, but organic farmers often rotate their crops to help maintain the soil's fertility.

Most experts agree that no one should avoid eating fruits and vegetables if they can't afford to buy organic. The benefits of eating fruits and vegetables outweigh the risks of any pesticide residue. If you are able to choose organic, as your budget allows, look for foods bearing the green-and-white "USDA Organic" seal.

One simple approach is to switch to organic for the 12 fruits and vegetables that are highest in pesticide residue when conventionally grown. They're called the Dirty Dozen, and they are the fruits and vegetables listed below. According to the Environmental Working Group, if your family eats these foods frequently, buying them organic could cut your intake of pesticides by a whopping 80 percent.

- Apples
- Celery
- Strawberries
- Peaches
- Spinach
- Imported nectarines
- Imported grapes
- Sweet bell peppers
- Potatoes
- Blueberries
- Lettuce
- Kale/collard greens

On the flip side, another list—the Clean 15—are the fruits and vegetables generally lower in pesticides.

- Onions
- Corn
- Pineapples
- Avocados
- Asparagus
- Sweet peas
- Mangoes
- Eggplant
- Domestic cantaloupe
- Kiwifruit

- Cabbage
- Watermelon
- Sweet potatoes
- Grapefruit
- Mushrooms

ᗞᑐ

I try to buy as much organic food as I can. If there's a choice between a conventionally grown food and an organically grown one, I will almost always buy the organic. Of course, organic foods are almost always more expensive. But for my kids' future, I believe that it's important to protect the health of the environment. I want my kids, and all kids, to have as much uncontaminated watershed and land as possible. If I had to choose the most important foods to buy organic, my priorities are produce and milk.

—*Ayala Laufer-Cahana, MD*

ᗞᑐ

Back when my kids were toddlers, there weren't a lot of organic options. Today organic foods are more readily available. I try to buy at least the Dirty Dozen fruits and vegetables organic. These are the 12 most contaminated fruits and vegetables.

I order food from a company called Nature's Garden. Every two weeks, they deliver a supply of fresh, organic, in-season produce to my home. Right now they deliver to Arizona and Georgia. Even if Nature's Garden isn't in your area, you might be able to find a farm nearby that sells fresh, local, in-season produce.

—*Susan Wilder, MD, a mom of a 17-year-old daughter and twin 13-year-old girls, a primary care physician, and the founder and CEO of Lifescape Medical Associates, in Scottsdale, AZ*

ᗞᑐ

The one food I think buying organic makes a big difference in is eggs, in both health benefits and taste.

There's a higher incidence of salmonella in cage-raised chickens. I also think there's a taste difference between eggs from convention-ally raised chickens and organically raised ones.

—*Amy Baxter, MD, a mom of 14- and 12-year-old sons and a 9-year-old daughter; the CEO of Buzzy4Shots.com; and the director of emergency research, Scottish Rite, of the Children's Healthcare of Atlanta, in Georgia*

I'm a vegetarian, but my daughter is not. When I buy meat for her, I usually choose organic, even things like organic, sulfite-free hot dogs.

I also buy organic fruits and vegetables when I can, especially for foods my daughter really likes and eats a lot of, such as strawberries.

—*Dina Strachan, MD*

∽

When my sons were toddlers, I bought as much organic food as I could. I still do. Living in the greater LA area, we're blessed with farmers' markets every week of the year.

When you buy organic, you know that the food hasn't been grown using pesticides, and it also hasn't been genetically modified. That is a huge concern for me. The majority of corn and soy grown in this country has been genetically modified. Studies show that animals that eat genetically modified foods have an increased risk of kidney and liver disease. That scares me!

—*Cathie Lippman, MD, a mom of 31- and 29-year-old sons and a physician who specializes in environmental and preventive medicine at the Lippman Center for Optimal Health, in Beverly Hills, CA*

∽

"Organic" refers to the absence of pesticides and additives. It says nothing about the food's nutritional value. Foods can be mass produced and not as nutritious, but still be "organic."

Food from local farms is usually grown with pride, and it travels a short distance to your table. It's likely to be more nutritious. Produce grown across the country, or on another continent, is usually picked before it's ripe, so it's less nutritious. There's nothing like picking a tomato grown in your own backyard.

I love going to farmers' markets. My daughter has gotten to know local farmers, and she's become more connected with the whole process of growing food. How sad, if her only exposure to food was to see it shrink-wrapped at the supermarket.

Conventional milk is a cocktail of hormones and antibiotics, so I try to always buy organic milk. But milk itself isn't always necessary. People in Asian cultures traditionally don't drink dairy products, and Asian diets are very healthy.

—Dora Calott Wang, MD, a mom of a nine-year-old daughter, a psychiatrist and historian at the University of New Mexico School of Medicine, and the author of The Kitchen Shrink: A Psychiatrist's Reflection on Healing in a Changing World, *in Albuquerque, NM*

Taking a First Aid Class and Preventing Choking

Moms are master jugglers of time—and money. Who among us ever has time—or money—to spare? But how much time and money would you spend to save your child's life? What if you could learn the basics in a few minutes—for free?

A website called FirstAidWeb.com offers free online CPR and first aid courses. Visit this site to take online, self-guided classes. You can take quizzes afterward to test your progress. These courses adhere to the American Red Cross and American Heart Association's guidelines. At the end, you receive CPR and first aid certifications, which are good for two years. Any more excuses? We didn't think so!

Of course, you can also take first aid and CPR courses at local hospitals, schools, and the Red Cross. It might be more fun to do this with your spouse, parent, or a friend.

One significant danger to toddlers, in fact up to age five, is choking. Ironically, food is responsible for most choking incidents. One reason why is because food—especially hard, smooth food—needs to be chewed with a grinding motion. You chew peanuts and baby carrots like that without even thinking about it! But children don't master this skill until around age four. A child might actually give up on chewing the food and try to swallow it whole.

Anyone can choke on any food at any time. That's why children should always have company when eating. (Really, that's why you should have company while eating too!) The following foods are particular choking hazards to children.

- Hot dogs and meat sticks
- Grapes, cherry tomatoes, and carrot sticks (unless they are chopped completely)

- Raisins, popcorn, and peanuts
- Hard candy and round candy such as jelly beans
- Gum

Many toddlers still explore the world by putting things into their mouths. So it's important to keep small nonfood items out of your toddler's reach. Particular choking hazards include the following.

- Popped balloons
- Pieces of plastic wrap and other thin plastic
- Small toys and magnets
- Marbles and other small balls
- Coins

A good rule of thumb is that if you can pass an object through a toilet paper roll, it's small enough for a child to choke on.

∽

I asked my mother and my mother-in-law to take a basic first aid class because they would be babysitting my daughter. I made sure all of our nannies took the classes too because I wanted them to know basic first aid. That's something I feel very strongly about.

You can take a basic first aid class at your local Red Cross and at many hospitals.

—*Lisa Campanella-Coppo, MD, a mom of a three-year-old daughter, an emergency physician, and the emergency department director of academic affairs at Monmouth Medical Center, in New Jersey*

∽

I didn't insist that my kids' caregivers take first aid classes. I thought it was more important to choose caregivers with common sense and calm temperaments. Freaking out at the sight of blood is not a great attribute in a caregiver. You want to find someone who remains calm, who broadcasts the sense that "everything is under control and it's not a big deal." That is 90 percent of first aid.

—*Amy Baxter, MD*

∽

When my kids were toddlers, I worried so much about them choking. They liked to eat grapes, and I cut those grapes into such tiny pieces that I think picking them up helped my kids develop their pincer grasps. We stayed away from things like M&M's and peanuts for a while because they are the perfect size to get stuck in a toddler's trachea!

—Ann Contrucci, MD, a mom of 13-year-old boy-girl twins who works as a pediatric emergency physician, in Atlanta, GA

By the time my babies were a year old, they were pretty well used to eating solid foods. They ate what the rest of the family ate. I remember Cheerios were always a favorite. I didn't really restrict their eating, although I was careful to avoid small foods, such as raisins, nuts, popcorn, and even hot dogs if they were cut into small circles instead of lengthwise. These foods can be choking hazards for kids.

—Susan Besser, MD, a mom of six grown children, ages 27, 25, 23, 21, 20, and 18, a grandmom of two, a family physician, and the medical director of Doctors Express-Memphis, in Tennessee

I liked to give my toddlers simple foods that were easy to eat. A favorite was canned Mandarin oranges. They taste great, and they're nutritious too.

I also liked Mandarin oranges because they were soft and weren't a choking hazard. I gave my toddlers a lot of soft foods that melted into mush in their mouths, such as canned green beans and Cheerios.

—Ann Kulze, MD, a mom of 23- and 17-year-old daughters and 22- and 20-year-old sons; a nationally recognized nutrition expert, motivational speaker, and physician; and the author of the best-selling book Dr. Ann's Eat Right for Life, *in Charleston, SC*

One of my biggest fears when my children were toddlers was that they might choke. I was very watchful anytime they were eating. Also we have a very firm rule in our house that anytime anyone is eating anything, they are seated upright at the table.

—Aline T. Tanios, MD, a mom of nine- and three-year-old daughters and a seven-year-old son and a pediatric hospitalist at Arkansas Children's Hospital, in Little Rock

I'm very nervous about my daughter choking, so I never allow her to eat alone. Quite frankly, I don't think anyone, of any age, should eat alone. Now that I have a daughter, I find myself avoiding eating while running up and down the stairs or driving in a car. I imagine myself choking to death when she is home alone with me, and then where would we be?

I cut round, hard foods, such as hot dogs and carrots, into small pieces before giving them to my daughter, and I never let her eat hard candy or chew gum.

Even with that neuroticism, my daughter had a choking episode. One day when we were in the grocery store, I opened a box of flavored Cheerios and gave her a few to eat. I didn't know, at the time, that the flavoring on the Cheerios keeps them from dissolving easily. My daughter started to choke, there was no air exchange, and her lips turned blue. I snatched her from the cart, flipped her upside down, pounded on her back, and the Cheerio popped out. When she finally caught her breath, she looked at me and said, "Mommy, that wasn't good." I didn't sleep for a week.

—*Lisa Campanella-Coppo, MD*

RALLIE'S TIP

When my youngest son was a toddler, he had a bad habit of putting entirely too much food in his mouth to chew and swallow comfortably. I told him over and over to chew and swallow each piece of food before putting another one in his mouth, and I warned him that if he didn't, he might choke. But because he had never experienced choking, he didn't know what all the fuss was about.

I tried everything I could think of to get my son to slow down and chew his food for more than a second or two, but nothing seemed to stick for very long. I was always worried that he would choke, so I never left him alone for a minute while he was eating.

Once when he was eating chicken at our kitchen table, I noticed that he got very still. His eyes began to water, and he started making gagging sounds. My heart stopped, because I knew he was choking! I pulled him out of his chair and performed the Heimlich maneuver on

*him. Fortunately, the mouthful of chicken came right out, and my son
was fine, but the experience of choking and not being able to breathe
scared him to death.*

*After that, my son was terrified of choking again. He started
chewing each bite of his food until it was watery mush and ran out the
corners of his mouth. He seemed to have developed a fear of swallowing
his food.*

*At first, I tried to reassure my son that there was a happy middle
ground. He needed to take just one bite of food at a time and chew it
properly, but he didn't need to chew each bite for five minutes. That
didn't help much. He was still a bit traumatized by the experience of
choking. His grandmother noticed that he was chewing his food exces-
sively, and when she asked him about it, he got really embarrassed. At
that point, I decided the best course of action was to just ignore my son's
excessive chewing and see if a little tincture of time would help.*

*It took about two months for my son to relax and begin chewing
and swallowing his food without fear. During that time, I made a point
of not saying a word about his odd eating behavior, and I made sure that
everyone else in the family avoided discussing it as well. I felt certain that
if we focused on it and made a big deal of it, we would only keep the
problem alive and make it worse.*

*Almost every child will choke on something at some point, so it's a
great idea for parents to take a first aid class so they'll be prepared to act
quickly and effectively. It's also important for parents to keep small
objects away from curious toddlers, and to keep a close eye on their
children when they're eating to make sure they can intervene if their child
begins to choke. Being present and knowing how to respond to a choking
incident could help you save your child's life.*

Watching for Allergies

If you have the sense that more and more kids are allergic to
foods, it's not your imagination. From 1997 to 2007, the prevalence of reported food allergies among kids under 18 years old
increased by 18 percent. In 2007, around 3 million kids younger

than 18—nearly four out of every 100 children in this age group—were reported to have a food allergy in the past year.

Considering how many foods there are, it's incredible to think that only eight types of foods account for 90 percent of food allergies. What are these common offenders?

- Milk
- Eggs
- Peanuts
- Tree nuts
- Fish
- Shellfish
- Soy
- Wheat

Food allergies can have other repercussions as well. Children with food allergies are two to four times more likely to have related conditions such as asthma and other allergies, compared to kids without food allergies. For example, 29 percent of children with food allergies also have asthma, compared to only 12 percent of children without food allergies, and 27 percent of children with food allergies have eczema, compared to 8 percent of children without food allergies.

But what is a food allergy, and what should you look for? A food allergy is a potentially serious immune response to eating a particular food or food additive. People with these allergies can have reactions ranging from a tingling tongue to death. The following are signs and symptoms to watch out for, especially when giving your toddler a new food for the first time.

- Tingling sensation around the mouth
- Tightness in the throat
- Wheezing
- Coughing
- Nausea and vomiting
- Stomach pain
- Diarrhea
- Hives
- Drooling
- Changes in behavior or mental status

Boys and girls have similar rates of food allergies. The good news is that children are slightly less likely to have food allergies after age five. Watching out for food allergies is another important reason to always keep your toddler company when she's eating.

◦⌇◦

When my son was a toddler, I often brought home strawberries for him as a sweet treat. After he ate them, his cheeks would get bright red. It took me about a month to realize he was having a reaction to the strawberries.

—Nancy Rappaport, MD, a mom of 22- and 17-year-old daughters and a 19-year-old son, an assistant professor of psychiatry at Harvard Medical School, an attending child and adolescent psychiatrist in the Cambridge, MA, public schools, and the author of The Behavior Code

◦⌇◦

As a pediatrician, I rolled my eyes at "allergy moms." Then I became one. Both of my girls have food allergies. It's really a challenge.

I discovered that my daughters had food allergies when they had blood in their stool. My older daughter was allergic to corn, wheat, sesame, dairy, and soy. We couldn't eat out, so we had to do all of our own cooking. I couldn't even pick up prepared meals at the grocery store for fear they might contain an allergen.

It was even scarier when our daughter went to preschool. We read a book to her about allergies called *Food Allergies and Me*. That helped her to understand why she couldn't eat the foods that everyone else could eat.

Now that my daughter is older, she's outgrown some of her allergies, except for sesame. That still really bothers her.

—Kate Tulenko, MD, MPH, a mom of four- and one-year-old girls, the author of Insourced: How Importing Jobs Impacts the Healthcare Crisis Here and Abroad, *and a pediatrician and global health specialist with IntraHealth, in Washington, DC*

◦⌇◦

One of my twins began to show signs of food allergies at birth. We did delayed food allergy testing, and we discovered she's allergic to almost all foods. Even lettuce!

Since then, we've tried many different treatments, including powerful steroid medicines. We have found the most success with naturopathic remedies.

—*Susan Wilder, MD*

My older son had food allergies when he was a toddler. Thankfully, he's outgrown them.

He was very allergic to eggs and milk. The poor kid didn't even know what cheese tasted like! Even if cheese was the 17th ingredient on a food label, he couldn't tolerate eating it. Whenever we ate out or at a friend's house, I took food along for my son to eat. I'd make it a special and fun snack so he wouldn't feel deprived or left out.

When a child has food allergies, it's hard to know if he has outgrown them. One day I was so tired, I was sacked out on the couch. I

When to Call Your Doctor

It's time to let your toddler try new foods, but the thought of discovering a possible food allergy can make mealtimes stressful. First, remember that only a handful of foods cause 90 percent of allergic reactions in children, and they include milk, eggs, peanuts, tree nuts, fish, shellfish, soy, and wheat.

When your child eats a food she's allergic to, her body's immune system reacts by releasing chemicals such as histamine to attack specific proteins in the food. She might have mild signs, such as a skin rash or a slight swelling of her lips, or she might experience very serious symptoms, such as trouble breathing or loss of consciousness. These signs and symptoms might begin immediately after eating a particular food, or they could develop a few hours after eating it.

Call your doctor if you suspect your child is having an allergic reaction. Watch for these early signs and symptoms.

- Runny nose
- Hives (red welts on the skin) or an itchy skin rash
- Tingling tongue or lips

heard my son in the kitchen, so I quickly went in to see what he was doing. He had gotten out the carton of eggs, broken them all, and finger-painted with raw eggs all over his body, including his face! I had his Epi-pen on hand, and I thought, *Well, let's see what happens next.* Fortunately, my son didn't have a reaction, so that's when we knew he had outgrown his allergy to eggs!

—*Kristie McNealy, MD, a mom of nine- and six-year-old daughters and four-year-old and 22-month-old sons and a blogger at KristieMcNealy.com, in Denver, CO*

When my kids were young, I knew the current guidelines of when to introduce foods that are common allergens, such as strawberries and peanuts. We didn't introduce strawberries until after my babies were a year old, and we didn't introduce peanuts until after they were two.

Other signs and symptoms of a food allergy include the following.
- Wheezing
- Coughing
- Feeling of tightness in the throat
- Hoarse voice
- Nausea and vomiting
- Stomach pain
- Diarrhea

Call 911 if your child has signs or symptoms of a severe allergic reaction, called anaphylaxis, which appear within minutes or hours after eating a particular food. They include the following.
- Skin rash, hives, or swollen lips or tongue
- Trouble breathing
- Drooling or trouble swallowing
- Weakness or loss of consciousness
- Gastrointestinal distress (such as vomiting, diarrhea, or cramping) along with another symptom of anaphylaxis

My oldest son has a mild allergy to tree nuts, by his own assessment anyway. He says that his tongue feels weird when he eats them. That can be a symptom of allergies, so I've taught him to read labels to know what to avoid. The symptoms of wheezing, mouth itching, and vomiting after eating particular foods should be taken seriously.

Even if no one in your family has severe food allergies, your child might still be susceptible to developing them if a close blood relative has allergies, eczema, and/or asthma.

—*Amy Baxter, MD*

❧

We don't have anyone with food allergies in my family, so I wasn't too worried about my daughter developing them. I introduced eggs, shrimp, and citrus (and garlic, onions, and cilantro) to my daughter before she was a year old. I gave her peanut butter when she was about a year old. Ironically, she doesn't like any foods made with nuts to this day!

I think that all of the focus we've put on food allergies has actually made the problem worse. Studies also suggest that the food avoidance we'd been practicing for years might have made the problem worse.

I recently overheard a mom at the playground say that her son was four years old, and she hadn't yet given him peanuts.

"We don't have allergies in the family, but we're being extra careful," she said.

That's just sad, I thought.

I see families who have so much anxiety about food issues. It makes parenting so much harder. Letting go of that anxiety makes for happier moms and happier babies.

If you do have a family history of food allergies, be sure to let your child's doctor know. Also, ask your doctor for recommendations about when to offer your child specific foods.

—*Katja Rowell, MD*

❧

When my son was a toddler, the American Academy of Pediatrics had recommended delayed introduction of certain solid foods.

Since January 2008, recommendations have changed dramatically. New studies indicate that delaying introduction of certain solid food to children is not helpful and might, in fact, be harmful, because it might actually promote the development of allergies to foods and other substances.

To help my children develop a healthy and well-rounded diet, I really tried to feed them anything and everything that they were interested in eating. I don't think parents should deny their toddlers nutritious foods due to excessive worry about the possibility of food allergy. I let my son eat fish when he was 18 months old, and I let my daughter eat a peanut butter cookie when she was 5 months old, and they were both so happy!

Although my son had an intolerance to milk protein when he was an infant, he outgrew it. This experience made me a little more cautious when it was time to introduce him to new foods. I think it's very important to watch children for obvious symptoms when they eat foods that can be highly allergenic, such as milk, soy, egg, wheat, peanuts and tree nuts, and shellfish. These foods account for the vast majority of food allergies. The signs and symptoms that parents should be most concerned about are the appearance of hives, drooling, difficulty swallowing or breathing, excessive vomiting, and changes in behavior or mental status. In some cases, food allergies can be severe and even life-threatening. If your child has any of these signs or symptoms, you should call 911 immediately.

—*Sigrid Payne DaVeiga, MD, a mom of a six-year-old son and a two-year-old daughter and a pediatric allergist with the Children's Hospital of Philadelphia, in Pennsylvania*

Dealing with the High Chair

If most moms were to name their favorite pieces of furniture in their homes, the high chair would probably not be at the top of this list. Or even on the list. High chairs are handy to keep toddlers safe and to contain their messes. But most moms won't be sad to see the high chair go!

When my daughter was about a year old, I got rid of her high chair tray. This way I could pull her high chair right up to the table, making her a part of our family meals. It made cleanup easier too!

—*Katja Rowell, MD*

⌇

When my kids were still eating in their high chairs, I put a huge plastic shower curtain on the floor underneath them. That way I wasn't as worried about them making a big mess.

After they were done eating, I'd take the shower curtain outside and shake it off.

—*Amy Baxter, MD*

Mommy MD Guides-Recommended Product
The Highchair Organizer

"When my kids were toddlers, I remember needing to hop up and get things at mealtimes, such as wipes or a clean spoon to replace the one that fell on the floor," says Amy Baxter, MD, a mom of 14- and 12-year-old sons and a 9-year-old daughter; the CEO of Buzzy4Shots.com; and the director of emergency research, Scottish Rite, of the Children's Healthcare of Atlanta, in Georgia.

"You don't have to get up and down as much with this clever new invention. It has storage compartments for extra utensils and wipes so that you don't have to interrupt the flow of dinner to retrieve them."

The Highchair Organizer attaches to the back of most brands of high chairs using adjustable straps. It has ample pockets to store everything you need to get through mealtime without interruption, including extra cups, bottles, spoons, wipes, baby food jars, treats, toys, plates, bowls, bibs, and pacifiers.

The Highchair Organizer comes in pink and green and costs $24.95. You can buy it at **THEHIGHCHAIRORGANIZER.COM**.

Cleaning my daughter's high chair can be such a chore. Luckily, we received a wonderful Fisher-Price high chair before my daughter was born. It wasn't expensive, and it has a really neat feature: You can take the seat cover off and wash it in the clothes washer. I love it. I wash the cover a few times each week, after especially messy meals. Between washings, I remove the cover and shake the crumbs off of it outside. It also has a removable tray that sits on top of the built-in tray, and I can throw that in the dishwasher.

—Jennifer Bacani McKenney, MD, a mom of a one-year-old daughter and a family physician, in Fredonia, KS

When my daughter was born, one of my business partners gave us a wonderful Peg Perego high chair. It looks super comfortable, and it's very functional. It's very easy to clean because you can wipe the whole chair down. The tray pops off, and it's dishwasher safe. Of course, the tray takes up one entire level of the dishwasher! But it's nice to have that option.

I try really hard to keep the high chair clean because my daughter doesn't know yet not to eat old food. If she's able to pick peas out of the crevices of the chair from earlier in the day, she'll eat them.

—Rachel S. Rohde, MD, a mom of a one-year-old daughter, an assistant professor of orthopaedic surgery at the Oakland University William Beaumont School of Medicine, and an orthopaedic upper-extremity surgeon with Michigan Orthopaedic Institute, P.C., in Southfield, MI

My older son sat in his high chair while eating when he was one and two years old. But once my younger son was old enough to sit in the high chair, we transitioned my older son to a regular chair. He sits on his knees so he can reach the table. Sometimes he sits on my lap to eat.

I didn't want to use a booster seat at home. I worried that my son would fall out of it onto the floor.

—Sharon Boyce, MD, a mom of three- and one-year-old sons and a family physician at DayOne Family Healthcare Clinic, in Battle Creek, MI

Quite frankly, I didn't care too much about keeping my daughter's high chair sterilized! It's plastic, and it's not going to have any pathogens growing on it that don't colonize our skin or household surfaces anyway. I simply washed the tray with soap and warm water. Of course, I wasn't mixing cookie dough with raw eggs or cutting up raw meat near her high chair, either.

I don't think common everyday germs are such a bad thing in small doses. I think we oversanitize our kids, doing them a great disservice. I agree with research that shows that the increasing prevalence of allergies that we are seeing in our children might be due to them being oversanitized early in life.

—*Lisa Campanella-Coppo, MD*

Cleaning Up Messy Eating

A neat-eating toddler is an oxymoron. Eating neatly requires dexterity, patience, and practice, and these are all in short supply for toddlers. But as your toddler grows and develops, she'll be better able to eat more neatly. Even better, she'll be able to help clean up the mess afterward!

When my older son was a little younger, I used to give him "clean" foods to eat so that I didn't have so much cleanup afterward! When I wanted him to eat something messy, like yogurt, I'd feed him myself.

—*Sharon Boyce, MD*

Both of my toddlers are messy eaters. I don't worry about it, though. I simply clean up the mess when they're done. I feel that the toddler years are a time to explore, and I accept the mess that goes along with it.

—*Shilpa Amin-Shah, MD*

Let the kids make a mess and don't freak out about stains on carpets, nor lost coats and broken toys. Mistakes are inevitable, and you and your kids will make them.

—*Elizabeth Chabner Thompson, MD, MPH, a mom of*

13- and 8-year-old daughters and 12- and 10-year-old sons, a radiation oncologist with 21 C. Radiation Oncology, and the inventor of the Mommy Bag, filled with supplies for moms-to-be having C-sections, in Scarsdale, NY

Even after my daughter turned one, most times, I still put her food right onto the (clean!) table, rather than on a plate. I found this to be neater because she didn't have a plate to knock onto the floor. We used those little sectioned-off plastic plates for saucier foods and put the plates straight in the dishwasher.

—*Katja Rowell, MD*

With toddlers, eating is a mess. My strategy has been to feed my kids in places where it doesn't matter if it gets messy and let them go at it.

I've kept all of my kids in high chairs through their toddler years, which helps to contain the mess too. After that, I moved them into a booster seat with a seat belt.

—*Kristie McNealy, MD*

To me, messy eating was a double whammy when my twins were toddlers. On the one hand, I wanted them to eat more food. And on the other hand, I wanted them to be more independent and feed themselves. Toddlers plus spaghetti equals an enormous mess.

I was determined to let my kids feed themselves, so I didn't worry about the mess. I just cleaned it up. This is not the time for parental OCD tendencies to come up! Let them learn how to eat on their own; the mess will soon enough be gone. Besides, it makes for some great photo ops!

—*Ann Contrucci, MD*

∽◦

I love the Swiffer. It's wonderful for quickly cleaning up small messes after meals.

Also, I bought a smocklike bib at Babies R Us. I put that on my daughter before she eats, and I don't have to worry so much about her spilling food on her clothes. This gives my daughter more freedom to eat.

—*Tanya Douglas Holland, MD, a mom of a two-year-old daughter, a women's health advocate, and a consultant in medical affairs to a pharmaceutical company, in Atlanta, GA*

∽◦

When my kids were a year old, of course they were messy eaters. Plenty of food got thrown around. I just expected it, and I cleaned it up. I decorated my home to make this less of a challenge. For instance, I didn't have carpet under my dining room table, and I didn't buy upholstered dining room chairs. Pretty much everything in my dining room was wipeable!

Messy eating is part of what you go through with babies. Then when they outgrow it, you miss it.

—*Ayala Laufer-Cahana, MD*

∽◦

When my kids were toddlers, I encouraged them to eat only at the kitchen table or kitchen counter. The rule was: No dragging food everywhere (except occasional car snacks). My husband and I also encouraged our toddlers to help us prepare foods and to participate in the cleanup by placing dishes in the sink or in the dishwasher. Much of the time, our toddlers "worked" alongside us in the kitchen.

—*Hana R. Solomon, MD*

Chapter 3
Introducing Table Foods

YOUR TODDLER'S DEVELOPMENT

Often when a child turns one year old, the baby who "ate anything" turns into a "picky eater." It's not just your child, and it's certainly not your imagination! A toddler's growth rate has slowed, and he needs only about 1,000 calories a day. If you think about how many calories you eat, you'll realize that 1,000 calories aren't a lot! Most toddlers should eat three meals a day and two snacks. By your toddler's first birthday, he's probably eating the same foods that you are. Consider this both a benefit—fewer things to prepare—and also a challenge—he's eating what you're eating, so make every calorie count!

TAKING CARE OF YOU

You're working hard to help your toddler to eat right. Why not help yourself to more nutritious food too? This is a great time to make an appointment with a nutritionist to have a diet checkup. Or you can do it yourself at home with websites such as MyPlate at LiveStrong.com and SparkPeople.com and apps like CalorieCamp by Calorie Count, MyFitnessPal, and Calorie Counter. (Many of these calorie trackers have both a website and an app.)

JUSTIFICATION FOR A CELEBRATION

Anytime that you serve a new food to your toddler and he responds with a smile and says, "I love it, Mommy!" give yourself a huge pat on the back and celebrate this tremendous success!

Making Meals a Family Affair

Family dinners were a regular occurrence for the Cleavers and that 1950s generation. Today, families race through their days at breakneck speed, and it can be hard to find the time to connect over a meal.

According to a Gallup poll, 28 percent of adults with children under the age of 18 report that their families eat dinner together seven nights a week. This is down from 37 percent in 1997. About half, 47 percent, of parents say their families eat together between four and six times a week. The last quarter, 24 percent, say they eat together three or fewer nights a week.

Interestingly, Canadian and British parents are more likely to have family meals every night: 40 percent of Canadian parents say they do, and 38 percent of British parents do.

But where's the beef? Experts say the benefits to family meals become more critical in adolescence. Studies show that the more often families eat together, the less likely kids are to smoke, drink, use drugs, get depressed, develop eating disorders, and consider suicide. Plus, experts say the more often families break bread together, the more likely the kids are to do well in school, delay having sex, eat their vegetables, speak with big words, and have better table manners.

What's for dinner? Hopefully some nutritious food and some family time.

I would love to eat our meals together as a family all of the time. My husband is an emergency physician, and he comes and goes at crazy hours. When we're all together in the house, we do try to eat together. If only one of us is home, we eat with our daughter, rather than watching her eat by herself.

—*Rachel S. Rohde, MD, a mom of a one-year-old daughter, an assistant professor of orthopaedic surgery at the Oakland University William Beaumont School of Medicine, and an orthopaedic upper-extremity surgeon with Michigan Orthopaedic Institute, P.C., in Southfield, MI*

When my children were young, my family really enjoyed mealtimes as a time to gather and talk. We used meals to communicate and to check in with everyone. Looking back, I think it was great that my family had those three meals a day together. Mealtimes were a wonderful opportunity for us to gather together as a family.

—Lisa Dado, MD, a mom of 23- and 20-year-old daughters and an 18-year-old son, a pediatric anesthesiologist with Valley Anesthesiology Consultants, and the cofounder and CEO of the nonprofit organization the Center for Humane Living, which teaches life skills with an innovative approach to traditional martial arts training in six centers in and around Phoenix, AZ

My husband and I do tag-team cooking: We take turns cooking each night, depending on who has had a less crazy day. Before we eat, we say a prayer. After the prayer, my daughter has started a tradition of yelling, "Ahhhhh" instead of "Amen."

We have a dining room, but we eat a lot of our meals in our kitchen. Our daughter's high chair pulls up perfectly to our kitchen island, and we sit around that. It's small and cozy, perfect to encourage conversation and sharing.

—Jennifer Bacani McKenney, MD, a mom of a one-year-old daughter and a family physician, in Fredonia, KS

I try to make meals a family affair as much as possible. But my kids would far rather sit and eat on our back porch than around our dining room table. My kids also love it when I pack our dinner up and we take it to the park for a picnic. We try to do that every so often. My kids aren't really that interested in eating big meals; they just want to have fun. I like to keep the focus on family more than on food.

Truth be told, my kids would also rather eat popcorn than dinner, but I have to draw the line somewhere!

—Jennifer Hanes, DO, a mom of a six-year-old daughter and a three-year-old son, an emergency physician, a certified forensic physician, and the founder of Empowered Medicine, PLLC, in Austin, TX

When my kids were toddlers, we tried to eat meals together as a family. One firm rule: No TV at mealtimes.

Family meals were actually easier to pull off when my kids were toddlers than it is today. When they're toddlers, you plop them into their high chairs, and they're not going anywhere. Now my kids have many activities of their own and busy schedules.

—*Amy Baxter, MD, a mom of 14- and 12-year-old sons and a 9-year-old daughter; the CEO of Buzzy4Shots.com; and the director of emergency research, Scottish Rite, of the Children's Healthcare of Atlanta, in Georgia*

I believe in making meals a family affair. However, I think we sometimes put too much pressure on ourselves to define a traditional meal as one with roast turkey, mashed potatoes, and green beans, and with every member of the family present.

My husband often worked late when our daughter was a toddler, and it wasn't practical to wait to eat until he got home. So I ate dinner with my daughter right after her nap when she was really hungry. Then when my husband got home a few hours later, our daughter sat at the table with him and maybe ate a snack or a few bites of his dinner. We stuck with the general structure of offering her food every two to three hours, and there was a lot of flexibility.

—*Katja Rowell, MD, a mom of a six-year-old daughter, a family practice physician, and a childhood feeding specialist with TheFeedingDoctor.com, in St. Paul, MN*

My husband and I work rotating shifts, so it's hard for us to eat together. When we do, we turn off the TV and the iPad and try to have a family meal. I really value family meals because I think meals are an important time to communicate. I always try to ask my husband and my daughter how their days were.

I remember one particular dinner when my 2½-year-old daughter asked me, "Mommy, how was your day?" I nearly fell off my chair and tried so hard not to laugh. She was such a little old lady! Of course, other days she looks at me and says, "Mommy, I hate conversation. I want to watch TV." Win some, lose some.

—Lisa Campanella-Coppo, MD, a mom of a three-year-old daughter, an emergency physician, and the emergency department director of academic affairs at Monmouth Medical Center, in New Jersey

Food is not as important to me as family time. We all eat for fuel. The company at the table is where we find comfort. We try to eat together. But most nights we eat in pairs because the kids have activities at different times.

On Sundays, we have our family dinners, and I try to cook a big meal. The most important thing is not leaving someone alone to eat. When our children were younger, they always ate together at the same time. Now they come in and out at all times. It's nice to share your day with someone over a meal and give that person your focused attention.

—Elizabeth Chabner Thompson, MD, MPH, a mom of 13- and 8-year-old daughters and 12- and 10-year-old sons, a radiation oncologist with 21 C. Radiation Oncology, and the inventor of the Mommy Bag, filled with supplies for moms-to-be having C-sections, in Scarsdale, NY

Getting Meals on the Table Fast

According to the Bureau of Labor Statistics, 64 percent of moms with children under age six work outside the home. (Of course we know that all moms work inside the home!) It can be very difficult to get a meal on the table fast. But the benefits to serving your toddler nutritious foods are so great that we encourage you to try your best!

When my kids were toddlers, I often got up really early in the morning before anyone else and started prep work for dinner that night, or even for several nights that week. For each meal, I planned ahead for foods with protein and starch, as well as a vegetable and a salad. That approach helped me to keep the meals balanced.

—Lisa Dado, MD

When my son was a toddler, he wanted to be carried around all of the time. This presented a big challenge when I was trying to cook dinner. When my son was a baby, I used to wear him in his BabyBjörn, but he had outgrown that.

One day, in desperation, I popped him into his hiking carrier, and I wore him on my back while I cooked. It worked great! I cooked many meals with him riding around on my back.

—*Eva Mayer, MD, a mom of an eight-year-old daughter and a six-year-old son and a pediatrician with St. Luke's Pediatrics Associates, in Bethlehem, PA*

Sometimes "fast" meal prep isn't fast enough for hungry toddlers. When I'm preparing a meal and one of my children wanders into the kitchen looking for something to eat, I make the vegetable course first and put it on the table. My kids can eat that as soon as they'd like.

If my sons eat their vegetables first and are a little less hungry for supper, that's okay! That makes me feel like a great parent.

—*Deborah Gilboa, MD, a mom of nine-, seven-, five-, and three-year-old sons, a parenting speaker whose advice is found at AskDoctorG.com, and a family physician with Squirrel Hill Health Center, in Pittsburgh, PA*

The half-hour or so before dinnertime is very challenging. All of my kids need something, all at once.

My Crock-Pot was the best tool for getting dinners on the table fast. In the morning, I'd put the ingredients for a beef roast or spaghetti sauce into my Crock-Pot, and I'd let it simmer all day. Sometimes I'd take a few minutes while my kids were napping to set the table and do some prep work such as tossing a salad. When it was time to eat, it took only a few minutes to actually get dinner on the table.

—*Jennifer Hanes, DO*

Even if meals needed to be prepared quickly, I tried not to feed my daughter processed food, especially from cans. There's no substitute for fresh, locally grown foods.

Many cans are lined with bisphenol-A (BPA), a chemical that is now banned from baby bottles in Canada and Europe. Even if the food is organic, if it comes from a can, it likely contains BPA, which might increase the risk for cancer and problems with brain development.

—*Dora Calott Wang, MD, a mom of a nine-year-old daughter, a psychiatrist and historian at the University of New Mexico School of Medicine, and the author of* The Kitchen Shrink: A Psychiatrist's Reflection on Healing in a Changing World, *in Albuquerque, NM*

My advice on cooking is to get as much help as you can. Many people like cooking. I am not one of them.

When I was pregnant with my second daughter, I gave myself a gift: I hired a woman to come to my house once or twice each week to cook our meals for the week. In two hours, she can prepare our suppers for the week! I've hardly cooked since. Each week, I set out the recipes I'd like her to prepare, and I shop for the ingredients. Then she comes and prepares the meals and puts some in the refrigerator and others in the freezer.

I found her on GoNannies.com. You can search there for different types of helpers, such as nannies, cooks, and housekeepers. The woman I hired isn't a professional chef. She's just a woman who likes to cook who needed a job. She doesn't prepare gourmet meals, just simple, healthy recipes. It's not expensive at all: I pay her $13 an hour, and she usually works only two hours each week. It's far cheaper than takeout, and it's much healthier to boot.

—*Kate Tulenko, MD, MPH, a mom of four- and one-year-old girls, the author of* Insourced: How Importing Jobs Impacts the Healthcare Crisis Here and Abroad, *and a pediatrician and global health specialist with IntraHealth, in Washington, DC*

Encouraging Healthy Choices

Right now, you're laying the foundation for your child's lifelong eating habits. No pressure. But it really is that important. Because your toddler wants to be just like you, modeling nutritious eating and snacking is probably the best thing that you can do. For example, if your toddler sees you eating yogurt, he's more likely to try it too. And of course you reap the health benefits of all of that healthy eating too while you're at it.

By offering your toddler nutritious meals and snacks that are filled with fruits, vegetables, protein, and whole grains, you're likely meeting all of his nutritional needs. The following are a few facts to consider talking with your child's doctor about.

- Toddlers need cholesterol and other fats for growth and development, so don't restrict these. Offer regular dairy products, not reduced-fat varieties, to your toddler.
- As many as 15 percent of U.S. children younger than age three aren't getting enough iron. The American Academy of Pediatrics suggests having one-year-olds screened for iron deficiency anemia with a simple finger prick. Also, offer your toddler iron-rich foods, such as green beans, peas, and sweet potatoes.
- Almost one in five children ages 1 to 11 might have low blood levels of vitamin D. The American Academy of Pediatrics recommends that children get 400 IU a day. Good sources of vitamin D are milk and eggs.
- Nine out of 10 U.S. children don't get enough fiber. Fruits, vegetables, and whole grains are good sources of fiber.

My healthy eating strategy is buying the right foods. This is especially important if you have a babysitter or nanny because she's going to feed your kids whatever you have in the house!

—*Heather Orman-Lubell, MD, a mom of 11- and 7-year-old sons and a pediatrician in private practice at Yardley Pediatrics of St. Christopher's Hospital for Children, in Pennsylvania*

When babies become toddlers, it's harder to control their eating habits. You're battling the sugar monster. The key is to control the access.

—*Dina Strachan, MD, a mom of a six-year-old daughter, a*

dermatologist and director of Aglow Dermatology, and an assistant clinical professor in the department of dermatology at New York University, in New York City

❧

Encouraging healthy choices is definitely a challenge. I try to make sure my kids eat a fruit or vegetable with every meal—even breakfast. While we limit sweets and fatty foods, we definitely enjoy them from time to time.

I count it as a major personal victory every time I succeed in making a wholesome meal that my son says he likes. The best reward is when my son asks, "Can we eat this every night?"

—*Sigrid Payne DaVeiga, MD, a mom of a six-year-old son and a two-year-old daughter and a pediatric allergist with the Children's Hospital of Philadelphia, in Pennsylvania*

❧

It's so critical that toddlers eat the proper foods. Their brains are developing so rapidly that proper nutrition is important for them to get the best start in life.

The toddler years are the last time you can really exert control over what your child eats. I handled this in the same way I handled family values. I told my girls, "This is the way that our family eats. Period. End of discussion." You can't get away with that with teenagers; you have to do this when they're toddlers.

—*Eva Ritvo, MD, a mom of 21- and 16-year-old daughters, a psychiatrist, and a coauthor of* The Beauty Prescription, *in Miami Beach, FL*

❧

One delicious, fun way to get a lot of fruits and vegetables into my daughter's diet is to make smoothies. She's loved them since she was a toddler. I toss fruits, vegetables, juice, and ice cubes into the blender and mix them all up. My daughter can help make smoothies too, and she loves that. She's a very hands-on type of girl.

—*Christy Valentine, MD, a mom of a six-year-old daughter, a specialist in pediatrics and internal medicine, and the founder of the Valentine Medical Center, in Gretna, LA*

My son is a good eater. I want him to enjoy eating nutritious foods. I don't like to give him a lot of sweets, but sometimes I'll add a bit of something sweet to encourage him to eat a nutritious food. For example, a tiny squirt of whipped cream makes a banana go down a lot easier!

—*Deborah Kulick, MD, a mom of two-year-old and eight-month-old sons, a child and adolescent psychiatrist at the Everett Teen Health Center, and an instructor in psychiatry at Harvard Medical School and the Cambridge Health Alliance, in Boston, MA*

I gave my toddlers lots of fresh fruit to eat. But sometimes fruits like strawberries can be tart, and my kids wouldn't want to eat them. Rather than sprinkling sugar on top, I drizzled a bit of agave nectar on them.

You can buy agave nectar at health food stores and even in the natural foods section of larger grocery stores. Nectar from the agave plant is all natural and not processed. It's sweeter than sugar, so you save calories by using only a tiny bit to sweeten anything.

—*Eva Mayer, MD*

My kids aren't picky eaters, but one thing I've found that helps them eat even better is having a backyard garden. We live in New York City; it's still possible in a city. Even if you only have room for a planter box, you can grow some of your own vegetables.

From very young ages, our kids would help us in the garden, planting the vegetables and also picking them. There's something about a kid picking a vegetable himself that makes him want to eat it. I think it makes our kids feel very connected to these wholesome foods. It's as if they think, *This is something I grew, something I took care of.*

—*Ann V. Arthur, MD, a mom of a 10-year-old daughter and an 8-year-old son, a pediatric ophthalmologist in private practice at Park Slope Eye Care Associates, and a blogger at WaterWineTravel.com, in New York City*

I feel very strongly about the importance of good nutrition. I was a working mother, and I wanted to make sure my daughter ate nutritious foods and a balanced, portion-controlled diet while I was at work.

I bought plenty of fresh fruits and vegetables, and each day I made lists for my nanny. It was like a Chinese menu: Choose one from column A, one from column B, etc. For example, one day my daughter could have a cup of strawberries, an orange, or a kiwifruit. And then she could have chicken, tuna, or shrimp.

To this day, my daughter eats a very balanced diet. She's also at a very healthy weight.

—*Debra Jaliman, MD, a mom of a 20-year-old daughter, a dermatologist in private practice, and an assistant professor of dermatology at Mt. Sinai School of Medicine, in New York City*

I had wanted my children to eat vegetarian like me. But one day my husband asked me to give our son a taste of beef. My son loved it! I thought, *Well, okay, I can't make him be a vegetarian.*

I definitely think that kids will learn to eat any food if you let them try it early enough. When my kids were toddlers, I made almost everything from scratch.

I used a lot of simple techniques to get my toddlers to eat nutritious foods. I'd give them silly names, like broccoli trees. I often arranged the food on their plates into funny faces. And I often taught my kids simple nutrition concepts, like "Green is good for growth."

—*Teresa Hubka, DO, a mom of a 14-year-old son and an 8-year-old daughter, an ob-gyn and the medical director of Comprehensive Wellness Care in Chicago, and an associate professor of obstetrics and gynecology and the chairman and residency program director of the department of obstetrics and gynecology at the Midwestern University/Chicago College of Osteopathic Medicine, in Downers Grove, Illinois*

I didn't have much trouble with feeding my children until they went to preschool. There they learned that vegetables were "yucky." My eldest child would eat an entire cup of mushrooms as a toddler at home, but once she went to preschool, she wouldn't touch them.

I think that if foods are cut and arranged to look beautiful, children are more likely to be interested in eating them.

My kids also loved to dip their food in things before eating it. I would use yogurt, ranch dressing, and pureed fruits (and sometimes I would sneak in vegetables) as a dipping sauce for cut fruits and vegetables.

I also found that my kids loved foods that were frozen cut-up. Frozen grapes are still one of their favorite snacks, and they're much better for them than popsicles! (Watch your children carefully while they're eating.)

As soon as my children could sit upright independently and manage their airways, I would give them bits of frozen fruits. I remember starting with mashed frozen blueberries. I learned about this from another mother who had given the frozen fruits to her children as they were teething. Her children were much younger than mine at the time and were able to manage these treats. I was more cautious, and I cut my children's grapes into smaller pieces and gave this to them when they were around 18 months old.

—*Laura M. Rosch, DO, a mom of a 12-year-old daughter and 7-year-old boy-girl twins, a board-certified internist who works at Central DuPage Hospital Convenient Care Centers in Winfield, IL, and an instructor in the department of family medicine at the Midwestern University/Chicago College of Osteopathic Medicine, in Downers Grove, IL*

◦⁄◦

When my kids were toddlers, I tried to cook as much as possible. For me, cooking is a joy, but if I don't have enough time to do it, it becomes a burden.

Cooking at home meant great smells from the kitchen and comfort foods, not fast food. At each meal, I tried to give our kids adult food and one carb, one protein, and one vegetable. I tried. I wasn't perfect. Sometimes we have "breakfast for dinner" and we eat scrambled eggs, waffles, or some other traditional breakfast food. It's fine, and the kids think it's fun. I'm human, and I run out of ideas like everyone else.

One of our boys is incredibly picky. He refuses to eat any vegetable other than broccoli (so I served it every night) or any fruit other than dried strawberries (which I dug out of the Special K, initially). Rather than focusing on what my son won't eat, I try to feed him the nutritious foods he will eat.

My son is healthy and off the charts in height, so I have no worries about malnourishment.

—*Elizabeth Chabner Thompson, MD, MPH*

I always keep a bowl of fresh fruit on the kitchen counter, and my sons can eat fruit anytime they want. Also, I have a "free" snack drawer stocked with nutritious snacks that they can eat anytime, such as apple crisps and other single-ingredient snacks.

My sons are only allowed to eat these snacks while they're sitting at the kitchen table. Wandering around snacking is not a good idea! First, it's a choking hazard. Second, it makes a mess. Third, it encourages a bad habit. If you need to eat, you should sit down and enjoy it.

I don't worry about good snacks "ruining" someone's dinner. I'd rather have my kids eat a nutritious snack before dinner than be cranky and hungry.

—*Deborah Gilboa, MD*

Imagine if someone dictated when and what you ate at every meal: I bet you'd resent it! Toddlers are trying to forge their own identities, and they're beginning to have strong preferences.

Eating became a power struggle between my son and me: He wouldn't eat certain foods just because I was hell-bent on making him eat them. So I started offering him little "courses," much like an Italian meal. There's the antipasti, the first course, the second course, then coffee and dessert. (Of course, they all involve some sort of fruit, milk, and vegetable combo.)

That way, my son felt like he got his pick of what he wanted to eat. The trick was that I had to present only one vegetable at a time, so if my son turned his nose up at it, I could then present a different course. The end result was that I needed to cook more food, but I definitely avoided the power struggle with my son.

When my son turned three, it was a whole different ball game. He became wise to my tactics and began to steadfastly refuse vegetables, just to be contrary. (My friends who have children the same age all corroborated—once our boys turned three, they all turned into mini-teenagers and did exactly the opposite of what we wanted.) I knew the importance of instilling a taste for healthy foods early, so I tried every method known to man to get my son to eat his veggies. You name it, I've tried it: bribery, reward, extortion, blackmailing, imploring, threats, using the check system, deception, scare tactics, dinner and a show, the happy face, anthropomorphizing food objects. I actually was quite proud of myself on the occasions when I came up with something that worked, such as telling him that there was a disco green bean party going on in his belly, and all the green beans wanted to go. I never saw him eat green beans so fast and with a smile on his face.

I can tell you that shortly after my son turned four, he just announced one day, "Mommy, when I was three, I didn't eat my vegetables; now I'm four, I'm going to eat veggies." I asked him, "You couldn't decide this last year to spare me a year's worth of torture?" But now when people ask me how I get my son to eat vegetables, I tell them it's all due to my unfailing persistence.

—*Cheryl Wu, MD, a mom of a four-year-old son, a pediatrician at LaGuardia Place Pediatrics in New York City, and a pediatric emergency physician at the Joseph M. Sanzari Children's Hospital of Hackensack University Medical Center, in New Jersey*

I fed my children the freshest, least processed foods possible. For example, I'd give them a homemade "popsicle" made from organic grape juice rather than store-bought popsicles.

It's important to give your children the food that their bodies need to thrive. The best foods are generally the ones that are the least processed.

—*Cathie Lippman, MD, a mom of 31- and 29-year-old sons and a physician who specializes in environmental and preventive medicine at the Lippman Center for Optimal Health, in Beverly Hills, CA*

Watching Out for Overeating

The statistics in the United States are sobering.

- Since 1980, obesity prevalence among children and adolescents has almost tripled.
- Approximately 17 percent of children and teens ages two to 19 are obese.
- Nearly one-third of low-income preschool children ages two to four are overweight, and 14 percent are obese.
- 12 percent of children ages six months to 23 months are overweight.

When to Call Your Doctor

A chubby belly or thighs on a baby are endearing, but it can be hard to know if your toddler's girth is healthy or cause for concern.

Weight can be particularly tricky for parents to judge. One study found that about a third of mothers with overweight kids underestimated their child's weight. For that reason, it's helpful to get guidance from your doctor. Pediatricians start calculating body mass index (BMI) at age two, and your doctor should tell you where your child falls on a growth chart. (If your doctor doesn't, ask for the information.)

If your child's BMI is at the 5th percentile to less than the 85th percentiles, don't worry. That's considered a normal weight for her age.

However, if your child's BMI is at the 85th to less than the 95th percentiles, she's considered overweight. Kids with a BMI in the 95th percentile or higher are considered obese. If that's the case, talk to your pediatrician about your child's eating habits and activity level, and brainstorm ideas for introducing healthy habits in your child's life that can help him get to a healthy weight. The doctor might even want to screen your child for diabetes or other conditions related to obesity.

This is also a good time to ask your doctor if it's worthwhile to see a registered dietitian for more advice about your child's diet.

Sadly, parents are often blinded by love for their children and might not see them as overweight. To make matters worse, doctors often don't speak up about a child's size until he has already become overweight.

It might be very helpful to keep in mind the portions that a toddler should eat. Don't go by the nutrition labels on packages! Those serving sizes are designed for adults. Realistic serving sizes for toddlers include the following.

- Bread: ½ slice
- Cereal: ⅓ cup
- Pasta: ¼ cup, cooked
- Cooked vegetables: ¼ cup
- Meat: 1 ounce
- Milk: ½ cup

A child-size divided plate, which often has three or four small compartments for food, can be a helpful tool to measure and balance your child's meals. Find one in his favorite color or adorned with his favorite cartoon character for bonus points!

I didn't worry about my twins overeating. I found that as they became toddlers, their appetites naturally slowed down in response to their slowing growth rate. I think that more parents of toddlers are worried about their toddlers not eating enough. I offered my kids a variety of foods to eat, and they grew and developed at a healthy rate.

—*Ann Contrucci, MD, a mom of 13-year-old boy-girl twins who works as a pediatric emergency physician, in Atlanta, GA*

I think there are only two foods my daughter doesn't like: avocados and pomegranates. Otherwise she's a very good eater, maybe too good.

My strategy to prevent overeating is that I serve my daughter the most nutritious foods of each meal first, for example, the vegetables and fruit. Then I give her the protein-rich food. And then finally I give her the grains or starch. This way my daughter doesn't fill up on pasta or bread, and then not have room for her vegetables.

Another trick I use to prevent overeating is putting any snack foods that my daughter loves, such as Puffs, in high cabinets so she can't see them. Out of sight equals out of mind.

—*Jennifer Bacani McKenney, MD*

My daughter's weight was above average, which was no surprise since I was a 9½-pound newborn, and my husband was over 10 pounds! At first, I did worry about my daughter's weight. This was about the time that the child obesity hysteria was really ratcheting up. Then I educated myself and really dug into the research. That reassured me that healthy growth is steady growth, even if it is a bit faster or slower than average.

Educating myself helped me relax and not worry about my daughter's weight, and I did a better job supporting her way of eating. I think we're born knowing how much we need to eat to grow in a healthy way. I had to learn to trust that for my family, and I am so grateful I did. I find that the less I worry about parenting in every way, the better my family does.

—*Katja Rowell, MD*

My children were all very good eaters. I never had any challenges getting them to eat. It was more of a challenge to prevent overeating. They were all in the high percentiles for weight. Fortunately, my kids were also tall, so their height kept pace with their weight.

I remember my son eating breakfast, holding a sausage in each hand! He was a big eater. I was just so happy that my kids were eating that I didn't worry too much about them overeating. I felt that I was doing a great job, getting them to eat.

Today, my kids are all very healthy. My son is an athlete, and he is incredibly disciplined about his diet. While most teens love to eat chips and cookies, my son won't eat anything like that. He takes a huge lunchbox to school, and it's filled with healthy foods like chicken, yogurt, and fruit.

—*Lisa Dado, MD*

It's ironic: Parents worry so much about their children being underweight their first two years, and then they worry about their children being overweight for the next 90 years. My girls have always been skinny, and that gives my husband no end of worry. But I'm not going to force them to eat. Right now, their appetites tell them when they're finished eating. That's a natural instinct, and we break that when we force kids to eat.

I want my girls to know that feeling of "I'm finished eating. I'm done." I hope that if I let them recognize it when they're one and four, they'll continue to recognize it when they're 20 and 24, and they won't struggle with weight problems.

I was fortunate that my family set good eating examples. My mom put food on our plates at the stove, and she put leftovers away quickly so second helpings were discouraged. She served fruit for dessert. My husband's family, on the other hand, ate family style with serving dishes on the table. His family encouraged second helpings and ate sweets for dessert. Guess which family has weight issues!

—*Kate Tulenko, MD, MPH*

RALLIE'S TIP

It's entirely possible for children to overeat, and it's not at all uncommon for parents to overfeed their kids. It might be hard to believe, but as parents, we aren't always good at determining whether our children are overfed, and thus whether they're overweight. We love our children completely—and often blindly!

When my oldest son was a toddler, he went through a phase of telling me that he was hungry several times a day, even shortly after he had just eaten a meal or snack. As a new mom, I was concerned that he was overeating and that he was at risk for becoming overweight. I asked my neighbor, who had five children, what she thought I should do, and she gave me some excellent advice. She told me that I should feed my son whenever he said he was hungry, but that didn't mean I should feed him exactly what he asked for. If he said he was hungry and he would only eat a cookie, then he probably wasn't really all that hungry.

If you are concerned that your child is overeating and gaining too much weight, take him to his pediatrician for a complete checkup and an evaluation of his eating habits. If his weight is in a good range for his height and age, he might be continually asking for food because he's actively growing and gaining weight as he should be. If the pediatrician finds that your toddler is underweight, his frequent requests for food could be a sign that he has a metabolic issue or a nutritional need that should be addressed. If he's overweight, he might have a physical or a behavioral issue that needs to be addressed.

Once your toddler has been evaluated by his pediatrician, it might be helpful to ask for a referral to a dietitian who specializes in childhood nutrition. Together, you can create a diet and feeding schedule that best meets your toddler's needs, and helps give you peace of mind.

Helping Picky Eaters

Picky eating is to toddlers what sleep deprivation is among mothers: very, very common. After a baby's first year of rapid growth, his growth slows, and so he naturally eats less. Plus, what toddler wants to stop to eat when there's a great big world out there to explore? And Thomas the Tank Engine is on TV to boot!

As a guideline, most toddlers should eat three meals and two snacks a day. But these aren't gargantuan-size meals and snacks! A toddler's meal or snack should only be about 200 calories, to reach the total goal of 1,000 calories a day. Here's what 100 to 200 calories looks like.

- One banana
- One cheese stick
- One cup yogurt
- One granola bar
- Six animal crackers
- One cup apple juice
- One cup milk

⌒

My son is a very picky eater. He likes shapes, so I found that when I cut his food into fun shapes, he's more likely to eat it. For example, I cut grilled cheese into triangles or stars. I use cookie cutters for other fun shapes.

Also, my son likes bright colors, so I put a few drops of food coloring into food to make it more colorful. For example, I might tint his pasta blue or green!

—*Shilpa Amin-Shah, MD, a mom of a two-year-old son and a one-year-old daughter and an emergency physician at Emergency Medical Associates, in Livingston, NJ*

My son and one daughter were very picky eaters. My philosophy is that it's disgusting to make a person eat a food he doesn't like. But unfortunately, that made me into a short-order cook, preparing many different foods at the same meal to keep everyone in my family happy.

In hindsight, it would have been better to say, "If you don't choose to eat what I've cooked, that's fine. But I'm not preparing you another meal!"

—*Dana S. Simpler, MD, a mom of 25- and 20-year-old girls and a 23-year-old son and a specialist in internal medicine in private practice, in Baltimore, MD*

∽

Practically all toddlers are picky eaters! It's important to remember that toddlers do better with smaller, more frequent meals than three square meals a day.

My strategy for my daughters was to give them plenty of snacks, but to make sure those snacks were nutritious foods, not empty calories. I'd pretty much offer the same foods as snacks as I did for meals. I had a round Tupperware container that held several pie-slice shaped containers. I'd fill these containers with nutritious snack options, such as carrots and cheese. I used to prepare a snack my kids loved: Spread whipped cream cheese onto thinly sliced deli meats and roll into spirals.

One temptation to avoid is crackers. They offer very little nutrition and fill kids up so they don't want to eat more nutritious foods.

—*Cathy Marshall, MD, a mom of 28-, 14-, and 11-year-old daughters and a pediatrician in private practice, in Encino, CA*

∽

Before my older son was 18 months old, he'd eat whatever I put into his mouth. But since then, he's become a pretty picky eater. My son knows that he has the power to refuse to eat certain foods. He eats whole grain pasta and bread. He likes bananas and grapes, but he has to be in the mood for apples.

Because my son doesn't eat a lot, I try to buy very nutrient- and calorie-dense foods. I want to make sure to get a lot of bang for my buck. So, for instance, I buy whole grain raisin bread. This way, my son eats some dried fruit with his bread. Plus, at 190 calories per slice, I know that my son is getting a lot of calories in a small amount of food.

—*Sharon Boyce, MD, a mom of three- and one-year-old sons and a family physician at DayOne Family Healthcare Clinic, in Battle Creek, MI*

✑

Like most toddlers, my daughter was often totally unpredictable about her tastes. For example, one day she'd like bananas, the next day she wouldn't. I tried to keep the big picture in mind and not worry about it. It's easy to get into the mind-set of "okay, she doesn't like bananas, so cross them off the list." But the next day if I tried again, she might eat them. Or maybe the next week, or the next month! Persistence paid off.

I just kept offering a variety of foods to my daughter, without pressure, and in time she'd give them a try. It took five years for her to learn to like lettuce, but she saw my husband and me enjoy salads for years. In the meantime she liked the cucumbers and tomatoes that were in the salads. The key with my own family has been repeatedly offering the foods that I want my daughter to grow up eating, and then biting my tongue about trying to make her eat them. Then patience, patience, patience!

—*Katja Rowell, MD*

✑

Picky eating is definitely a challenge. My daughter is very headstrong, and she knows what she likes and what she doesn't like. She's a very picky eater.

I try to give my daughter nutritious foods that she likes, such as applesauce and yogurt, but I've had to get a little creative in getting her to eat vegetables. I've made Jessica Seinfeld's spinach brownie recipe, and my daughter enjoyed it. I also give my daughter foods like Veggie Wedges (e.g., carrot fries), which she likes.

My daughter is a fan of the Dr. Seuss book *Green Eggs and Ham*. I often use that book to encourage her to try new things.

"Try it. You might like it," I tell her.

—*Tanya Douglas Holland, MD, a mom of a two-year-old daughter, a women's health advocate, and a consultant in medical affairs to a pharmaceutical company, in Atlanta, GA*

My daughter refused to touch meat between ages 1½ and 2½. She readily ate yogurt and cheese, vegetables mixed with cheese, rice cereal, and all kinds of fruit.

I was worried sick that my daughter wouldn't get enough protein. However, by 2½, she was back to eating everything the rest of us ate. She was an extremely healthy eater from then on. In fact, in high school she worried about putting on too much weight. My daughter had a dairy intolerance that became worse during adolescence. This meant she had to give up cheese and yogurt as well as milk. A few years ago, she also developed gluten intolerance, and she's now on both a gluten-free and dairy-free diet.

—*Stuart Jeanne Bramhall, MD, a mom of a 31-year-old daughter and a child and adolescent psychiatrist in New Plymouth, New Zealand*

Feeding toddlers is tricky; they can practically live on air. The way I look at it is that toddlers eat by the week. At any one meal, or even on any one day, they might not eat much. But if you look at the bigger picture of an entire week, hopefully you'll see that it all evens out.

I think parents get into trouble when they worry too much that their toddlers aren't eating enough, and this causes them to cave to toddlers' requests for not-so-nutritious food. They think, *Well, at least he's eating something*, even if that something is Goldfish crackers for breakfast.

No toddler ever starved himself. Take the long view, and be sure to offer healthy choices to your toddler.

—Victoria McEvoy, MD, a mom who raised four children; a grandmom of six-, four-, and two-year-old grandsons; an assistant professor of pediatrics at Harvard Medical School; the medical director and chief of pediatrics at Mass General West Medical Group; and the author of 24/7 Baby Doctor, *in Boston, MA*

? When to Call Your Doctor

A baby's weight triples during the first year of life, but you'll notice your child's growth slowing quite a bit after blowing out the candle on his first birthday cake. That can make it hard to know if he's gaining enough weight during the toddler years.

The best way to know if your child is underweight is by plotting his weight on a growth chart, which your pediatrician should do during his well-child visit. If your child's BMI falls below the 5th percentile, he's considered underweight.

The first thing to do is to talk about your family history with your pediatrician. If your or your spouse's family tends to be small, your child might follow suit. Your child's doctor might also consider performing tests to see if a medical condition is affecting your child's weight, and she might start monitoring your child's growth more often than she was before. If your pediatrician suspects a growth disorder, she might recommend seeing a pediatric endocrinologist.

My second child was a notoriously poor eater. I literally pulled my hair out trying to get him to eat. I learned that it didn't help matters if I became frustrated. Time and time again, when I got frustrated, it backfired, and he ate less, not more.

I finally accepted the fact that my son didn't have a hearty appetite. He was growing, and his pediatrician wasn't concerned. So I took my cue from him. Once I was able to let go and I stopped fussing at my son to eat, the stress level went down. My son and I were both much happier.

Looking back, I wonder if some of my son's eating challenges were related to an underlying health issue. He had chronic sinus problems and frequent sinus infections. If a child is a really picky eater, it's wise to talk with a pediatrician to make sure there isn't a health issue that's causing the diminished appetite. A smoldering infection, such as an ear infection, can make a child less interested in eating. Along the same lines, a sinus infection can make it more difficult to smell and taste food, making it less palatable.

My other children were all hearty eaters with welcoming palates, even as toddlers. I didn't exploit their tastes early on by giving them foods like French fries and ice cream. I knew I couldn't keep those foods away from my kids forever, but I sure could while they were toddlers. I gave them only nutritious foods, such as green beans, spinach, and squash.

—*Ann Kulze, MD, a mom of 23- and 17-year-old daughters and 22- and 20-year-old sons; a nationally recognized nutrition expert, motivational speaker, and physician; and the author of the bestselling book* Dr. Ann's Eat Right for Life, *in Charleston, SC*

⤬

I definitely noticed my daughter became a picky eater in her toddler years. Before my daughter turned two years old, she would eat anything and everything—all variety of fruits, veggies, meats, fish, and even spicy foods. Suddenly, when my daughter was around two years old, she decided that she would eat only certain foods and not others. Veggies were in the "not" category, that's for sure!

My husband and I had to use different forms of motivation to get our daughter to eat better. For instance, we would tell her that she could only have her favorite food (like a peanut butter sandwich) if she first ate four carrots. Or she could only have a cookie if she first ate five bites of the chicken that the rest of the family was having. It was like we had to find the "button" to push to get her to eat the right things!

We also learned that persistence and patience pay off. One day our daughter would hate a certain food, but the next day she would love that same food!

—Melody Derrick, MD, a mom of a two-year-old daughter who's expecting another baby and a family physician in private practice with Cadence Physician Group, in Winfield, IL

Each of my sons has gone through a crazy picky eating phase. My husband and I have a three-pronged approach to deal with this. First, although we often like to try new foods, we introduce only one new food at a meal. For example, if we're trying a new vegetable, we prepare familiar protein foods and starches that we know our kids love.

Second, my sons know that they don't have to eat everything on their plates. However, if they want seconds of any one thing, they have to finish everything else first.

Third, no matter what we're eating, our sons can always request a few nutritious foods in addition. I'm not a short-order cook, but they can always have hummus and pita, carrots and ranch dressing, or peanut butter and bread.

The key with toddlers is to offer them choices with limits. I don't have any kids who are seriously underweight, so I've never been concerned about any of them starving.

—Deborah Gilboa, MD

RALLIE'S TIP

During the toddler years, children often develop rather erratic eating behaviors. They're so busy at this stage of life that they often feel that they have far more interesting things to do than eat!

The toddler and preschool years are a very important time in terms of developing healthy eating habits. It's helpful for parents to remember that growth for toddlers normally occurs at a much slower pace than it did during infancy. Because babies are growing so rapidly, they spend much of their time eating. A slower rate of growth explains why many toddlers seem to have less than hearty appetites and display less interest in food and eating. This causes many moms to worry that their children aren't getting enough to eat.

My middle son wasn't a big eater as a toddler, and I often wondered if I should push him a little harder to eat more often or to eat more at meals and snacks. I tried to get him to eat when he didn't really want to once or twice, and the results were not good. Mealtime quickly became unpleasant, and he probably ended up eating less than he would have if I had just left him alone. Plus, I think the stress of the battle gave us both indigestion.

As mothers, our job is to provide our children with a variety of wholesome, nutritious foods at meals and snacks in a relaxed, comfortable environment. The decisions about whether to eat—or how much to eat—at a particular time belong to your toddler. Allowing him to respond to his own internal cues of hunger and satiety will help your toddler develop a healthy attitude toward food and eating. Forcing children to eat when they don't feel hungry, on the other hand, increases the risk that they'll develop unhealthy eating behaviors.

The best way to determine if your toddler is getting enough to eat is to check with your pediatrician to make sure that he's growing and gaining weight at an appropriate rate. If he is, you can relax and enjoy these busy toddler years!

In spite of my concerns about my son's eating habits, he continued to grow and gain weight appropriately. As it turned out, he was a much better regulator of his appetite and his food intake than I was.

While some toddlers refuse to eat certain foods or at certain times, others can become very attached to one food or another. It's not a good idea to habitually give in to your toddler's demands for a particular food whenever he insists on having it. As a parent, you know what's best for your child. If he cries and demands a cookie and a soda right before dinner, he'll fill up on sugar and empty calories, and he'll be less likely to eat the more nutritious foods that you serve at the evening meal. If your child really is hungry, you can offer him a choice of nutritious items, such as apple slices or cheese cubes instead of a cookie.

It's not advisable to punish a child for undesirable eating behaviors, because it can lead to more problematic eating behaviors and attitudes toward food. It's also unwise to "force" a child to eat. Your best bet is to create a consistent routine. Start by preparing a nutritious breakfast, lunch, and dinner plus at least two snacks for your toddler at roughly the same time each day. Put the food on the table or on his high chair, and sit down with him to eat. Even if he says he's not hungry, ask him to sit down while you and the rest of your family eat your meal. If he hasn't been joining the family for meals before now, start by asking him to stay seated for three to five minutes, and gradually increase the amount of time he's required to stay at the table.

Make sure that there's at least one nutritious food on your toddler's plate that you know he likes. That way, you'll know that he won't go hungry because he doesn't like what you've served, and you won't feel obligated to jump up from the table and prepare another food. If he asks for—or demands—something that isn't on his plate, gently but firmly let him know that it's not on the menu right now, without making a big deal about it. As long as you're consistent, it doesn't take long for toddlers to learn to sit at the table and eat and enjoy the foods that the rest of the family eats and enjoys.

Teaching Kids a Love of Cooking

You are what you eat. But maybe more importantly, you eat what you cook. So what better way to help kids eat better than to teach them how to cook better?

Toddlers are often eager to help, and they find many cooking tasks fun: mixing, rolling, and, best of all, tasting! To kids, cooking is all fun and games.

My older son really loved cooking, even as a toddler. He helped me in the kitchen, for example by helping me mix things or find things in the refrigerator.

I also wanted to buy my son a kitchen play set. But every one we could find was pink! Finally my in-laws found a child's cooking set that was blue and white with gold stars. My son loved to play with that cooking set, and we have passed it around to other boys in the family since.

—*Leena Shrivastava Dev, MD, a mom of 15- and 11-year-old sons, a general pediatrician, and an advocate for child safety, in Philadelphia, PA*

My older son loves to help me cook. I try to make him a part of the process. He puts on a little apron, and he can mash potatoes or bananas with a masher. I admit I have to set the bowl onto our very clean kitchen floor, so it doesn't fall off the counter.

—*Deborah Kulick, MD*

My kids are all pretty good eaters. I think that it helps that since our kids were toddlers, my husband and I have engaged them in the preparation of food and let them taste it as we cooked.

My husband loves to make bread, and we have developed a bit of bread snobbery. Our kids like homemade bread fresh, warm, and buttered. Wonder Bread won't cut it in our house.

—*Brooke A. Jackson, MD, a mom of 4½-year-old twin girls and a 2½-year-old son, a dermatologist, and the founder and medical director of the Skin Wellness Center of Chicago, in Illinois*

When my daughters were toddlers, I gave them age-appropriate "jobs" in the kitchen, such as pouring measured ingredients into bowls, spooning cupcake batter into the cups, and even cleanup duties.

With teaching kids to cook comes the importance of teaching kids to cook safely. All of my knives have black handles. I taught my daughters very early on not to touch black handles, so they wouldn't accidentally grab a sharp knife.

—*Marra S. Francis, MD, a mom of eight-, seven-, and five-year-old daughters and a gynecologist, in San Antonio, TX*

I encouraged my toddlers to hop on the stool and help me in the kitchen. If I was cutting tofu, I would give a small piece to my toddlers and allow them to use a butter knife to cut their piece. If I was washing spinach, their hands were in the sink along with mine.

When tasting, I would allow the kids to taste and make appropriate noises, such as "yummy" or "blow first, hot." We also would make "pictures" with veggie pieces, and then eat the drawings.

Another fun toddler task was blending smoothies. My toddler would help pour the milk into the blender, drop the berries in, and press the button. This was a great opportunity to repeat single words to increase vocabulary. Cooking with kids is a schoolroom opportunity in your kitchen.

I feel like I accomplished my goal of encouraging my kids to eat well. My adult kids now ask for tofu when they come home, for example.

—*Hana R. Solomon, MD, a mom who raised four children, a grandmom of three, a board-certified pediatrician, the president of BeWell Health, LLC, and the author of* Clearing the Air One Nose at a Time: Caring for Your Personal Filter, *in Columbia, MO*

In the past, I didn't like cooking and always resisted my mother's attempts to teach me. But I realized that my picky toddler would always eat his grandmother's Asian dishes. So I said to myself, *Well, I guess I now need to learn how to make Chinese food!* After a year of cooking at least three days a week and subjecting my son and myself to charred food and at times nauseating culinary experiences, I can now say I'm a pretty good cook, at least for the under-five set. And a pretty great thing happened along the way: I now actually enjoy cooking!

Since my son was about two years old, I've let him help me prepare meals. For example, he can cut tofu with a butter knife. It's really not that much different than cutting Play-Doh! It helps him with his hand-eye coordination, and it also keeps him busy. Now that my son is four, he's quite proficient at peeling garlic. It must have something to do with those little fingers. (I keep joking that working at a garlic factory could be his fallback career.) He also helps me by snapping green beans, squeezing lemon juice, and beating eggs. I can't wait until he can finally cook by himself. That way, I get to ask him what's for dinner!

—*Cheryl Wu, MD*

Learning to Use Utensils and Dishes

By age one, young toddlers are eager to exert their new independence and pick up food all by themselves. By about a year and a half, most children can use a spoon to get the food into their mouths, when they want to. Otherwise, it winds up who knows where.

By about 2½, most toddlers have mastered the art of the fork. At around this age, many toddlers become fastidious, not wanting to get food on their hands nor on their adorable little faces! The end of the mess is in sight: By age five, children should be using utensils all of the time. Hurrah!

When my kids were toddlers, I bought an assortment of plastic cups, bowls, and plates. I stored them in a low cabinet that my kids could reach themselves. This way, my kids would help themselves to the dishes, without fear of breaking one. They could help me set the table and even empty the dishwasher. This also gave my kids a bit of independence, which toddlers crave.

—*Dana S. Simpler, MD*

My youngest son has been the least messy eater of all of my children. He sees what his big sisters and brother do, and he wants to be like them. He's always wanted to feed himself, and he's been eating with a fork and spoon practically forever.

One thing that makes it easier for children is to let them use child-size utensils with chunky, rubber handles. They're easier to hold onto. I also have a large supply of unbreakable plastic dishes.

—*Kristie McNealy, MD, a mom of nine- and six-year-old daughters and four-year-old and 22-month-old sons and a blogger at KristieMcNealy.com, in Denver, CO*

My daughter is just starting to use a fork and a spoon. But when she gets frustrated, she resorts to eating with her fingers.

I have found that even if the utensils decorated with cartoon characters are more expensive, they're worth the price because my daughter is more willing to use them! So we have Elmo forks and spoons and Dora the Explorer cups. Having the familiar characters on the dinnerware makes my daughter more interested in using them.

—*Rachel S. Rohde, MD*

⁓

At two, my younger son is very comfortable using a fork and spoon. He's so adept that he can twirl his spaghetti on his fork!

I didn't buy any new toddler silverware. We had some left over from my older son, but usually we just give our younger son our regular-size silverware.

—*Rebecca Reamy, MD, a mom of seven- and two-year-old sons and a pediatrician in emergency medicine at Children's Healthcare of Atlanta, in Georgia*

⁓

I am not a big fan of plastic dishes and utensils. I used them when my girls were one and two, but by the time my younger daughter turned three years old, I transitioned her to using grown-up glass plates and bowls. It's been fine!

—*Cheri Wiggins, MD, a mom of six- and three-year-old daughters, a specialist in physical medicine and rehabilitation at St. Luke's Magic Valley, and the cofounder of the Mommy Doctors Bakery (makers of Milkin' Cookies), in Twin Falls, ID*

⁓

In addition to giving my daughter utensils at each meal, I also always give her a napkin or paper towel too. That way, she's able to dab a bit at any mess she makes!

—*Tanya Douglas Holland, MD*

Eating Out with Your Toddler

According to a Gallup poll, 60 percent of Americans eat out at least once a week. Forty-two percent say they eat out twice a week, and 18 percent eat out three or more times a week.

Parents, of course, are no exception to this. In fact, according to the National Restaurant Association, some of the biggest restaurant trends have parents straight in their crosshairs. Five of their top 20 trends for 2012 involve kids. These trends include the following.

- "Healthful" kids' meals
- Children's nutrition as a culinary theme
- Whole grain items in kids' meals
- Fruit/vegetable kids' side items
- Children's mini-meals (smaller versions of adult menu items)

But most important is your answer to the question: Do you want fries with that?

〰

At home, my daughter uses toddler-size utensils. When we go out to eat, rather than having to bring those along, I often ask for plastic silverware. It's smaller than regular silverware, and it's easier for my daughter to manage.

—*Tanya Douglas Holland, MD*

〰

My husband and I have taken our daughter to a couple of restaurants. But as a toddler, she can be a little unpredictable, so it's easiest to stick with places where there are a lot of families. If we are at the mall, we'll go to the food court, where a quick exit is possible if needed.

—*Rachel S. Rohde, MD*

〰

When I took my toddlers out to eat, I was careful to give them clear direction up front. Rather than saying, "Be a good girl," which is vague and really meaningless to a toddler, I'd say, "Remember our two restaurant rules: Stay in your seat and use your inside voice."

My girls could understand those simple rules, and they were able to follow them. You can't, of course, give a toddler 49 rules to follow. Keep the rules simple and short.

—*Cathy Marshall, MD*

When my husband and I took our toddlers out to eat, they knew we expected them to behave. If one of our sons didn't behave, one parent would take him to the car.

You don't have to do that many times before kids realize that you really mean it. If one of my sons had to go to the car, he knew that his brother was having a good time and he wasn't. Pretty soon, my husband and I would only have to ask, "Do you need to go to the car?" and our boys would shape up.

—*Carrie Brown, MD, a mom of eight- and six-year-old sons and a general pediatrician who treats medically complex children and specializes in palliative care at Arkansas Children's Hospital, in Little Rock*

When my sons were one or two years old, our meals were chaotic. Sometimes I had no idea what I was even eating! But by the time my sons were three and four years old, they were able to sit through a meal, and we could all enjoy a nice family dinner. My husband and I could safely take our kids to restaurants because they knew that "restaurant-grade" behavior was expected. Eating out became a pleasure again.

—*Ayala Laufer-Cahana, MD, a mom of 16- and 14-year-old sons and a 12-year-old daughter, a pediatrician, and the founder of Herbal Water Inc., in Wynnewood, PA*

When we go out to eat, I always ask the waiter to bring four servings of the kids' vegetable of the day first—one for each of my sons—before we even crack open the menus. That way, when my kids are hungry and bored, they eat all of their vegetables first, while they're coloring on their placemats and playing with their straws. With any luck, after they've eaten their vegetables, they might be a little less starving for the sweet drinks and mac 'n cheese.

Also we keep kosher, and the way we are able to go out to eat is we eat vegetarian in restaurants. Vegetables and meatless pasta are great choices.

—*Deborah Gilboa, MD*

Chapter 4
Breastfeeding

YOUR TODDLER'S DEVELOPMENT

Around the world, many children older than age one are still breastfeeding. In fact, the World Health Organization and UNICEF both recommend that babies breastfeed for at least two years.

According to the Centers for Disease Control and Prevention, at one year old, 23 percent of babies in the United States are still breastfeeding. The American Academy of Pediatrics states that breastfeeding should be continued for at least the first year of life and beyond for as long as mutually desired by mother and child.

But by age one, almost all children in the United States are eating solid foods as well. Breastfeeding might serve as a complement to that and also be a source of comfort.

TAKING CARE OF YOU

What better way to protect your breasts than by having a mammogram? If you're on the north side of 40 and you haven't had your annual mammogram, schedule it today! The National Cancer Institute recommends that women age 40 or older have screening mammograms every one to two years.

JUSTIFICATION FOR A CELEBRATION

If you are still breastfeeding after your child is one year old, the day you stop is bound to be bittersweet. Treat yourself with kindness, and take some time to reflect on and even celebrate this milestone.

84

Breastfeeding an Older Baby

It can be challenging for moms to continue to nurse an older baby, but it's rewarding as well. Here are some of the benefits to nursing.

For your toddler:

- Breast milk continues to offer vitamins and other nutrients and helps improve immunity.
- Nursing offers close, skin-to-skin contact.
- Taking time to breastfeed gives toddlers a respite in their busy days.

For you:

- A number of studies have shown health benefits, including a reduced risk of certain cancers. Ovarian and uterine cancers have been found to be more common among women who didn't breastfeed.
- Making milk requires 200 to 500 calories a day. To burn that many calories, you'd have to swim 30 laps in a pool or bicycle uphill for an hour!
- Despite concerns that breastfeeding pulls calcium from a mother's bones, studies find that after weaning their children, breastfeeding mothers' bone density returns to pre-pregnancy levels, or even higher levels.
- Breastfeeding provides a skin-to-skin closeness with your toddler.
- Prolactin, the hormone produced when making milk, appears to have a calming effect on moms. And who couldn't use a little more of that?

My twins still breastfed until they were about 15 months old, each morning and then again in the evening. I think that they enjoyed that special time they each had me all to themselves. I didn't want to make them give that up until they were ready. It turned out to be a very natural weaning process; one day it was just done.

—*Ann Contrucci, MD, a mom of 13-year-old boy-girl twins who works as a pediatric emergency physician, in Atlanta, GA*

My goal was to breastfeed my older daughter until she turned a year old. But my daughter turned one over the winter, and I didn't want to stop breastfeeding her during flu season. I wanted her to continue to get the immunity-boosting benefits of nursing. So I breastfed my older daughter until she was about 20 months old.

The challenge was that as my daughter got older, she nursed less frequently. And as she nursed less frequently, my milk supply went down. Along with a friend of mine, Lennox McNeary, MD, I created a line of lactation cookies called Milkin' Cookies, which help to increase milk supply.

You can buy Milkin' Cookies at Milkin-Cookies.com for about $21 for a two-week supply.

> —*Cheri Wiggins, MD, a mom of six- and three-year-old daughters, a specialist in physical medicine and rehabilitation at St. Luke's Magic Valley, and the cofounder of the Mommy Doctors Bakery (makers of Milkin' Cookies), in Twin Falls, ID*

Encountering Criticism and Breastfeeding in Public

In our culture, breastfeeding isn't always encouraged. And the older the child grows, the less encouraged it is. A grandmother who chose formula, an employer not supportive of pumping, or well-meaning friends might not encourage, or even actively discourage, moms who breastfeed their toddlers.

I nursed my twins after they were a year old. I didn't hear any direct criticism about it, but no doubt there was talk. Nursing my twins was very important to me. I had encountered criticism about it from the very beginning, even from family members who simply didn't understand that breastfed babies ate more frequently. It was something I really wanted to do for my babies, and I didn't really care what anybody else thought about it. By this time, my twins were nursing only once or twice a day, and it was more for comfort than anything else. I knew this time was precious and fleeting, and I just enjoyed it while it lasted.

> —*Ann Contrucci, MD*

I encountered some criticism for breastfeeding my son after he turned one year old. I believe it's still perfectly natural for a one-year-old to be breastfeeding a few times a day if both mom and baby want that. After my son turned a year old, even my own family members made comments like, "Isn't he too old to nurse?" I just ignored everyone because I knew both my son and I loved breastfeeding.

As my son got older, I would definitely still breastfeed him in public, but I did so much more discreetly (before, I would just sit in the corner and breastfeed my infant with a nursing cover). I hid inside the car, in the dressing room of a store, or in the back storage room of a restaurant, and I made sure to carry my nursing cover with me, especially on long trips and when we attended large gatherings, where a meltdown was almost guaranteed. Fortunately, I bought a nursing cover with a design I love! I still have it, because I associate

When to Call Your Doctor

Mastitis is an infection of the tissue of the breasts. It's more common in moms nursing younger babies, but it is still possible to get it after your baby is one year old.

When self-care techniques such as applying moist heat don't make the painful swelling of mastitis go away, you might need to get a prescription for an antibiotic from your doctor.

Call your doctor if you have the following symptoms of mastitis.

- Breast pain
- A breast lump
- Swollen, tender, and red breasts
- A feeling of warmth on the breasts
- Fever or flulike symptoms such as nausea or vomiting
- Unusual nipple discharge, such as pus
- Changes in nipple sensation
- Swollen or tender lymph nodes in your armpit on the side of your body as the breast that's painful

such sweet memories with it. I used one from Peanut Shell.

—*Cheryl Wu, MD, a mom of a four-year-old son, a pediatrician at LaGuardia Place Pediatrics in New York City, and a pediatric emergency physician at the Joseph M. Sanzari Children's Hospital of Hackensack University Medical Center, in New Jersey*

My oldest and youngest children both lost interest in breastfeeding when they started to eat solid food. My middle child would have nursed through college. I had to cut him off when he was about 18 months old, and I was pregnant with my youngest child.

My husband's family thought I was an unbathed hippie freak for nursing my son for so long. I ignored them. At one point, I told them that I'd stop nursing my son when he could ask for it by name. But then when he was able to do so, I wasn't ready to stop. I told them I was sure he'd quit nursing by the time he graduated from high school.

—*Amy Baxter, MD, a mom of 14- and 12-year-old sons and a 9-year-old daughter; the CEO of Buzzy4Shots.com; and the director of emergency research, Scottish Rite, of the Children's Healthcare of Atlanta, in Georgia*

I breastfed my son until he was almost three years old. I encountered some criticism, but I took heart in the knowledge that breastfeeding boosted my son's immunity. When my son would get sick, he'd have mild symptoms for a day or two. I'd catch the same bug and feel awful for over a week. I tried to nurse as long as I could to keep him as healthy as possible.

My son was born prematurely, so breastfeeding was a challenge. That struggle to breastfeed meant that I was less willing to allow pressure to impact my decision to do what I felt was best for my son. Being armed with the information about the benefits of breastfeeding makes it easier to ignore people who don't understand its importance.

—*Lennox McNeary, MD, a mom of a three-year-old son, a specialist in physical medicine and rehabilitation at Carilion Clinic, and a cofounder of the Mommy Doctors Bakery (makers of Milkin' Cookies), in Roanoke, VA*

I stopped nursing in public when my daughter was around 18 months old. By that time my daughter was really only interested in nursing in the mornings and the evenings at home.

—*Cheri Wiggins, MD*

A lot of times people don't understand the huge time commitment of breastfeeding. It takes many hours each day! Who wants to spend all of those hours alone, or in some tiny, cramped room? It's important for moms, hopefully early on, to become comfortable breastfeeding in public. You shouldn't have to feel you have to find a restroom or a broom closet in which to nurse your baby! The breast isn't a sex organ; it was designed to feed a baby!

I wouldn't have been able to breastfeed as long as I did without becoming comfortable nursing my baby around both family and friends, and also in public, in a café or a restaurant. Otherwise I would have felt so isolated that I would have given up. I learned how to breastfeed modestly, and breastfeeding in public felt more natural over time.

—*Ayala Laufer-Cahana, MD, a mom of 16- and 14-year-old sons and a 12-year-old daughter, a pediatrician, and the founder of Herbal Water Inc., in Wynnewood, PA*

Weaning Your Toddler

Stopping breastfeeding is likely to be an emotional event for you, or your baby, or both! You'll likely know in your heart when the time is right.

We started transitioning to a cup around eight to nine months, and we finished breastfeeding just before my babies turned a year old. The rule at our house is that when you can verbally ask for "boobies" (what my kids called the breast), you don't get any more boobies.

—*Carrie Brown, MD, a mom of eight- and six-year-old sons and a general pediatrician who treats medically complex children and specializes in palliative care at Arkansas Children's Hospital, in Little Rock*

When my daughter was 21 months old, I was ready to stop nursing. She wasn't. By that point, though, I needed to stop for my own sanity. Although I was fortunate that nursing came very easily physically, by that point I was emotionally ready to be done.

Weaning went much more smoothly than I had expected, though. Two months later, I got pregnant again. So I was pretty much pregnant or nursing for five years straight! After I weaned my younger daughter when she was 22 months old, it felt really, really good to have my body back!

—*Cheri Wiggins, MD*

⌇

I breastfed my first son until he was one. I planned on doing the same for my second child. Weaning was tough for both my first child and me. I stopped nursing him during my lunch initially and then stopped the nighttime feeds. I anticipated that weaning my second son would be even tougher, and I was right. I weaned him at 15 months. I had the most painful breast engorgement, and he cried for hours on end for about two weeks.

—*Bola Oyeyipo-Ajumobi, MD, a mom of four- and one-year-old sons, a family physician in private practice, and the owner of SlimyBookWorm.com, in Highland, CA*

⌇

I breastfed each of my three children, and the experience was different with each of them. My older daughter weaned herself at six months. My son was happy with bottle and breast. My younger daughter was stubborn, and she refused to take milk except from the breast. I guess we could have starved her, but there was something very tender about her insistence.

—*Nancy Rappaport, MD, a mom of 22- and 17-year-old daughters and a 19-year-old son, an assistant professor of psychiatry at Harvard Medical School, an attending child and adolescent psychiatrist in the Cambridge, MA, public schools, and the author of* The Behavior Code

⌇

I nursed both of my sons. I weaned my older son when he was

14 months old because I was pregnant with my younger son. It seemed like too much to ask of my body to be pregnant and nursing at the same time!

It wasn't difficult to wean my older son. He was already using a sippy cup by then, and he was nursing only a few times a day. He was ready to give it up.

My younger son weaned himself when he was 10 months old. I wasn't ready, and I was really devastated by it.

—*Sharon Boyce, MD, a mom of three- and one-year-old sons and a family physician at DayOne Family Healthcare Clinic, in Battle Creek, MI*

I nursed my sons for a long time. When they were each around two years old, I wanted to stop the middle-of-the-night nursings. We all slept in a family bed, so for about a month, I slept in another room, and my husband soothed the boys if they woke in the night. It took several weeks of protest, but I needed to stop those nighttime feedings. At that point, I needed to take care of myself. There's a time for everything, and sometimes you just have to say no, even it hurts a little. It's important to listen to your inner voice.

—*Lauren Feder, MD, a mom of 18- and 14-year-old sons, a nationally recognized physician who specializes in homeopathic medicine, and the author of* Natural Baby and Childcare *and* The Parents' Concise Guide to Childhood Vaccinations, *in Los Angeles, CA*

I weaned my son from breastfeeding when he was about 20 months old. Over time, I dropped from nursing him three times a day, to twice, then only once a day. One fortunate thing was that I didn't nurse him to sleep, which could cause tooth decay. His last nursing session to give up was the one before dinner. When I got home from work, we'd have some bonding time on the couch. It was hard to give that up because it was such a relaxing time for both of us.

As my son got older, he was spending less and less time nursing and more and more time doing acrobatics on my breasts, to the point that I got bruises over my chest. His restlessness and the abuse I endured actually made it easy to wean him. Afterward, I did miss it a little, but he certainly didn't. (The kids who have a hard time weaning are often the night nursers, those who wake up at night and need to nurse to go back to sleep.) The really bizarre thing was that I continued to lactate for another six months if I squeezed hard enough. (The things they never teach you in medical school!)

—*Cheryl Wu, MD*

❧

When my babies were around a year old, I stopped breastfeeding, and I gave them whole cow's milk to replace breast milk.

I think that the transition was harder on me than on my babies. While I was at work, they got pumped breast milk in a bottle anyway, so daytime feedings were an easy switch to cow's milk. I breastfed them in the morning and at night. The morning nursing wasn't too hard to stop because I was rushing around to get to work. I'd just hand the baby a sippy cup with milk.

Giving up that before-bedtime feeding was harder, though. I have to admit, I hung on to that one a little longer. It was more for my babies' comfort than anything else. I gradually stopped breastfeeding them before bed, but I continued to hug them so they still fulfilled their touch quotient.

—Susan Besser, MD, a mom of six grown children, ages 27, 25, 23, 21, 20, and 18, a grandmom of two, a family physician, and the medical director of Doctors Express-Memphis, in Tennessee

RALLIE'S TIP

As babies grow into toddlers, they're likely nursing less and less. Like many things in life, a mother's production of breast milk operates according to the law of supply and demand. In the majority of cases, the more milk our babies demand, the more milk our bodies produce for them. Anytime we nurse our babies less or they demand less milk, our production and supply of milk begin to diminish. So naturally, you produce less milk, and because your child nurses even less, you produce even less milk. This is nature's way of helping the weaning process along!

To wean my sons, I simply nursed less often and for shorter and shorter periods of time. If you're nursing your baby three times a day for 20 minutes at a time, you can start by nursing just twice a day for 10 to 15 minutes at a time for a couple of days. Then you can keep reducing the duration and frequency of nursing even more until your baby is completely weaned from the breast. By doing this, you'll produce less and less milk, and that will make weaning more comfortable for you. It will also make weaning more pleasant for your baby, because she'll be progressively adjusting to nursing less and drinking more from her sippy cup.

Chapter 5
Bottlefeeding

YOUR TODDLER'S DEVELOPMENT

It's not uncommon for one-year-olds, even two-year-olds, to be still drinking from a bottle. But that doesn't mean it's advisable. Most physicians recommend starting to phase out your child's bottle at age one, if you haven't started to do so already.

Children are developmentally ready to drink from a sippy cup as early as six months. As your toddler is seeking independence, you might find that transitioning him from a bottle to a sippy cup is easier than you imagined!

TAKING CARE OF YOU

As you're transitioning your toddler away from bottles and formula, why not take some time to think about your own calcium needs and bone health? Women should get at least 1,000 milligrams of calcium each day. However, most women get only between 748 and 968 milligrams each day—not enough.

Calcium is important for many reasons, including preventing osteoporosis, which is a condition of gradual bone loss that can lead to fractures.

Good sources of calcium include milk, fortified orange juice, yogurt, and cheese. Milk: It does a mom good.

JUSTIFICATION FOR A CELEBRATION

The day you stop bottlefeeding is bound to be a happy one. No more bottles to make, clean, and store! Happy day!

Bottlefeeding an Older Baby

If your baby still takes a bottle after age one, you have plenty of company. The American Academy of Pediatrics recommends phasing out the bottle between 12 and 24 months of age.

Here's one very compelling reason why: A study published in *Pediatrics* found that babies who were still given bottles past two years old were around 30 percent more likely to be obese at age 5½ years. The scientists think that drinking a bottle past infancy might encourage the child to drink too many calories.

It's fascinating to think that only a few generations ago, formula wasn't nearly the big business it is today. The first formulas were developed in the mid–1800s. But they were so terrible that pretty much all parents stuck with breastfeeding. The first true formula was created in 1867. It was a goopy combination of wheat flour, malt flour, cow's milk, and bicarbonate of potash. But that didn't deter its marketers from billing it as "the perfect infant food."

The first non–powder baby formula hit store shelves in 1951. In the 1950s, the developed world really embraced formula, and for a generation or two it was the feeding method of choice.

Both of my kids still were drinking some from a bottle past one. My son actually still takes a bottle.

I did stop their nighttime feedings when they were around a year old. I weaned them off the bottle slowly. Truth be told, I think it was harder for me to give up the bottle than it was for them.

—*Jennifer Hanes, DO, a mom of a six-year-old daughter and a three-year-old son, an emergency physician, a certified forensic physician, and the founder of Empowered Medicine, PLLC, in Austin, TX*

I cringe when I hear people talk about any absolute cutoffs, like "your baby has to be off the bottle by 12 months." Every family and child is different. I didn't let the last bottle of the night go until my daughter was almost 18 months. I just needed that cuddle time with my not-so-cuddly baby! Other toddlers who may be developmentally delayed may need the bottle longer, or may need to have their nutrition supported with formula or breast milk while they learn to eat solids. Moms should always be encouraged to do what is right for their children.

—*Katja Rowell, MD, a mom of a six-year-old daughter, a family practice physician, and a childhood feeding specialist with TheFeedingDoctor.com, in St. Paul, MN*

Mommy MD Guides–Recommended Product
Similac SimplySmart Bottle

"My daughter tends to be picky with her bottles and sippy cups, but she is able to grip the SimplySmart bottle well, and she is comfortable with the size of it," says Jennifer Bacani McKenney, MD, a mom of a one-year-old daughter and a family physician, in Fredonia, KS. "The first time my daughter tried it, she would have drank every drop, but she actually fell asleep with it toward the end!

"I like the large size of the bottle's opening, which prevents me from spilling formula everywhere," Dr. McKenney says. "I find with other bottles that it's often difficult to get the powdered formula into the top of the bottle without some getting on the counter because the opening is usually the same size as the formula scoop.

"I also like the SimplySmart On-the-Go Powder Cap. It attaches to the bottle so I can easily take a serving of formula on the go, and I don't have to go digging through my diaper bag to find the formula dispenser."

Eight-ounce Similac SimplySmart bottles cost $7.49 or $14.49 for a pack of two. You can buy them at Walmart and Target and online at **AMAZON.COM**, **BABIESRUS.COM**, **DIAPERS.COM**, and Abbott Nutrition at **ABBOTTSTORE.COM**.

Rallie's Tip

When I was ready to wean my oldest son from his bottle, I worked really hard to make it as stress free as possible for him, but he just didn't want to give it up. He'd already had to give up breastfeeding. I hadn't given him a pacifier when he was a baby, and he'd never been a thumb-sucker, so he didn't have any kind of backup plan. He was really attached to his bottle, but the pediatrician insisted that babies should stop bottlefeeding around their first birthdays.

A few weeks after I weaned my son from the bottle, all my hard work was nearly undone while we were visiting some friends. My son swiped their son's bottle and held on to it for dear life! If I had it to do over, I wouldn't have rushed my son's weaning. I'm sure that a few more weeks of holding on to his beloved bottle wouldn't have hurt him a bit.

Cleaning Nipples and Bottles

By now, you're likely a pro at cleaning your baby's bottles and nipples. Most likely you just run them through the dishwasher cycle with the rest of your dishes. If you have well water, though, some experts suggest it might be a good idea to continue to sterilize bottles and nipples. In any event, the end of all of this bottle cleaning and sterilizing is in sight!

∽

I buy all dishwasher-safe bottles and nipples. I just put all of my kids' bottles and nipples into the dishwasher to clean them. The dishwasher caddies for nipples make this a very easy task.

—Jennifer Hanes, DO

∽

I never sanitized anything. There's so much bacteria in the air and on your hands that it seemed silly to me to sterilize bottles and nipples. I simply washed everything in the dishwasher.

—Lisa Campanella-Coppo, MD, *a mom of a three-year-old daughter, an emergency physician, and the emergency department director of academic affairs at Monmouth Medical Center, in New Jersey*

I have a simple method for cleaning my sons' bottles and cups. I keep a small plastic container in my sink, and I fill it each morning with soapy water. Through the day, I toss my son's bottles and cups in there. Then at the end of the night I fill the container with hot, soapy water and hand wash them. I just let them air dry.

I wash other dishes in the dishwasher. I've found the best detergent is one called Dapple. You can buy it on Amazon.com.

—*Michelle Davis-Dash, MD, a mom of a one-year-old son and a pediatrician, in Baltimore, MD*

Weaning Your Toddler

The American Academy of Pediatrics recommends weaning a child from the bottle between his first and second birthdays. Sometimes that's easier said than done! Babies and young toddlers often associate the bottle with comfort and security—and with you.

Interestingly, some experts believe that the longer babies stay on formula the better, because they fear that many parents feed their toddlers such terrible food, such as French fries and cookies.

But when the time is right for you to wean your toddler, keep the following in mind. First, when a baby gets a bottle, Mom takes the bottle away after he's finished with it. Toddlers, on the other hand, are more on the go than babies. They can carry their bottles around with them and drink whenever they wish. This gives their teeth more exposure to whatever is in the bottles, and this can create an acidic mouth environment that leads to cavities.

Second, toddlers drinking from bottles tend to drink more milk than toddlers weaned from the bottle, 32 ounces a day, compared with 16 to 24 ounces a day. Drinking more formula or milk means taking in more calories, plus the toddler probably isn't eating as much solid food. He can be missing out on important nutrients.

It's time to say bye-bye, bottle!

I took away my kids' bottles when they turned a year old. Before that, though, I got them used to drinking through a straw. My kids were breastfed, and because drinking from a straw comes naturally to breastfed babies, they took to it quickly. That helped to ease their transition from bottle to cup.

—*Amy Baxter, MD, a mom of 14- and 12-year-old sons and a 9-year-old daughter; the CEO of Buzzy4Shots.com; and the director of emergency research, Scottish Rite, of the Children's Healthcare of Atlanta, in Georgia*

To wean my daughters from their nighttime bottles, I switched one bottle at a time from milk to water. My daughters slowly lost interest in wanting the bottle and waking up for it when they knew it was only water.

—*Jeannette Gonzalez Simon, MD, a mom of three- and one-year-old daughters and a pediatric gastroenterologist in private practice, in Staten Island, NY*

My daughter is still transitioning from her bottle to a cup. She loves her bottle, and she carries it around with her. She never took a pacifier, and I think that sucking on her bottle is comforting to her, especially at night before bed. We are trying to wean her, but she's been sick! We have started giving her water in her bottle at night, which is better for her teeth.

My daughter is starting to like to drink from a big cup. When I give her water, she'll gulp, gulp, gulp, then she'll say, "Mmmmmmmm" and smile. I find that she does well drinking from an open cup with a straw.

—*Rachel S. Rohde, MD, a mom of a one-year-old daughter, an assistant professor of orthopaedic surgery at the Oakland University William Beaumont School of Medicine, and an orthopaedic upper-extremity surgeon with Michigan Orthopaedic Institute, P.C., in Southfield, MI*

I feel that because I'm a doctor, I don't always get the same advice from my pediatrician that she would give to a mother who's not a doctor. I think she sometimes assumes that I know things that I don't.

Weaning from the bottle is a great example of this. My daughter was still merrily drinking from a bottle at 18 months. When I took her in for a checkup, her pediatrician scolded me for it! I felt bad, but I honestly didn't realize that I should have weaned her already. After that, I weaned my daughter from the bottle pretty quickly.

—*Lisa Campanella-Coppo, MD*

∽

I switched my older daughter from a bottle to a sippy cup when she turned one year old. The before-bed bottle was the last one to go.

I have to admit that my triplets were still drinking from a bottle at age two. It was a lot harder for me to give that up, partly because I was being lazy. Switching three kids at once was a lot harder than switching one. But when I did switch my triplets over, I found it wasn't a big deal. They changed to a cup very willingly.

—*Sadaf T. Bhutta, MD, a mom of a six-year-old daughter and four-year-old triplets and an assistant professor and the fellowship director of pediatric radiology at the University of Arkansas for Medical Sciences and Arkansas Children's Hospital, both in Little Rock*

∽

My sons were still bottlefeeding in their early toddler years. I tried to wean them, especially from nighttime feedings because I know how having that lactose in their mouths at night promotes baby bottle tooth decay. But what I knew as a doctor and what I did as a mother were sometimes two different things. As any mom knows, sometimes you can't help it.

My sons were very little, and I didn't want to force them to eat more at dinner so they didn't need a snack before bed. So I did still give them a bottle before bed so that they could last through the night. I had them rinse their mouths out with water before they went to sleep.

Fortunately, it wasn't too long before my sons were able to give up that pre-bed bottle. They'd have one bottle in the morning when they first got up. When they were around 2½, they gave up bottle-feeding for good, thankfully.

—*Leena Shrivastava Dev, MD, a mom of 15- and 11-year-old sons, a general pediatrician, and an advocate for child safety, in Philadelphia, PA*

Bottlefeeding worked for all of my family. My husband, my mother, even my father could feed the children. It was wonderful to share this, and it was completely practical for our lifestyle.

Crazy as it seems, all of my kids soon gave up the bottle when I switched from formula to milk. They went to a covered toddler cup, and our youngest went directly to an open two-handled cup. There were sippy cups or juice and milk boxes when we were on the go, but I taught them to drink out of a cup and not spill. I have never been a fan of constant bottling just to keep a child quiet. My children drank when they were thirsty and not for comfort or oral gratification.

—*Elizabeth Chabner Thompson, MD, MPH, a mom of 13- and 8-year-old daughters and 12- and 10-year-old sons, a radiation oncologist with 21 C. Radiation Oncology, and the inventor of the Mommy Bag, filled with supplies for moms-to-be having C-sections, in Scarsdale, NY*

RALLIE'S TIP

After age one, it's time to start weaning most babies from the bottle. And of course you can do it! Mothers have been doing this since bottles were invented, and we all know that it takes a little tough love and a lot of determination. Unfortunately, there's no magic method. When you take away your baby's bottle, he'll probably miss it at some point, and if he cries for it, you might be tempted to give it back. But once you make your decision, stick with it. Remind yourself that you're doing it for his own good. He'll miss his bottle only for a day or two, but his beautiful teeth will last a lifetime!

Parents have heard over and over about the potential health consequences of prolonged bottlefeeding and especially the bedtime bottle, even if they don't allow their babies to take a bottle to bed. It can promote erosion of tooth enamel and tooth decay, and it can contribute extra calories that lead to excess weight gain. Still, denying your baby a bedtime bottle can be incredibly challenging for moms and dads. It makes it far more difficult to get babies to sleep, and when babies don't sleep, neither do their parents.

There are two ways to break the bedtime bottle habit. You can do it gradually, or you can do it cold turkey. With my youngest son, I knew how challenging weaning was going to be, because I'd already gone through it twice with my older children. I had gradually weaned my middle son from the bedtime bottle in a stepwise fashion. I started by serving the bedtime bottle chilled rather than warm, which made it much less enticing. Then I replaced the milk with water, which he liked even less. When I finally took the bedtime bottle away, he wasn't all that crazy about it anyway, so it wasn't a big deal.

When it was time to wean my youngest son, my life was so hectic that I didn't do the gradual weaning. I decided that we would go cold turkey. To make sure that I didn't cave, I threw away all of his bottles so there would be no turning back. The first couple of nights were a little stressful for both of us, and it took my son about an hour longer than usual to get to sleep, and I felt pretty guilty about upsetting him.

Looking back, I think it's better to gradually wean babies from the bedtime bottle. Make sure your baby has had enough to eat and drink a couple of hours before bedtime. It's helpful if you have established a predictable bedtime routine to comfort and soothe your baby, so that you're not 100 percent dependent on the bottle. A nice warm bath, rocking while reading a story, and snuggling with a lovey can be great sources of comfort, security, and relaxation before bedtime, even when the bedtime bottle is no longer a part of the routine.

Chapter 6
Transitioning to the Cup

YOUR TODDLER'S DEVELOPMENT

Most children are ready to start drinking from a sippy cup by about six months. So by now, your child is really able to master this transition skill, on her way to drinking from an open cup. Sippy cups can be helpful to ease this transition. They can also make your life easier because they help to prevent spills!

TAKING CARE OF YOU

When you're thirsty, you get a drink. It's as simple as that, but did you ever think about how many calories you're drinking? It's surprising how many calories are in beverages. For example, 12 ounces of apple juice contains 192 calories, 12 ounces of lemonade contains 168 calories, and 12 ounces of cola contains 136 calories. Then there's the venti peppermint white chocolate mocha with whipped cream at our favorite coffeehouse. It tips the scales at 680 calories!

To make calorie counting even more of a conundrum, manufacturers can be sneaky, saying a bottle of juice, for instance, contains two, or even three, servings.

Fortunately, plenty of beverages have no calories at all: water and unsweetened coffee and tea. Take some time to rethink what you drink!

JUSTIFICATION FOR A CELEBRATION

It can be a challenge to find a cup that your child will use. Celebrate when you find your child's cup of choice, the one that she will love to use!

Choosing a Cup and Timing It Right

If you take a trip to the sippy cup section of your local Walmart or Target, you'll be greeted by a dizzying array of sippy cups. Brace yourself because you'll have a lot of decisions to make: Straw or spout? Soft spout or hard spout? Insulated or not insulated? Handles or no handles? Through a little bit of fun trial and error—and with a hefty dose of patience—you'll be able to find a cup that your toddler will love.

∽

I transitioned my toddlers from bottles to sippy cups before they were one year old. This is very important to avoid any dental problems like caries.

> —*Aline T. Tanios, MD, a mom of nine- and three-year-old daughters and a seven-year-old son and a pediatric hospitalist at Arkansas Children's Hospital, in Little Rock*

∽

My daughter was easier to transition to a cup than my son was because she saw her big brother drinking from a cup, so she wanted to do that too. She started to drink from a sippy cup when she was around 10 months old, and now she drinks from a regular cup.

My daughter likes to drink her milk with a straw. I think that sucking sensation is comforting to her. She drinks her juice sans straw, straight from the open cup.

> —*Shilpa Amin-Shah, MD, a mom of a two-year-old son and a one-year-old daughter and an emergency physician at Emergency Medical Associates, in Livingston, NJ*

∽

I had a lot of difficulty transitioning my daughters to a cup because they were both born prematurely. They had a lot of trouble sucking.

My best advice is not to go out and buy six of one type of sippy cup and hope for the best! I had to try a bunch of different styles until finally I found one my daughters could use. My daughters did better with cups that didn't have valves. You can take the valve out of most cups, but then they make a mess. I found the best type was the Take & Toss cups because they don't have valves, but the holes are so small they don't make a mess either.

Once you find a cup your toddler likes, don't expect that your other kids will like it too. My girls each preferred different types of cups!

—*Kristie McNealy, MD, a mom of nine- and six-year-old daughters and four-year-old and 22-month-old sons and a blogger at KristieMcNealy.com, in Denver, CO*

∽◌∾

When my older son was ready to drink from a sippy cup, I bought one. Then I bought another. And another. And another, until I finally found one that my son liked.

It turns out that my son preferred the sippy cups with soft spouts, such as Nuby and Munchkin. They worked out very well until my son discovered that he could bite the tops off. That's a choking danger, so I quickly switched my son to the hard-spouted sippy cups.

—*Sharon Boyce, MD, a mom of three- and one-year-old sons and a family physician at DayOne Family Healthcare Clinic, in Battle Creek, MI*

∽◌∾

It wasn't hard to transition my babies to drinking from a sippy cup. But it was messy! Toddlers do love to sling their sippy cups around! Mostly I just cleaned up the messes. I tried to restrict their walking around with food and drink to the kitchen, dining room, and play-room, but as every mom knows, kids are great at "escaping," and they move fast! So occasionally I would find food and cups in all sorts of places.

—*Susan Besser, MD, a mom of six grown children, ages 27, 25, 23, 21, 20, and 18, a grandmom of two, a family physician, and the medical director of Doctors Express-Memphis, in Tennessee*

∽◌∾

I pretty much tried to skip the sippy cup stage entirely. Sippy cups are fine at home, but if you go to visit a friend or to a restaurant, they probably won't have sippy cups.

Instead, I transitioned my kids from the bottle to drinking from an open cup with a straw. Restaurants are far more likely to have straws, and you could even carry a stash of them in your purse.

To entice my kids the first time, I used a large straw and would suck up a smoothie into it and then touch it to their lips to show them that straws are worth the effort to get the yummy drink.

—Jennifer Hanes, DO, a mom of a six-year-old daughter and a three-year-old son, an emergency physician, a certified forensic physician, and the founder of Empowered Medicine, PLLC, in Austin, TX

Switching to Cow's Milk

Physicians recommend transitioning children after they turn one year old to drinking cow's milk instead of formula. But how much cow's milk does your toddler need? Around two cups per day is about right for two- and three-year-olds.

Clear out some space in your fridge because toddlers should drink whole milk, while you are probably buying fat-free milk or at least reduced-fat milk for yourself and the rest of your family. One- and two-year-olds need the dietary fat from whole milk for normal growth and brain development. Not to worry, this is a temporary situation. Once your child is three years old, you can transition her over to the same type of milk that you drink.

Milk offers calcium and vitamin D, which helps your growing toddler build strong teeth and bones. The American Academy of Pediatrics recommends that all children, including infants, get at least 400 international units of vitamin D a day. (Talk with your toddler's doctor before giving this or any supplements.)

Some children are allergic to cow's milk. In fact, it's one of the most common allergies in children. Some children who are allergic to cow's milk are also allergic to soy milk. Talk with your child's doctor if you're concerned about this. She might suggest an alternative such as almond milk or goat's milk. (Though of course consider if your family has a history of tree nut allergy before introducing almond milk.) Fortunately, most children outgrow milk allergy by age three.

After I weaned my kids from breast milk to iron-fortified formula, I moved on to cow's milk. I almost always buy organic milk because my kids drink so much of it. I feel it's better for them, and also I want to support organic farming.

—*Ayala Laufer-Cahana, MD, a mom of 16- and 14-year-old sons and a 12-year-old daughter, a pediatrician, and the founder of Herbal Water Inc., in Wynnewood, PA*

When my kids were toddlers, organic milk wasn't commonly available. But I did try to buy milk that was hormone free. It wasn't too much of a concern because my daughters don't drink much milk. Now that they're older, they drink almond milk or soy milk, and they eat a lot of yogurt.

—*Susan Wilder, MD, a mom of a 17-year-old daughter and twin 13-year-old girls, a primary care physician, and the founder and CEO of Lifescape Medical Associates, in Scottsdale, AZ*

After children turn one, they don't need to drink milk. They do need vitamin D and calcium, though, so I give my daughters vitamin supplements. Or you could give kids orange juice that's fortified with vitamin D and calcium.

Milk is also a good source of protein, so if your children are not drinking milk, you do need to ensure they are getting enough protein in their diets through meat, eggs, or beans.

—*Kate Tulenko, MD, MPH, a mom of four- and one-year-old girls, the author of* Insourced: How Importing Jobs Impacts the Healthcare Crisis Here and Abroad, *and a pediatrician and global health specialist with IntraHealth, in Washington, DC*

I am not a fan of giving children cow's milk. Instead I gave my kids almond milk to drink. Almond milk has fewer calories than dairy milk and it's very healthy. It's much more commonly available today, and it is even sold in many grocery stores. Many children (and adults) get abdominal pains or increased mucus production from milk, so avoiding it can be a healthy practice, and if they drink almond milk, they still get protein and calcium.

—*Dana S. Simpler, MD, a mom of 25- and 20-year-old girls and a 23-year-old son and a specialist in internal medicine in private practice, in Baltimore, MD*

A lot of kids don't like milk. Mine didn't. Instead of giving them milk to drink, I gave them dairy foods to eat, such as yogurt and cheese, so they would still get enough calcium in their diets.

—*Victoria McEvoy, MD, a mom who raised four children; a grandmom of six-, four-, and two-year-old grandsons; an assistant professor of pediatrics at Harvard Medical School; the medical director and chief of pediatrics at Mass General West Medical Group; and the author of* 24/7 Baby Doctor, *in Boston, MA*

My daughter loved her bottle. But after she gave it up, she never wanted to drink milk again. When she was a toddler, I started to give her calcium supplements. To this day, my daughter barely puts milk in her coffee! Fortunately, she still takes calcium supplements.

—*Debra Jaliman, MD, a mom of a 20-year-old daughter, a dermatologist in private practice, and an assistant professor of dermatology at Mt. Sinai School of Medicine, in New York City*

When my twins were a year old, I started to give them whole cow's milk. Toddlers' brains are growing so rapidly that they need the fat in the whole milk to help their brains to develop appropriately. They also need the extra calories in whole milk to fuel their growth.

Once children are two years old, it's okay to change them over to the type of milk that the rest of the family drinks. In my case, my twins have always been small, so I continued to give them whole milk.

—*Ann Contrucci, MD, a mom of 13-year-old boy-girl twins who works as a pediatric emergency physician, in Atlanta, GA*

I weaned my daughter rather late from the bottle, when she was around 18 months. After that, my daughter boycotted milk. Now I give her yogurt smoothies, and she drinks them happily.

I make our smoothies with leftover organic Stonyfield yogurts that she doesn't finish, bananas, and organic skim milk. I feel very strongly about keeping synthetic hormones and antibiotics out of her diet, so I buy all organic dairy. I have started buying the premade Stonyfield organic smoothies for her, but I still prefer to make them from scratch with fruit when I can. That helps keep the sugar content down.

—*Lisa Campanella-Coppo, MD, a mom of a three-year-old daughter, an emergency physician, and the emergency department director of academic affairs at Monmouth Medical Center, in New Jersey*

When I switched my daughter to cow's milk, she developed serious eczema all over her thighs and groin area. Her pediatrician, who could give me no explanation for why she developed this problem, gave me steroid cream to treat it. Fortunately, a book I found in a health food store talked about milk protein causing eczema in sensitive individuals. I stopped giving my daughter the cow's milk, and her rash cleared up.

Unfortunately, soy milk and formula gave my daughter diarrhea. The pediatrician encouraged me to try yogurt and cheese, because the protein in them is "denatured." My daughter had no problems with yogurt and cheese, and I supplemented these foods with chewable child calcium/vitamin D tablets.

—*Stuart Jeanne Bramhall, MD, a mom of a 31-year-old daughter and a child and adolescent psychiatrist in New Plymouth, New Zealand*

RALLIE'S TIP

Cow's milk is a good source of protein and calcium for babies, but there are other sources of these nutrients that your child might enjoy. Even if your toddler doesn't like the taste of milk or if she doesn't tolerate it well, she might love cottage cheese, yogurt, or another dairy food. Some brands of orange juice are fortified with calcium.

My oldest and youngest sons loved milk, and they drank plenty of it as toddlers. My middle son couldn't wait to be done with it. After he gave up his bottle, he never seemed to want milk again. Because milk is the leading source of calcium in the American diet, I was concerned that he might not be getting enough of the mineral to stay healthy. Fortunately, he loved other calcium-rich foods, including cheese, yogurt, fortified orange juice, and broccoli, and I made sure that he got some of these foods every day. I also gave him a children's multivitamin and mineral supplement every day.

If you discover that your toddler isn't willing to drink or eat any type of dairy food, ask your pediatrician for a referral to a pediatric dietitian. This professional can help you design a diet for your child that will meet her nutritional needs, so that she'll be healthy, and you'll be happy.

Choosing a Juice

Among physicians, juice is a hot-button issue! Some physicians are morally opposed to giving kids juice; other physicians feel there is a place in a child's diet for some juice.

The American Academy of Pediatrics (AAP) has such strong feelings about juice that they published a paper dedicated just to it: "The Use and Misuse of Fruit Juice in Pediatrics." (You can probably guess where this is going!) The AAP reminds that "Fruit juice offers no nutritional advantage over whole fruit. In fact, fruit juice lacks the fiber of whole fruit." They recommend that children ages one to six years old drink no more than four to six ounces of juice each day.

When you're standing at the grocery store, confronted by the imposing wall of juices, check the labels carefully. Choose 100 percent fruit juice, with no added sugars. Some of those bottles contain an alarming amount of sugar—and very little juice.

☙❧

I'm happy to say that my daughter has never really liked juice. I'm not a huge fan of juice because it's fruit without the fiber. I give my daughter mostly water to drink, and I give her plenty of fruit to eat.

—*Rachel S. Rohde, MD, a mom of a one-year-old daughter, an assistant professor of orthopaedic surgery at the Oakland University William Beaumont School of Medicine, and an orthopaedic upper-*

*extremity surgeon with Michigan Orthopaedic Institute, P.C., in
Southfield, MI*

⟨≈⟩

A challenge with a lot of toddlers is that they want to fill up on juice and milk, and then they don't want to eat. I did give my toddlers juice, but really I don't think kids need to drink juice at all. If you do give them juice, water it down considerably.

—*Victoria McEvoy, MD*

⟨≈⟩

I think that the sugary drink habit is one of the worst things for kids' nutrition. So many kids grow from babies who drink only breast milk to teens who guzzle 300 calories of soda a day.

After I weaned my kids from breast milk, I gave them water and milk to drink, not juice. On occasion, if I wanted them to have fruit juice, I squeezed fresh juice myself and served it in a cup. I believe that a sweet drink in a baby bottle leads to poor nutrition habits and craving sweets, and it ruins those brand-new teeth. Sugary drinks don't register in the brain as food, and drinking them leads to overconsumption and weight gain.

—*Ayala Laufer-Cahana, MD*

⟨≈⟩

I never gave my daughter juice. It's awful. Instead, I gave her whole fruits to eat and water or sparkling water to drink.

I actively sought out interesting, exotic fruits and vegetables to give my daughter. I purchased these foods at a local gourmet store. Her favorite now is persimmons.

When my daughter was two, she loved artichokes, and she even knew how to eat them. At restaurants, she'd order sautéed mushrooms! I introduced unusual fruits to her as if they were perfectly normal, so she'd love to eat them.

—*Debra Jaliman, MD*

⟨≈⟩

My son gets juice at day care, and the only stipulations I have are that it must be 100 percent juice and the day care teachers must mix it with an equal amount of water, so that it's half water and half juice.

My son doesn't know the difference because he's always drank his juice diluted. It gives the water a little flavor. He's good with that.

—*Michelle Davis-Dash, MD, a mom of a one-year-old son and a pediatrician, in Balitmore, MD*

RALLIE'S TIP

Drinking nothing but orange juice or apple juice can cause some problems for babies and toddlers, including an increased risk for obesity, tooth decay, diarrhea, and other gastrointestinal problems, such as excessive gas and abdominal discomfort. Instead of drinking more juice, children should be encouraged to eat whole fruits. When children are thirsty, it's usually best to offer them water to drink.

Juice is extremely sweet, and as a result, most children love the taste of it. But when kids drink too much juice, their stomachs get filled up, and they might not have a good appetite for other nutritious foods. While toddlers might be getting plenty of calories from orange juice or apple juice, these calories come from sugars, rather than from fat and protein, which are critical for your toddler's good health and for her proper growth and development.

My middle son didn't care for the taste of milk, and he always asked for a cup of juice when he was thirsty. I'd tell him that he could have some juice if he was still thirsty after he drank some water. When I did offer him juice, I diluted it with an equal amount of water, so that he wasn't getting so much sugar and as many calories with every serving. Diluted juice is still plenty sweet and delicious, and most children love the taste of it.

Keeping Cups Cold and Clean

Sippy cups are filled with tiny little crevices, and they're often warm and wet. They're perfect little petri dishes worthy of any sixth-grade science project. It's important to clean sippy cups thoroughly and let them dry out well, so that your toddler isn't drinking mold and bacteria along with her juice. (Ick.)

To prevent tooth decay, toddlers shouldn't be carrying their sippy cups along all day, sipping from them at will. But here in the real world, sometimes the cups might be out of the fridge for an extended period of time. You might consider buying insulated sippy cups. They are better at keeping drinks colder and safer—longer.

✑

I only buy dishwasher-safe cups! I also usually only put water in them, so that they're not so hard to clean. My daughter received some cups that aren't dishwasher safe as gifts. I give those to her to play with in her play kitchen, so they still get plenty of use.

—*Rachel S. Rohde, MD*

✑

Anything that is dishwasher safe, I run through my dishwasher. Fortunately, most of my sons' toddler cups, utensils, and plates were dishwasher safe.

When my sons were toddlers, if there was leftover juice in their sippy cups, I would try to put it in the refrigerator right away. If that didn't happen and juice sat out for more than a couple of hours, I would throw it out.

—*Leena Shrivastava Dev, MD, a mom of 15- and 11-year-old sons, a general pediatrician, and an advocate for child safety, in Philadelphia, PA*

✑

It's such a challenge to clean all of those sippy cup parts. I keep a small plastic basin in my sink filled with warm, soapy water. As the day goes on, I toss my daughter's sippy cups, the parts, and her pacifiers in there to soak. At the end of the day, I hand wash them.

I look forward to the end of the sippy cups. Even though they're not supposed to leak, my daughter manages to get milk or juice all over. My house seems to become sticky everywhere! Soaking the sippy cups and parts allows me to clean them inside and out and take care of some of that stickiness!

—*Jennifer Bacani McKenney, MD, a mom of a one-year-old daughter and a family physician, in Fredonia, KS*

✑

My daughter had some sippy cups with straws, and they were such a pain to clean. I'd run everything through the dishwasher, but I generally had to wash the straws by hand.

I bought a Munchkin dishwasher basket. I washed the small parts of the sippy cups and bottles in that.

—Lisa Campanella-Coppo, MD

◌

I am not a fan of sippy cups. They get dirty and they stink, which makes me suspicious about the germs they harbor. Instead, I taught my kids to drink from an open cup with a straw. The straws are disposable, so you never have to clean them.

—Jennifer Hanes, DO

◌

I gave my daughter a sippy cup, but I was pretty firm that she drank from it only at the table. I've seen kids who wander around with juice in sippy cups all day. That's a hard habit to break, and also it's messy. In between meals, my daughter only had water in her sippy cup, and I cleaned it out after she was finished drinking from it. If she had some milk or diluted juice left after a snack, I popped it in the fridge, and tossed it if she didn't drink it at the next meal or snack.

—Katja Rowell, MD, a mom of a six-year-old daughter, a

Mommy MD Guides-Recommended Product
Foogo Cups

Rallie's Tip: Foogo, by Thermos, is a great choice for sippy cups. The cups are designed to keep beverages at the right temperature longer to prevent bacteria from multiplying. The cups come in metal or plastic, and both types have soft plastic spouts. The metal cups are designed to keep beverages cold for up to six hours. All Foogo cups are BPA free and can be put in the dishwasher.

A seven-ounce metal cup with double-wall vacuum insulation costs $16.99, and an eight-ounce plastic cup with removable handles costs $7.99 at **SHOPTHERMOS.COM**. You can also find the cups at Target, Walmart, Walgreens, and **AMAZON.COM**.

family practice physician, and a childhood feeding specialist with TheFeedingDoctor.com, in St. Paul, MN

༄

Cleaning is not one of my attributes. I never sterilized anything. I simply rinsed out my children's sippy cups or ran them through the dishwasher. I'm sure my children ate their pound of dirt well before they were three years old. Perhaps because of this, and the colds they got during preschool, they almost never get sick now!

It could also be that I was nursing while I was exposed to all kinds of illnesses during my pediatric residency and that boosted my kids' immunity. Continue to breastfeed, especially when you get a cold, so you can give the antibodies to your children.

—Amy Baxter, MD, a mom of 14- and 12-year-old sons and a 9-year-old daughter; the CEO of Buzzy4Shots.com; and the director of emergency research, Scottish Rite, of the Children's Healthcare of Atlanta, in Georgia

༄

I started to give my older daughter milk or water in a sippy cup when she was around seven months old. I question how well most sippy cups are insulated to keep drinks cold enough to protect against spoiling. Luckily, we live in a small town, so we only have a few minutes' drive to get anywhere, so the drinks weren't out of the fridge long.

Some sippy cups are such a pain to clean! I often had to hand wash them to get them clean. I was very happy when my younger daughter was old enough to transition to a Clean Canteen instead. They are easier to clean. I just run them through the dishwasher.

Better yet, as soon as my girls were able to drink from an open cup, I started to give them milk and water in Duralux glasses. They're made of tempered glass, so they're very sturdy, practically kid-proof.

—Cheri Wiggins, MD, a mom of six- and three-year-old daughters, a specialist in physical medicine and rehabilitation at St. Luke's Magic Valley, and the cofounder of the Mommy Doctors Bakery (makers of Milkin' Cookies), in Twin falls, ID

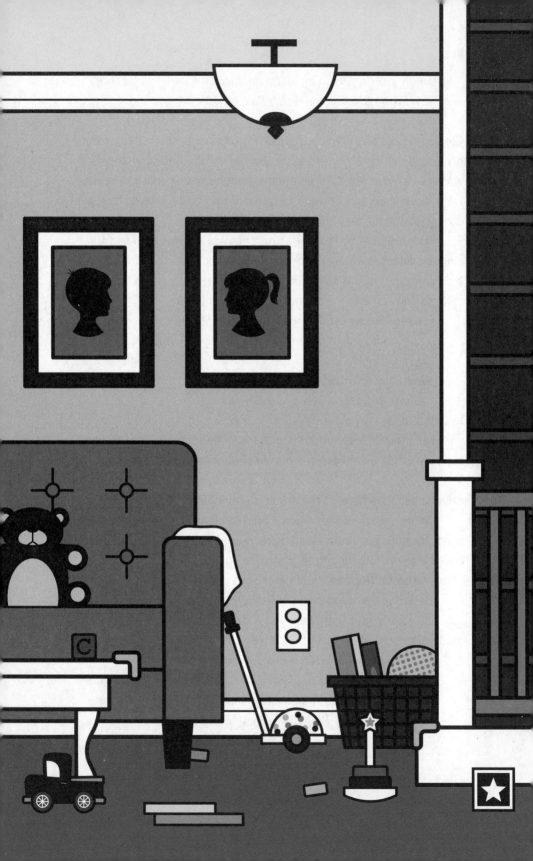

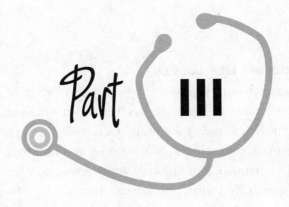

Part III

HEALTH AND SAFETY

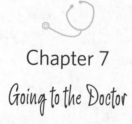

Chapter 7

Going to the Doctor

YOUR TODDLER'S DEVELOPMENT

It makes sense that during your baby's first year, when he's growing and developing the fastest, he has the most frequent well-child visits. He likely had well-baby visits at a few days or a few weeks old, one month, two months, four months, six months, and nine months. The frequency of visits will slow down now, and you're probably scheduling visits for 1 year, 15 months, 18 months, 2 years, and then 3 years.

These well-child visits are wonderful opportunities to check in with your child's doctor, track your toddler's growth and development, ask questions, and gain a little reassurance. You're doing a great job, Mom!

TAKING CARE OF *YOU*

You take your child to the doctor for regular visits like clockwork. But when was the last time you checked in with *your* doctor for a checkup? Schedule an appointment today, and consider asking for some simple tests, such as blood pressure, cholesterol levels, and thyroid function. (Check with your insurance company first to make sure the cost will be covered.)

JUSTIFICATION FOR A CELEBRATION

Anytime your toddler receives a clean bill of health from his doctor is cause for a celebration indeed!

Working with Your Pediatrician's Office

Your child's doctor is an expert in children's health, but *you* are the expert on your child. Together you're a powerful team to help your child stay healthy. At your child's well-child visit, you can expect your child's doctor to weigh and measure your toddler. It's also a great time to seek the doctor's advice on any issue that's troubling you, such as your child's potty training or eating and sleeping habits.

❧

My kids aren't scared to go to the doctor. I think it's largely because I'm a doctor, and they know that doctors are nice people!

But I did buy my kids a book about going to the doctor, and I've read it to my toddlers often. It tells kids what to expect when they go to the doctor.

—*Shilpa Amin-Shah, MD, a mom of a two-year-old son and a one-year-old daughter and an emergency physician at Emergency Medical Associates, in Livingston, NJ*

❧

One of the many things I love about my daughter's pediatricians is that they have separate waiting rooms for sick kids and for well kids. I really appreciate that my daughter isn't sitting next to a child with the flu while she's waiting for her well visit!

—*Rachel S. Rohde, MD, a mom of a one-year-old daughter, an assistant professor of orthopaedic surgery at the Oakland University William Beaumont School of Medicine, and an orthopaedic upper-extremity surgeon with Michigan Orthopaedic Institute, P.C., in Southfield, MI*

❧

I met my children's pediatrician through a friend. I like that practice so much that we continue to go there, even though we've moved to a house much farther away. I don't want to be the expert for my kids, and once I found a doctor I trusted, I didn't want to lose that.

One interesting thing about our practice is that the doctors are teamed up with nurse practitioners. Each visit, they alternate, so one visit you see the doctor, the next time the nurse. I find it benefits my children to have two experienced clinicians getting to know them (and us) well.

—*Deborah Kulick, MD, a mom of two-year-old and eight-month-old sons, a child and adolescent psychiatrist at the Everett Teen Health Center, and an instructor in psychiatry at Harvard Medical School and the Cambridge Health Alliance, in Boston, MA*

A lot of toddlers are afraid of strangers and going to unfamiliar places, but my kids have never been scared of going to see the doctor. That might be because they've always gone to the *same* doctor.

—*Heather Orman-Lubell, MD, a mom of 11- and 7-year-old sons and a pediatrician in private practice at Yardley Pediatrics of St. Christopher's Hospital for Children, in Pennsylvania*

When to Call Your Doctor

Your child's doctor is there to answer questions and give advice about sicknesses, medications, injuries, and behavior issues.

As a general guideline, call your pediatrician's office and ask if the doctor should see your child if he has any of the following symptoms.

- A cough or cold that doesn't get better after several days, or if a cold gets worse and leads to a fever
- A severe sore throat or swallowing problems
- A rash, particularly if there's also a fever
- Ear discomfort with a fever (or if your child can't sleep or drink, is acting sick, and has diarrhea or is vomiting)
- An ear that's draining
- Diarrhea or vomiting that lasts more than three hours
- Bloody diarrhea
- A fever combined with repeated vomiting
- Blood in the urine
- Sharp pains in the abdomen or stomach
- Deep cuts that may need stitches, puncture wounds, or large abrasions

As best I can, I always try to make things fun, for my kids and for my patients. Here's an example of something I do with my patients, which parents could adapt when they take their kids to the doctor. When a toddler comes for a visit, I start the visit off lightheartedly.

"What did you bring for me today?" I'll joke as I peek in his throat.

"Are you cooking something down there in this ear?" I'll ask as I look in an ear.

Toddlers are full of fun, and they love to laugh. Starting a visit off with a giggle instead of a grimace sets the tone for a positive experience.

—*Cathy Marshall, MD, a mom of 28-, 14-, and 11-year-old daughters and a pediatrician in private practice, in Encino, CA*

- Your child is limping or can't move a leg or arm
- Pain that worsens or doesn't go away after several hours
- Your child has refused to drink for more than 12 hours

Call 911 if your child has any of these very serious signs or symptoms.

- Persistent bleeding that doesn't stop when you apply pressure
- You think your child has ingested something poisonous
- Seizures
- Breathing trouble
- Blue, purple, or gray skin or lips
- Neck stiffness or a rash with a fever
- A head injury followed by loss of consciousness, confusion, vomiting, or poor skin color
- A sudden lack of energy or your child can't move
- A large, deep cut or burn, or a cut or burn on the head, chest, abdomen, hands, groin, or face
- Your child is unconscious or doesn't respond
- Your child becomes withdrawn or is less alert

My only rule of thumb about going to the pediatrician is never to treat my own child! I always checked my assessments of my child with our pediatrician to make sure I knew what I was doing!

I think that the Internet can add unnecessary anxiety for mothers. I don't think it's a problem for parents to ask the doctor about something that they read online. As physicians, it's our job to educate patients about health concerns and address all of our patients' questions. Sometimes, the Internet can be more detrimental to anxiety-prone parents (like me).

—*Mona Gohara, MD, a mom of five- and three-year-old sons, a dermatologist in private practice, an assistant clinical professor in the department of dermatology at Yale University, and a cofounder of K&J Sunprotective Clothing, in Danbury, CT*

People say that physicians should never treat their own children. I never heeded that advice, and it backfired every time.

One time, I tried to look in my daughter's ear because she had an infection. I tried to take out some earwax, and her ear started to bleed. Another time, my daughter had a strep infection that came back after treatment, and I gave her a shot. I hit a nerve in her leg with the needle, and she couldn't walk for a week. A third time, she had a wart on her finger. I treated it with acid, and she developed a big keloid scar.

I learned from these misadventures, and I stopped treating my own children. This advice is also valid for mothers who aren't physicians who might research medical concerns on the Internet and try to take matters into their own hands. It's important to choose a pediatrician you trust and just go with it.

—*Victoria McEvoy, MD, a mom who raised four children; a grandmom of six-, four-, and two-year-old grandsons; an assistant professor of pediatrics at Harvard Medical School; the medical director and chief of pediatrics at Mass General West Medical Group; and the author of* 24/7 Baby Doctor, *in Boston, MA*

Toddlers often need to go to the doctor a lot. I think it's important to choose a pediatrician you like and convey that feeling to your child.

Going to the doctor can be scary for toddlers. When my daughters would say they didn't want to go to the doctor, I explained that there are things in life we don't want to do that we have to do. We have to sleep. We have to eat. We have to go to the doctor. That's life.

"I understand that you don't want to go," I'd say. "I don't like to write medical chart notes either, but I have to do it. There's no way around it. That's how it is with going to the doctor."

When you take your toddler to the doctor, it helps to be calm yourself. Don't be anxious about taking your toddler to the doctor. Children pick up on how you are feeling. Also, after the visit is over, quickly change the mood. Go do something fun. My teen just reminded me that after a doctor's visit, we would go to the dollar store that was right next door. Or give your toddler a reward such as a sticker. You want to change his or her mind-set as quickly as possible. Later if he or she protests going to the doctor, you can say, "I know you don't want to go, but remember last time, how much fun we had after?"

—Eva Ritvo, MD, a mom of 21- and 16-year-old daughters, a psychiatrist, and a coauthor of The Beauty Prescription, in Miami Beach, FL

Getting Shots

Probably the only person less happy about getting a shot than your child is you. It's hard to see a child frightened or in pain, even for a second. Babies today get a lot of shots. Back in 1983, children got around seven vaccinations. Today, by the time a child is two years old, he might receive up to 23 vaccinations. We've come a long way though. Today's vaccines deliver fewer antigens and come with fewer side effects than those given 30 years ago.

Fortunately, by age two, your child should have received most of his childhood immunizations. Put on your bravest face, knowing your child will take his cue on how to react to the vaccination from you.

෴

I am a big believer in the importance of vaccinations. Even if my toddlers cried when they got shots, I knew that the shots were for their own good. Getting your child vaccinated is one of those things you just have to do.

—*Victoria McEvoy, MD*

My toddlers didn't like to get shots, of course. I found it helpful to put a little numbing spray on the area first or some EMLA cream, which is used to numb the skin. It might have been more for emotional support than actual pain relief, but it helped get us through the shots.

—*Eva Mayer, MD, a mom of an eight-year-old daughter and a six-year-old son and a pediatrician with St. Luke's Pediatrics Associates, in Bethlehem, PA*

I cried the first time my daughter got vaccines—probably because of my postpartum hormones. After that, my husband took her to the doctor for her shots. He still hasn't forgiven me for the two times he had to take her to get blood tests for allergies. I love him for it. I hate holding her down and watching her cry. He does it for me.

—*Lisa Campanella-Coppo, MD, a mom of a three-year-old daughter, an emergency physician, and the emergency department director of academic affairs at Monmouth Medical Center, in New Jersey*

Of course, toddlers hate shots and don't want them. But shots are a rite of passage. When my girls were toddlers, I used to draw a bunny on their arms where the shots were going to go. We called the shots "bunny shots" to soften the blow.

The message to toddlers should be simple and clear: We don't have to like everything we have to do. That's an important message for kids to hear. Life isn't fun and giggles 24/7. Remaining calm and reassuring is important. Help them to feel better as soon as the shot is done.

—*Eva Ritvo, MD*

A big pet peeve of mine is when a mother tells her toddler, "The mean nurse is coming in to give you a shot." That's horrible!

When a toddler has to have a shot, it's best to hold him, cuddle him, and help to get him through the experience. Five minutes after the shot, kids are generally over it.

I don't recommend giving children pain medicines such as acetaminophen (Tylenol) or ibuprofen (Motrin) before they have their shots because some studies suggest they could interfere with the desired immune response. But if your child is cranky or has a fever after the shot, you could give an age- and weight-appropriate dose of the medicine. (Talk with your toddler's doctor before giving him this or any medication.)

—*Heather Orman-Lubell, MD*

∽

When my son was a toddler, I'd take a cold juice box to his well-child visits. I'd hold the box on the skin where the shot would go beforehand, and then while my son got his shots, I'd let him take a big slurp of very cold juice. That numbed the pain and also distracted him!

Later, I invented Buzzy4Shots. It's simply a palm-size vibrating device shaped like a bee with ice pack wings. When it's pressed on the child's skin above the needle stick, the combination of the two sensations—cold and vibration—blocks the sting of the shot. You can buy Buzzy at the store on Buzzy4Shots.com for $39.95.

While some nurses do know how to use Buzzy correctly, many either don't or don't want to take the time. Bringing your own doesn't interfere with the way nurses normally give shots, and I've found that when my kids know they have Buzzy, it dramatically decreases their fear of needles.

—*Amy Baxter, MD, a mom of 14- and 12-year-old sons and a 9-year-old daughter; the CEO of Buzzy4Shots.com; and the director of emergency research, Scottish Rite, of the Children's Healthcare of Atlanta, in Georgia*

∽

One of my daughters was terrified of shots. One time when she got a flu shot, she howled so loud I thought she'd bring down the house.

I find that putting an ice pack on the area before and after the shot helps ease the pain. It might be mainly the placebo effect, but if it helps, that's great. Even better is to buy an ice pack shaped like your child's favorite cartoon character. My office keeps a whole stash of these on hand, and we let the children choose which one they'd like to use each visit. But a parent could simply keep one at home in the freezer and bring it along in a small lunch cooler.

Also, it's critical that parents are on the same team as the physician. Take the time to gently explain to your toddler that, "Shots are important. One second of pain protects you from a long illness. The nurses and doctors are here to help."

—*Cathy Marshall, MD*

Waiting Patiently

Patience is a virtue. But it's a virtue that is likely in short supply after you've been waiting at the doctor's office for 40 minutes. With a wriggling, wailing toddler. You likely feel like doing some wailing of your own!

When my daughter was about six months old, I bought an iPad. I bring it anywhere that we might have to wait, such as at the doctor's office. Lots of educational apps are suitable for toddlers. I find it to be both educational and fun for her.

—*Lisa Campanella-Coppo, MD*

I keep a stash of coloring books and crayons in my bag at all times. They are so helpful to keep kids busy when you're waiting, such as at the doctor's office. I've found that even kids who don't particularly like to color will gladly color if there's nothing else to do.

—*Aline T. Tanios, MD, a mom of nine- and three-year-old daughters and a seven-year-old son and a pediatric hospitalist at Arkansas Children's Hospital, in Little Rock*

Taking my daughter to the doctor's office was a miserable experience until she was around two years old. When my children were toddlers, I found that blowing bubbles was a great distraction. I even brought a small bottle of bubbles to the doctor's office. If we had a long wait in the exam room or if my daughter was crying while the doctor tried to examine her, I'd blow a few bubbles. The doctor didn't mind a bit!

—*Eva Mayer, MD*

I've been very fortunate that we haven't had long waits at the pediatrician's office. The pediatrician doesn't have any toys in the waiting room, but there is a nice fish tank in the waiting room that my daughter loves to look at. I bring books and toys along in case we have to wait.

Once we get into the exam room, my daughter likes to play with the paper on the exam table. I know that's not what it's there for, but it's a great alternate use!

—*Rachel S. Rohde, MD*

When my twins went for their well-child visits, I scheduled both visits for the same time. This was efficient, but challenging. While the doctor

Mommy MD Guides–Recommended Product
Bee-Stractor Cards

"When my kids were toddlers and we had to wait anywhere, such as at the doctor's office, we played Eye Spy," says Amy Baxter, MD, a mom of 14- and 12-year-old sons and a 9-year-old daughter; the CEO of Buzzy4Shots.com; and the director of emergency research, Scottish Rite, of the Children's Healthcare of Atlanta, in Georgia. "A few years later, I created Bee-Stractor cards. These are five picture cards on a ring with related counting and finding questions on the back. For example, the questions include: How many stars do you see? Can you find an astronaut? Which cow has a plunger on its head?"

Bee-Stractors are a quick and handy way to distract bored kids, break a behavior spiral, or take a child's mind off a painful procedure. They're actually proven to decrease pain while getting an IV. You can buy them at the online store on **BUZZY4SHOTS.COM** for $6.95.

was examining one twin and talking to me, I had to keep the other twin strapped in the stroller. This way I didn't have to worry that this twin was climbing up on the exam table or crawling around on the floor. I also brought along things to keep my kids occupied, such as board books.

I know this is a challenge for other parents as well. Even if you don't have twins, you might have another child who needs to tag along to the doctor's visit. Keeping a sense of humor, staying calm, and, maybe most importantly, having a bountiful supply of Cheerios or Goldfish is probably the best advice there is. We've all been there!

—*Ann Contrucci, MD, a mom of 13-year-old boy-girl twins who works as a pediatric emergency physician, in Atlanta, GA*

Asking Questions

Such a cliché, but the dumbest question truly is the one that's not asked. People become pediatricians and family physicians because they love children and they want to help. How can your toddler's doctor help to answer your questions if you don't ask?

෴

When I take my daughters to the pediatrician, I always bring a list of questions to ask. I also bring lots of toys so the waiting is easier.

—*Kate Tulenko, MD, MPH, a mom of four- and one-year-old girls, the author of* Insourced: How Importing Jobs Impacts the Healthcare Crisis Here and Abroad, *and a pediatrician and global health specialist with IntraHealth, in Washington, DC*

෴

When I take my son to the doctor, I like to ask my questions up front. But I make sure to tell the doctor he doesn't have to answer right away, but rather he can answer anytime during the visit. It's also very helpful to bring along a pad of paper and something to write with!

—*Michelle Davis-Dash, MD, a mom of a one-year-old son and a pediatrician, in Baltimore, MD*

As a first-time mom, I ask a lot of questions at the doctor's office. But as a physician, I know that's perfectly normal! What other first-time moms might not realize is that physicians are used to first-time moms asking a lot of questions. And they are balanced out by veteran moms, who ask much fewer questions. So ask away!

Physicians sometimes assume that moms automatically know certain things, so if you don't ask, we might assume you already know! I try to remember all the questions I asked my own family doctor at my daughter's visits and help spark some questions for my patients.

—*Jennifer Bacani McKenney, MD, a mom of a one-year-old daughter and a family physician, in Fredonia, KS*

If I have a lot of topics to cover with the doctor (usually this is with specialists), I will write the questions down and go through the list with the doc. Most doctors, especially specialists, know that you have waited a while to get the appointment, so they will answer the questions on your list, however long it might seem. It can be helpful to wait to ask the questions until the end of the visit. This way, many of your concerns have already been addressed during the initial part of the visit, and you might have only a handful of concerns left on your list.

—*Jeannette Gonzalez Simon, MD, a mom of three- and one-year-old daughters and a pediatric gastroenterologist in private practice, in Staten Island, NY*

My husband and I learned very early on that it was better if I said nothing at the well-child visits and let him talk with the pediatrician to be sure his questions got answered. Otherwise, there was a lot of doctor talk between me and the physician, and my husband did not get the information he needed. So we started making a list of questions before we arrived and letting him ask them.

The few times that there has been a more complex issue that I thought the pediatrician would need more time to look into, I sent an e-mail in advance to save time in the office.

I try not to provide medical care to my own kids (even though I am a pediatrician, I still don't think it is a good idea), so my husband calls the after-hours number to get advice. In either case (when we're calling or in the pediatrician's office), I try to be sure we have a list of my son's signs and symptoms and when they occurred, for example, when a symptom such as nausea started, how many times my son vomited, and how high his fever was before and after giving a dose of acetaminophen (Tylenol). That is the kind of information I would want if I were seeing the patient.

—*Carrie Brown, MD, a mom of eight- and six-year-old sons and a general pediatrician who treats medically complex children and specializes in palliative care at Arkansas Children's Hospital, in Little Rock*

I never brought a list of questions to the doctor's office. On the flip side, I always forgot to ask one or two questions. I didn't hesitate to call, e-mail, or text my pediatrician after the visit with follow-up questions. He always got back to me promptly with the answers.

—*Sadaf T. Bhutta, MD, a mom of a six-year-old daughter and four-year-old triplets and an assistant professor and the fellowship director of pediatric radiology at the University of Arkansas for Medical Sciences and Arkansas Children's Hospital, both in Little Rock*

RALLIE'S TIP

I feel very fortunate that my boys have been healthy since they were born, but there were lots of times that I had questions that I wanted to ask their pediatrician. To make sure that I didn't forget my questions, I'd write them down in my datebook on the page that marked the date of our next appointment.

Our pediatrician was a very kind and patient man, and at the beginning of each of our well-child visits, he would ask me if I had any concerns about my child's health or behavior. I'm sure he had learned from years of experience that every mom—including moms who are also doctors—has plenty of questions about her children.

By asking me about my concerns at the beginning of the checkup, he made it easy for me to ask questions, and it also helped him do a more effective examination. If I told the pediatrician that my son had been pulling at his right ear recently, for example, he could pay special attention to my son's right ear during his examination.

During a well-child visit, I think it's generally best for you, the doctor, and your toddler if you ask questions before the examination begins. Toddlers normally need a few minutes to relax in the doctor's presence, and it's very helpful if they see mom and the doctor chatting comfortably. Asking your questions early in the visit also helps doctors conduct a more effective physical exam because it allows them to look for clues that might help explain the signs or symptoms you've described. And when you ask your questions up front, you're most likely to get the information and explanations that you want.

I think the worst time to ask doctors questions is after they've completed their examination and they're wrapping up the visit. That's why it's really helpful to keep a running list of the issues that you'd like to discuss with the doctor. As soon as you've said hello to each other and chatted a bit, you can whip out your list and get down to business.

If you have several questions about your child's health and behavior, or if you feel that your concerns will require a lengthy discussion with the physician, it's helpful to tell the receptionist or the person making the appointment that you'd like to schedule a little extra time to talk to the doctor at your next visit.

As physicians, taking time to discuss health-related concerns is a very important part of our job, so you should never feel bad about asking questions. If you feel that you're being brushed off or rushed, or if you don't feel comfortable asking your doctor questions about your child's health, you might be better off finding a physician whose communication style is better suited to your needs.

Giving Medicines and Supplements

"A spoonful of sugar helps the medicine go down." Mary Poppins probably meant that quite literally, which isn't such a great idea. (But then flying by umbrella probably wasn't such a great idea either.) But if by "sugar" you mean a hefty dose of hugs, kisses, and good wishes, then by all means, a spoonful of that sugar really will help the medicine go down.

As with babies, don't give your toddler any medications without the A-OK of your child's doctor. Along the same lines, don't give your toddler any nutritional supplements, such as multivitamin and mineral supplements, without checking with his doctor first. Some pediatricians and family physicians discourage giving supplements to toddlers. But it's wise to check in on your family's situation first.

∽

The only medication I've given to my daughter is acetaminophen (Tylenol) for a fever. It's really important to measure infant and children's Tylenol very carefully. The infant formula is very concentrated, so you want to make sure to give the right amount.

It's best to give medications according to the baby's weight rather than the baby's age because all babies grow at different rates. It's important not to give too much because it can harm the baby, but it's important to give enough or you won't get the fever down.

—*Jennifer Bacani McKenney, MD*

∽

I would only give my kids medicine if I thought it would truly ease their symptoms. If they were sick, but weren't feeling bad, there was no need for medicine. But if they were sick and were feeling bad because they had a high fever, for example, then I would give an age- and weight-appropriate dose of acetaminophen (Tylenol) or ibuprofen (Motrin) to bring the fever down.

It seems most of the time toddlers just want acknowledgment of an ailment. Usually this can be achieved with an ice pack or a cool cloth.

—*Jennifer Hanes, DO, a mom of a six-year-old daughter and a three-year-old son, an emergency physician, a certified forensic physician, and the founder of Empowered Medicine, PLLC, in Austin, TX*

As quickly as I could, I transitioned my kids from liquid medications. They are harder to give an exact dose, and they're easier for kids to spit out or to spill. That's a problem because you don't know how much of the medicine the child got into his body.

For example, acetaminophen (Tylenol) is sold as Children's Meltaways, which melt in the child's mouth. You can buy Tylenol Children's Meltaways at stores and online. Of course, you need to keep them far away from children, such as in a high, locked cabinet.

—*Cheri Wiggins, MD, a mom of six- and three-year-old daughters, a specialist in physical medicine and rehabilitation at St. Luke's Magic Valley, and the cofounder of the Mommy Doctors Bakery (makers of Milkin' Cookies), in Twin Falls, ID*

I try to minimize the amount of medicine I give to my daughter. I use medication as a last resort.

Some children's medicines are flavored like bubble gum or grape to get kids to take them. But the problem is that they taste *too* good. I stress to my daughter that you should only take medication when you need it.

Also, when my daughter needs to take medicine regularly, such as allergy medicine, I give it to her at the same time each day. I think this helps to emphasize to her that you take this only once a day, as directed.

—*Tanya Douglas Holland, MD, a mom of a two-year-old daughter, a women's health advocate, and a consultant in medical affairs to a pharmaceutical company, in Atlanta, GA*

It's critical to memorize the phone number for Poison Control (800-222-1212), program it into your phones, or at least write it somewhere very handy. Most parents have to call Poison Control with a question at least once during their kids' childhoods.

One day, I accidentally left the Children's Motrin (ibuprofen) sitting out, and my son got it. I was able to estimate about how much he drank because I remembered about how much was in the bottle. (It's always a good idea to make a mental note of how much of any medicine is left in the bottle.) I knew that my son had gotten about triple his one-teaspoon dose. I called Poison Control, and thank goodness, they said he would be fine, no treatment needed. I knew that, but the reassurance from an objective source was helpful. I wasn't a doctor at that time, but a parent!

Any time that a child ingests something potentially harmful, don't hesitate to call Poison Control immediately. That's what they're there for, and they're kind and helpful. Depending on what the child has ingested, it might be critical to get medical attention immediately for the child to make a full recovery. Also, there are certain substances that we don't want a child to vomit because this can lead to even more problems. Poison Control can help a panicked parent sort through the best course of action to take.

—*Ann Contrucci, MD*

❧

Even though my kids were good eaters, I still gave them a multivitamin each day. My dentist said that gummy vitamins are bad for their teeth because they get stuck in the grooves. I gave my kids the harder, chewable vitamins instead, such as Flintstones. My kids protested about the taste, so I crumbled them into applesauce or yogurt.

—*Eva Mayer, MD*

❧

I avoided giving my sons medicine as much as possible. But I did give them a daily multivitamin and mineral supplement.

I now recommend IntraKID liquid multivitamin from Drucker Labs to my patients. I've had kids tell me that they remind their moms to give it to them because they feel better when they take it.

—*Cathie Lippman, MD, a mom of 31- and 29-year-old sons and a physician who specializes in environmental and preventive medicine at the Lippman Center for Optimal Health, in Beverly Hills, CA*

❧

I didn't give my toddlers any vitamins. They were eating a very balanced diet. However, in some cases it might be warranted, especially concerning vitamin D and breastfeeding or prematurity. Check with your pediatrician regarding your particular situation.

—*Ann Contrucci, MD*

RALLIE'S TIP

My children didn't take many antibiotics growing up, but when they did, they invariably got diarrhea. Antibiotics (anti = against, biotic = life) don't discriminate when it comes to killing bacteria. These drugs kill the bad bacteria that are causing the ear or sinus infection, and they also kill the good bacteria called probiotics (pro = for, biotic = life) in the gut that play a critical role in immunity. Probiotics help break down food to improve digestion and absorption of nutrients, and they also help detoxify the gut.

After taking a round of antibiotics, many children experience minor to major GI upset, including stomach cramps and diarrhea. Studies show that nearly a quarter of people taking antibiotics end up developing diarrhea, and as many as one in five people discontinue antibiotic therapy due to this unpleasant side effect.

While a person is taking antibiotics, the probiotic bacteria in the gut end up dying by the millions and being eliminated in the stool. The food that is eaten isn't digested properly because the probiotic bacteria population isn't strong enough or healthy enough to do its job. Both factors contribute to diarrhea and abdominal discomfort.

One of the best ways to offset this negative chain of events is to give children probiotics while they're taking antibiotics, and continue to give the probiotics for a week or two after the antibiotic treatment has ended.

Probiotics are generally beneficial for kids whenever they have diarrhea or stomach upset from any cause. When my sons were young, I would open up a capsule of probiotics (I always kept a bottle in the fridge) and sprinkle them on their tongues. I'd also give them yogurt with live and active cultures of probiotic bacteria. When my children were little, I had to get these products from a health food store, but now you can buy several varieties of probiotics-containing yogurt at just about any supermarket.

Literally hundreds of studies from some of the leading academic and medical institutions in the world document the safety and efficacy of probiotics in promoting improved GI health in children and adults.

Chapter 8
Toddler Proofing

YOUR TODDLER'S DEVELOPMENT

Every new step of development requires you to also step up your toddler-proofing efforts. Now that your toddler can walk, run, and climb, she's much more able to get herself into a heap of trouble! Your goal: Try to stay one step ahead.

TAKING CARE OF YOU

Do you smoke? If so, quitting is a giant leap you can take to improve your health, and the health of everyone around you.

A recent study found that long-term smoking and exposure to secondhand smoke might increase a woman's chances of developing breast cancer after menopause. Plus, women who smoke are 25 percent more likely to develop heart disease than men who smoked. Another recent study found that women who are regularly exposed to smoke are more likely to have an abnormal Pap test than women who aren't. Really, just say no to cigarettes.

JUSTIFICATION FOR A CELEBRATION

You'll know when the time is right to actually start to take down all of those babyproofing devices. The day you can ditch the baby gates for good will be a great reason to celebrate!

Toddler Proofing the Nursery

It's a scary stat: Every minute, 17 children go to the emergency department with unintentional injuries. That's 9.2 million visits each year.

Your toddler's bedroom is an especially important room to toddler proof because it's the one room she probably spends quite a bit of time alone in. Here are some simple safety steps to take.

- If you haven't already, remove any mobiles from the crib.
- Keep the crib mattress at its lowest setting.
- Keep the crib far away from any window treatments, such as miniblind cords and drapes.
- Make sure that all furniture is far enough away from the crib that your toddler can't use it to climb out of her crib.
- If you haven't secured furniture such as dressers to the wall or floor, do so without delay. (According to a Home Safety Council survey, 71 percent of parents say their toddlers have climbed on a piece of furniture. Yet only 28 percent of parents have anchored heavy furniture to walls or the floor to prevent tip-overs.)
- Make sure outlet protectors are securely in place.
- Be careful which toys you leave in the nursery. Soft stuffed animals are okay. Small pieces like Legos are not!
- Never leave plastic bags or other suffocation hazards in your child's room.
- Keep your toddler's room warm, but not too warm. Aim for a room temperature between 68°F and 72°F.
- Remove your toddler's bib before putting her in her crib. And never tie a pacifier around her neck.
- Buy flame-retardant sleepwear. Also dress your toddler in snugly fitting sleepwear. It's less likely to catch on fire and won't burn as rapidly because there's less air between the clothing and the skin.

While we're on the topic of fire prevention, you hopefully have working smoke alarms in place on each floor and outside all sleeping areas. And hopefully you diligently replace the batteries at least once a year. (Fall back, change your batteries!) But did you know that in a recent study, 90 percent of small children slept through a smoke alarm going off for 30 seconds? The best protection is to have interconnected smoke alarms, so that if one goes off, they all will go off. Even if your children don't hear them, you will. Also, hold regular fire drills with your family, practicing getting out of the house safely and meeting at a designated place outside your home. Conduct some of your practice sessions at night because most home fires blaze after dark.

Babyproofing is a very big, very important job. I hired a babyproofing service to come to my house. It wasn't expensive, especially because it bought me tremendous peace of mind.

I don't buy new cars or expensive shoes. I'd rather spend money on something like having an expert babyproof my house.

—*Dina Strachan, MD, a mom of a six-year-old daughter, a dermatologist and director of Aglow Dermatology, and an assistant clinical professor in the department of dermatology at New York University, in New York City*

When my son was about a year and a half old, we transitioned him from his crib to his mattress on the floor. Of course, then he could get out of his room any time he wanted. So we put a baby gate in the doorway.

My son quickly learned how to climb over the gate, so we put another baby gate in the doorway, an inch or two above the first. He couldn't climb over them both!

—*Carrie Brown, MD, a mom of eight- and six-year-old sons and a general pediatrician who treats medically complex children and specializes in palliative care at Arkansas Children's Hospital, in Little Rock*

My husband and I used to use a baby gate in my son's nursery doorway. One of the many challenges with toddlers, though, is that sometimes the babyproofing devices that were so helpful when they were younger actually become a danger when they're older. For example, now my son is perfectly capable of climbing over the baby gate to get to the other side. I worry that he might lose his balance on the way over, fall, and get hurt. So we stopped using the baby gates, and instead we lock the doors.

—*Rebecca Reamy, MD, a mom of seven- and two-year-old sons and a pediatrician in emergency medicine at Children's Healthcare of Atlanta, in Georgia*

When toddler proofing, it's very important to get down on all fours and crawl around anywhere your toddler might go. Try to reach anywhere and everywhere; if you can reach it, you can be certain the toddler will try to reach it too!

My husband did most of this hard work. We covered all of the outlets, used baby gates, used the playpen a lot to keep our kids out of trouble, and, of course, kept a watchful eye on them. We kept cleaning products as well as medications up high where our sons couldn't reach them. We also made sure we kept the cords for our window blinds tied up and out of reach. I had a friend who had a tragedy in her home from this, so we were particularly attentive to this issue. In addition, we made sure that the kids' cribs were nowhere near a window or cord.

—*Leena Shrivastava Dev, MD, a mom of 15- and 11-year-old sons, a general pediatrician, and an advocate for child safety, in Philadelphia, PA*

Toddler Proofing the Bathrooms and Kitchen

Water, hot stoves, knives—no doubt about it, there are plenty of ways for a toddler to harm herself in the bathroom or kitchen. Here are some simple safety steps to take.

- Keep bathroom doors closed or at least install baby gates to keep your toddler out.
- Turn the temperature of your hot water down to 120°F. To test it, run your hot water until it's as hot as it gets. Fill a ceramic mug, and then take your water's temperature

with a meat thermometer. If you live in an apartment or can't adjust your water temp, install an anti-scald device on the faucet. Because kids have thinner skin than adults, their skin burns more quickly. Just three seconds of exposure to 140°F water can give a child a third-degree burn.

- Place a cover over the tub faucet to protect your wriggly toddler from bumps.
- Install nonslip mats in your bathtub and on the floor next to the tub.
- Check the temperature of the tub water before letting your toddler get in.
- Never leave your toddler unattended in the tub.
- Immediately after your toddler is out of the bath, drain the tub water completely.
- Don't use bags to line wastebaskets because they are a suffocation hazard.
- Install finger guards on doors so they can't accidentally slam shut on your toddler's fingers.
- Wipe up puddles of water immediately. Teach your toddler that wet floors are slippery floors and to "walk gently." Because toddlers can't always react quickly enough to break their falls with their arms, they often fall onto their heads or faces.
- Put a toilet lock on all toilets. Keep the lids down and latched so your toddler can't play in the water or drown.
- Move all medications and vitamins to high, locked cabinets. This includes items you might not think of as dangerous, but can be, such as Visine and iron tablets.
- Be mindful of the many small items in the bathroom that can be choking hazards, such as contact lens case caps and medicine container lids.
- Keep hair dryers and curling irons unplugged and, better yet, stowed away.
- Make sure your hair dryers and other appliances in the bathroom have large, rectangular plugs. Inside those spe-

cial plugs is a circuit that senses water and, in milliseconds, shuts off the power, keeping your child safe if the appliance accidentally falls into water.

- Keep kitchen doors closed or at least install baby gates to keep your toddler out.
- Move cleaning chemicals to high, locked cabinets. This includes dishwasher detergents, furniture polish, and pretty much anything you'd use to clean your home.
- Load the dishwasher with knives pointing down and keep the dishwasher closed, locked if possible.
- Push everything as far to the back of counters as possible, and never leave cords to appliances dangling off the edge where your toddler could grab them.
- If your stove's knobs are on the front, within reach of your child, remove them or install knob locks.
- Train yourself to cook on the back burners whenever possible and to turn pot handles toward the back of the stove.
- Before you take a hot pan or pot off the stove, for example, to drain cooked pasta in the sink, scan the room to see where your toddler is. Then say a simple warning like, "Hot stuff, stay back!"
- Establish a "no toddler" zone about four feet in front of your stove.
- Don't hang dish towels on the bar of your oven door. Your toddler could use the towel to pull the oven door open.
- Explain often to your toddler that the stove and oven get hot and that knives are sharp.
- Stash stools in another room so your toddler can't push them to gain access to the counter or cabinets.
- Consider installing a latch on your fridge so your toddler can't open it and pull something heavy down on herself or grab choking hazards such as grapes.

෴

When my twins were little, I moved all of our medication into high, locked cabinets. Kids will climb! Out of reach is not good enough. One thing that's critical to move is vitamins and minerals. Iron is one of the deadliest things a child can ingest. Another one is too much acetaminophen (Tylenol), an overdose of which can cause liver failure.

—*Ann Contrucci, MD, a mom of 13-year-old boy-girl twins who works as a pediatric emergency physician, in Atlanta, GA*

My daughter is very happy and inquisitive. It's difficult to keep up with her and to keep her out of the places we don't want her to go, such as the shower. I just keep a really good eye on her, and I try to divert her attention when she's headed toward something I don't want her to do.

I put locks on the kitchen and bathroom cabinets and the toilets. I moved all of the cleaning fluids to higher cabinets that are also locked. Now, if we could just keep her from toilet papering the house!

—*Rachel S. Rohde, MD, a mom of a one-year-old daughter, an assistant professor of orthopaedic surgery at the Oakland University William Beaumont School of Medicine, and an orthopaedic upper-extremity surgeon with Michigan Orthopaedic Institute, P.C., in Southfield, MI*

It's so hard to keep my eyes on my toddler all of the time. At some point, you have to go to the bathroom or grab something from another room. But you really can't leave a toddler alone for even a moment. Toddlers understand "no," but they don't always understand the consequences of their actions.

We had a disaster a couple of months ago. We have a Whirlpool tub in our master bathroom, and my son got into the bathroom. He turned on the water, and he was standing outside the tub, splashing in the water. So much water splashed out of the tub that it soaked through the floor and began dripping through the ceiling below! It damaged the drywall so badly that we had to hire someone to fix it. After that, we've been certain to keep our bathroom door locked so my son can't get in there unattended.

—*Rebecca Reamy, MD*

I put adhesive bathtub stickers on the bottom of my tub. This prevents my toddlers from slipping. They're also so much easier to clean than tub mats because nothing can grow underneath them.

I put a spout guard on the tub faucet. My toddlers are always bouncing around in the tub, and I don't want them to whack their heads on the sharp, hard faucet.

When I get my kids' bath ready, I turn the cold water on first, and then I add hot. This way, I can titrate the warm water more carefully.

—*Shilpa Amin-Shah, MD, a mom of a two-year-old son and a one-year-old daughter and an emergency physician at Emergency Medical Associates, in Livingston, NJ*

I found that if I gave my toddlers clear direction on where they could and could not go, they listened very well. For example, in my kitchen, I kept the items that my kids were allowed to play with in different drawers than the things they weren't allowed to play with. My kids understood that they could play with the plastic dishes and containers and bang some pots and pans in the drawers next to the sink, but they couldn't play with the breakable dishes in the drawer next to the stove. Toddlers understand yes and no really well, even at age one!

>—*Ayala Laufer-Cahana, MD, a mom of 16- and 14-year-old sons and a 12-year-old daughter, a pediatrician, and the founder of Herbal Water Inc., in Wynnewood, PA*

When my kids were toddlers, my husband and I installed those plastic latches to keep the cabinet doors closed. That was easy and effective.

Today, I've babyproofed my home for my grandkids, but my mother-in-law also lives with us. With her stiff, arthritic hands, she can't open those plastic latches. Instead, I bought magnetic locks. You can buy sets of a key and two locks online and in baby supply stores for around $16. This works great to both keep our "grandtoddlers" out of cabinets and let my mother-in-law get into them!

>—*Susan Besser, MD, a mom of six grown children, ages 27, 25, 23, 21, 20, and 18, a grandmom of two, a family physician, and the medical director of Doctors Express-Memphis, in Tennessee*

Mommy MD Guides-Recommended Product
Safety 1st Oven and Refrigerator Locks

Your toddler is now tall enough to reach the oven door and strong enough to pull open the refrigerator, so it's time to start making these appliances safe. It's particularly important if you have an extra fridge or freezer in your basement or another out-of-the-way place where your toddler might decide it's a good spot to play hide and seek.

Safety 1st offers oven and refrigerator locks to prevent injuries, but remember when you install them that the surface has to be very clean before you put them in place. The Safety 1st Oven Door Lock (Model HS035) retails at $5.49 and can be found at Walmart, Babies R Us, and online retailers. The Safety 1st Refrigerator Door Lock (Model HS187) retails at $5.49 and can be found at Walmart and online retailers. Visit SAFETY1ST.COM for more information.

The best babyproofing for toddlers is constant vigilance. Even if you have done great babyproofing, you have to keep your eyes on your toddler practically all of the time. For example, I had moved all of the medication and cleaning supplies in my kitchen far out of my kids' reach into a high kitchen cabinet. One day, my younger daughter pushed a kitchen chair over to the counter, climbed up onto the counter, grabbed a bottle of Children's Benadryl, opened up the childproof cap, and drank it. Unfortunately, my nanny was occupied with my other children at the time, and she didn't discover this until my daughter had ingested a lot of medicine. My husband raced home from work and took our daughter to the pediatrician. Thank goodness she was fine. She was pretty sleepy though!

—Lisa Dado, MD, a mom of 23- and 20-year-old daughters and an 18-year-old son, a pediatric anesthesiologist with Valley Anesthesiology Consultants, and the cofounder and CEO of the nonprofit organization the Center for Humane Living, which teaches life skills with an innovative approach to traditional martial arts training in six centers in and around Phoenix, AZ

My younger son is very happy and energetic. He's also a climber. One day, I came into the kitchen to find my son standing up on the counter! He had pushed a kitchen chair over to the counter and climbed up onto the counter. Of course, if he fell from there, he could be seriously hurt, so I locked the kitchen chairs in the office to prevent him from doing that again.

Next, my son figured out how to push a chair from our dining room into the kitchen, so that he could use that chair to climb up onto the counter. I moved those chairs to the office too. So now we have no place to sit in our dining room or kitchen! Fortunately, my son can't push the couch from the living room into the kitchen!

—Rebecca Reamy, MD

I was very careful to babyproof the cabinets under the sinks in our bathroom and kitchen. My husband and I keep things in there, such as medicines and cleaners, that I don't want my sons to have access to.

Rather than buying the cabinet latches or magnets that you have to install, I bought the plastic ones that secure the knobs from the outside. They're so much easier to use, and my son can't open them.

All of the babyproofing in the world isn't a substitute for watchful parenting, though. You never know what day your toddler will figure out how to open those cabinet locks. When that day comes, you want to be standing by to keep him out of the potentially dangerous things inside.

—*Sharon Boyce, MD, a mom of three- and one-year-old sons and a family physician at DayOne Family Healthcare Clinic, in Battle Creek, MI*

It's critical to always have the Poison Control number (800-222-1212) on hand. You'll need it at a time that you'd never imagine. For example, one day I was in the kitchen with my son, emptying the dishwasher. My son was happily "drumming" on the open dishwasher door. Suddenly, I noticed that he had white powder around his mouth! I realized that he had scooped up—and tasted—the dishwasher detergent residue. I called Poison Control and, luckily, found out that we use the "irritating but nontoxic" dishwasher detergent!

—*Deborah Gilboa, MD, a mom of nine-, seven-, five-, and three-year-old sons, a parenting speaker whose advice is found at AskDoctorG.com, and a family physician with Squirrel Hill Health Center, in Pittsburgh, PA*

Keeping my toddlers in their high chairs was a challenge. It seemed horrible to have to strap them in, but that's what we had to do to keep them seated.

I remember one awful day, I was at work, and my daughter stood up in her high chair and fell out and hit her head. Because she blacked out briefly, she had to go to the hospital for a head CT. Thank goodness she was fine. But it was scary! It gave me a whole new respect for high chairs to know how easily a little one could stand up and fall right out onto her head.

—*Siobhan Dolan, MD, MPH, a mom of 16- and 13-year-old daughters and an 11-year-old son, a consultant to the March of Dimes, and an associate professor of obstetrics and gynecology and women's health at Albert Einstein College of Medicine/Montefiore Medical Center, in Bronx, NY*

Toddler Proofing the Living Areas

Living rooms and toy rooms offer so many opportunities for fun and games with your toddler. Here are some simple safety steps to take.

- Install doorknob covers or lock doors to any dangerous areas, such as down basement steps.
- Keep baby gates at the top and bottom of stairs securely closed.
- Teach your toddler to stay away from heaters, vents, and fans.
- Keep electrical cords and power strips out of reach.
- Make sure outlet covers are inserted securely.
- Keep candles and matches far out of reach.
- Move glass picture frames and breakables to higher ground. The glass from a picture frame, for instance, could quickly cut a child. Move glass tables to another, locked room.
- Slide TVs back from the edge of cabinets, or better yet mount them to the cabinet or wall.
- Secure heavy and tall furniture, such as bookcases, to the

wall or floor. Each year, nearly 15,000 kids visit emergency departments for furniture-tip-over-related injuries.
- Pad sharp edges of fireplaces and tables.
- Be on the lookout for choking hazards on the floor or on low tables, such as coins, paper clips, and buttons.
- Watch your toddler's fingers carefully when you're reclining and putting up chairs and sofas.
- Secure miniblind cords and draperies high out of your toddler's reach.
- Keep latex balloons completely away from kids younger than eight years old. If a child puts a popped balloon in his mouth, the balloon can drape itself over the entrance to his larynx, suffocating him.
- Along the same lines, tie up and discard plastic shopping bags, keeping them far out of your toddler's reach.
- Keep art supplies high out of your toddler's reach. Even things like crayons can be snapped in two and become a choking hazard.

～∽

As an emergency physician, I'm neurotic about safety! I started baby-proofing very early, before my son could even crawl. So by the time my son was a toddler, we had plenty of safety measures in place. We had locks on the cabinets, and I had moved all dangerous substances such as dishwashing detergent up to high cabinets far out of my son's reach.

The challenge of babyproofing for toddlers, though, is that you have to give them some freedom to learn and grow. So, for instance, they have to learn to go up and down stairs. My husband and I left the baby gate on our main staircases. But we have two carpeted steps that lead down to our family room. We left that ungated, so that our son could practice going up and down those safer steps.

—*Shilpa Amin-Shah, MD*

～∽

You can't babyproof every single thing. I did put gates at the top and bottom of our stairs. I padded the hard edges of our fireplace with a hearth guard, adhesive-backed foam that's sold at buybuy Baby or other stores, and added a few body pillows in front of the fireplace. We don't use the fireplace yet because we are afraid our daughter will want to touch the glass, and it gets very hot.

We have a piano, and my daughter was drawn to that like a magnet. I was afraid that she'd climb up onto the bench, fall off, and hit her head on a sharp corner. I wrapped my pregnancy Snoogle pillow around the bench to deter my daughter from climbing up on it.

—*Rachel S. Rohde, MD*

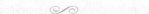

Some things you just can't babyproof for. My older son would run so fast through our house that he'd smack into things. Once he hit the wall so hard it left a dent. He didn't injure himself, but it did make me realize how cheaply our house was made.

We played outside a lot after that. Also, my husband and I worked hard to babyproof our house. We padded everything, including putting foam edges on tables and down the corners of walls. By the time our second son was a toddler, we had moved to a new house. We didn't do nearly as much babyproofing for him. We saved a lot of money on foam, and he survived anyway.

—*Carrie Brown, MD*

I've seen so many kids come to the emergency department with lacerations and gashes from falling onto sharp corners of furniture and fireplaces. I put padding on the corners of our fireplace and coffee tables. We didn't have any glass-topped tables, but if we had, I would have put them far away from my toddlers, in the basement or attic. Those can be a hazard.

I also put outlet covers into my outlets. Some people now advise against this because the outlet covers can be small enough to be choking hazards. I was careful to buy the covers that are very difficult to pull out. In fact, they were so hard to get out that *I* couldn't even get them out. There was no way my toddlers could pry them out of the outlets.

—*Ann Contrucci, MD*

Two weeks ago, my younger son figured out how to open the doors in our house. As luck would have it, the doorknobs are oval shaped, not traditional round knobs, so babyproofing doorknob covers don't fit on them.

My husband and I started to lock the doors to the rooms that we don't want our son to go into, such as the bathroom. We keep the keys on the molding above the doors. The problem is that our older son isn't tall enough to reach them! He has to carry a key around in his pocket. Fortunately, this won't last forever. We did later find a latch that attaches to the door frame that our older son can reach but our younger son can't.

—*Rebecca Reamy, MD*

I don't get really wrapped up in babyproofing. My philosophy is that you have to protect your kids from the dangers that will kill them. So I put guards on the windows, gates at the top and bottom of stairs, and protectors in outlets.

Once those major dangers are covered, I've found that you really can't predict or prepare for all of the ways kids will injure themselves. One of our most serious near-injuries happened one day when I came down my stairs to find my toddler balanced precariously on our heater register, clinging to the curtain! There's just no way to babyproof to prevent that from happening!

—*Deborah Gilboa, MD*

Babyproofing for a toddler is an oxymoron. I don't think you really can babyproof for a toddler. You can try, but mainly you just have to stay one step ahead of her. And you shouldn't take your eyes off your toddler. If she's in another room and she's quiet, you know you're in trouble.

It's important to make sure your toddler can't open the doors to your house and get outside by herself. We had a scare with one of my sons.

We had a guest one day, and I thought our son was with my husband. But my husband thought our son was with me. We realized our son wasn't even in the house.

We all frantically searched the neighborhood for him. We found there was a swamp near our home that we didn't even know about. It's critical to know where all bodies of water are near your house, such as which neighbors have pools, if there are any streams or ponds, and even if there are places where water collects after storms. If a child is missing, search those areas first.

It turns out that my son had wandered into the middle of a busy road. A passerby stopped, whisked our son to safety, and waited on the sidewalk with him for us to arrive. Thank goodness, our son was fine.

—Victoria McEvoy, MD, a mom who raised four children; a grandmom of six-, four-, and two-year-old grandsons; an assistant professor of pediatrics at Harvard Medical School; the medical director and chief of pediatrics at Mass General West Medical Group; and the author of 24/7 Baby Doctor, in Boston, MA

Keeping Your Toddler Safe in the Car

Probably the most important safety device you own is your child's car seat. Your toddler depends upon you using it correctly, each and every time you put her in the car. Properly used car seats slash an infant's risk of dying in a car crash by 71 percent.

Interestingly, the American Academy of Pediatrics' guidelines regarding toddlers in car seats recently changed. They now urge parents to keep kids rear-facing to age two years, or until they reach the height or weight limit of the car seat itself. A rear-facing seat better protects a child's head, neck, and spine in a crash.

A 2007 study published in the journal *Injury Prevention* found that toddlers younger than age two are 75 percent less likely to be severely injured or die in a car crash if they are rear-facing. Another study found riding rear-facing to be five times safer than riding forward-facing.

Another critical safety factor to consider is completely within your control. Never ever talk on the phone or text while your child is in the car. A recent study showed that you're six times more likely to get into a crash if you're texting. No text or call is more important than arriving safely at your destination.

For babyproofing, I believe in having a few very firm rules. One of them is all children ride in car seats. Always.

—*Siobhan Dolan, MD, MPH*

Going from two kids in car seats to three kids in car seats is a challenge. I bought one of the narrowest car seats on the market at the time—the Sunshine Kids Radian 65—so I could get three car seats across in my car's backseat.

—*Kristie McNealy, MD, a mom of nine- and six-year-old daughters and four-year-old and 22-month-old sons and a blogger at KristieMcNealy.com, in Denver, CO*

When my youngest child fought getting in her car seat, I instituted the car seat game. When we got to the car, we sang a song. If my daughter was in the seat by the end of the song, she received a small sticker. (I kept a sticker stash under my car visor.) With this game, our mornings started with smiles instead of fighting.

—*Cathy Marshall, MD, a mom of 28-, 14-, and 11-year-old daughters and a pediatrician in private practice, in Encino, CA*

With my toddlers, there were some rules that were 100 percent concrete, no fudging around. One of them was that as soon as we got into the car, they got buckled into their car seats and they behaved properly while I was driving. If they started fighting, I simply pulled off the road until everyone had settled down.

—*Eva Ritvo, MD, a mom of 21- and 16-year-old daughters,*
a psychiatrist, and a coauthor of The Beauty Prescription, *in*
Miami Beach, FL

When my daughter was a toddler, it was very challenging when she had a tantrum when I was driving. I would turn the radio up, and the tantrums would usually stop.

—*Stuart Jeanne Bramhall, MD, a mom of a 31-year-old daughter*
and a child and adolescent psychiatrist in New Plymouth, New
Zealand

I worry a lot about choking. I never let my daughter eat in the car. If she chokes, I fear I would have a hard time pulling over to get her out of the car.

—*Lisa Campanella-Coppo, MD, a mom of a three-year-old*
daughter, an emergency physician, and the emergency department
director of academic affairs at Monmouth Medical Center, in
New Jersey

One of the greatest dangers in the car is distracted driving. When I'm driving and my kids are in the car, it's tempting to look back to check on them, to interact with them, or worse to try to pass things back and forth to them. I try to keep all of this to a minimum and focus on my driving. Everything else can wait until we arrive safely at our destination.

—*Jennifer Hanes, DO, a mom of a six-year-old daughter and*
a three-year-old son, an emergency physician, a certified forensic
physician, and the founder of Empowered Medicine, PLLC,
in Austin, TX

I believe it's critical to keep kids rear-facing in the car as long as possible. It's much safer for a child's head and neck to ride in a rear-facing seat. In some countries, kids ride in rear-facing seats until they're five or six years old.

I carefully researched which car seats can remain rear-facing longer. This was an important factor for me when I purchased my daughters' car seats.

It's important to check the car seat to see how long the child can ride rear-facing. My older daughter reached the upper limit for rear-facing in her car seat before she turned three years old, and I was very disappointed to have to turn her seat around.

—Cheri Wiggins, MD, a mom of six- and three-year-old daughters, a specialist in physical medicine and rehabilitation at St. Luke's Magic Valley, and the cofounder of the Mommy Doctors Bakery (makers of Milkin' Cookies), in Twin Falls, ID

One of the biggest problems with car seats is that people don't install them properly. My husband went to a car seat installation class. His was offered by a local car dealership, but various police departments and even hospitals now offer workshops on how to install car seats properly.

It was very important to me to make sure that I was following all of the rules for putting children in car seats properly. I especially had to pay attention to the weight recommendations because my children were on the smaller side, so they weren't 20 pounds when they turned one, and the recommendation then was that they needed to weigh more than 20 pounds and be at least 12 months old before you should turn the car seat forward-facing. Now the recommendation is to keep your child rear-facing as long as possible—until your child reaches the top height or weight limit allowed by your car seat's manufacturer.

I didn't let my sons eat in the car until they were much older. Of course, when my older son was in the back, he was able to watch his baby brother and give him a bottle in an emergency, but usually we didn't resort to this. Only when they were able to protect their own airways and I was able to watch them were they allowed to eat in the car—but the downside is the car looks way dirtier after that!

—Leena Shrivastava Dev, MD

Keeping Your Toddler Safe Outside

Chances are, your child isn't allowed out of the house by herself. That's a good rule to follow because there are so many ways for a child to get hurt outside. It's a great idea to have childproof locks on the doors leading outside, or even alarms so you know if your toddler has made a break for it.

Here are some simple safety steps to follow when your toddler is outside.

- If your toddler will be outside for more than 10 minutes, apply sunscreen.
- Dress your toddler in layers and encourage her to wear mittens and a hat to keep warm enough in winter.
- In summer, if it's hot outside, offer your toddler plenty of shade to play under and water to drink.
- Bring a cordless phone or your cell phone outside when your kids are playing outdoors.
- Anytime your toddler is crossing a street, teach her to hold a grown-up's hand.

～

When my girls were toddlers, we played outside a lot. Because children have limited judgment, you have to protect them from the elements. So I put sunscreen on my girls each morning, and I reapplied it as needed, especially after they had been in the water.

—*Eva Ritvo, MD*

～

When my son was a toddler, I always put sunblock on him whenever he went outside in the summer months. I also made sure to reapply sunblock on the surface areas of his skin where the sun directly hits, which increases the chances of burning. These include the face, the back of the neck, the top of the ears, the top of the shoulders (he loved tank tops and still does!), and the lower legs, which were exposed during long strolls in the stroller.

There are two types of sunscreen, physical and chemical, but there is no direct evidence that chemical sunblocks cause harm in infants. So I asked a dermatologist friend of mine which sunblock he uses on his own two kids. He said he uses the physical kind, which has active ingredients such as titanium dioxide or zinc oxide. However, he and his wife use chemical sunblock on themselves. This type of sunblock includes active ingredients such as avobenzone, oxybenzone, etc. My friend explained that unlike chemical sunblocks, which get absorbed into the skin (and might even be absorbed systemically into an infant, because their skin is so much thinner, and their skin-surface-to-body-volume ratio is so much larger than an adult's), physical sunblocks sit atop the skin to block out the sun's rays.

I used California Baby brand sunblock when my son was younger, and as he got older, I switched to Neutrogena and Aveeno. I also loved the Neutrogena sunblock stick, which I threw in my wallet for quick reapplication. (I was that mom who would forget to bring a change of clothes when we went to the sprinklers at the local park!)

—*Cheryl Wu, MD, a mom of a four-year-old son, a pediatrician at LaGuardia Place Pediatrics in New York City, and a pediatric emergency physician at the Joseph M. Sanzari Children's Hospital of Hackensack University Medical Center, in New Jersey*

Most adults understand the importance of routinely applying sunscreen when outside, but toddlers often resist being completely coated in lotion. You have the option of dressing your toddlers in sun protective (UV protective) clothing. I usually dress my two sons in light-colored, long-sleeved shirts and longer shorts. This UV protected attire minimizes the amount of skin exposed to the sun. Less exposed skin means less sunscreen—and less arguing.

Also, I encourage my sons to wear hats, but my younger son is fond of immediately removing his hat. I have tried to persuade my sons to wear sunglasses, but compliance is low. I try to keep my sons out of the midday sun, and I apply broad-spectrum sunscreen to their ears and faces. I reapply the lotion at least every two hours.

With my sons, I do the best I can. My husband and I dress in sun protective clothing and protect ourselves with sunscreen too so we'll be good role models.

—*Amy J. Derick, MD, a mom of three-year-old and 19-month-*

old sons who's expecting another baby and a dermatologist in
private practice at Derick Dermatology, in Barrington, IL

One strategy I've found helpful to encourage my girls to wear safety equipment while playing outside is to focus on "good sportsman" behavior. For example, I say, "Good sportsmen wear their helmets" or "Good sportsmen wear their safety goggles." Our girls know that it's not an option: If you're biking, wear a helmet. If you're skating, wear your knee pads.

Also, if we're reading a book and see a picture of a child wearing a helmet—or not—I always point that out to my daughters. I try to consistently get across the message of the importance of safety.

—*Kate Tulenko, MD, MPH, a mom of four- and one-year-old girls, the author of* Insourced: How Importing Jobs Impacts the Healthcare Crisis Here and Abroad, *and a pediatrician and global health specialist with IntraHealth, in Washington, DC*

Keeping Your Toddler Safe in the Water

Kids are drawn to water like moms are drawn to Pringles potato chips. It's totally irresistible. No toddler should be anywhere near any water without a responsible parent or grown-up within arm's length. Nearly 1,000 kids die each year by drowning. Most drownings occur in home swimming pools, but young children can drown in as little as two inches of water.

Here are some simple safety steps to take to keep your toddler safe around water.

- If you don't know how to swim, it's a good idea to learn.
- Consider taking your toddler to swimming lessons. But know that at the toddler stage, swimming lessons are no replacement for constant, direct supervision near water.
- Know where all of the bodies of water are around your home. Does your neighbor have a pool? Is there a stream across the street? Is there a fish pond down the block? Does water collect in a parking lot after a storm? If your child is

ever missing, *run* to these water-collecting spots first.

- Invest in proper-fitting, Coast Guard–approved life vests. For toddlers, the best ones have a strap between the legs and also head support. Water wings and rings are toys, not safety devices.
- Teach your toddler that wet feet are slippery feet and to "walk gently" around water.
- If the weather turns bad, especially if you hear thunder or see lightning, get everyone out of the water immediately.
- Don't let your toddler swim in very cold (below 70°F) or very warm water.
- If you have a pool, hot tub, or decorative pond, know this is a huge responsibility. The pool should be enclosed by a fence at least four feet tall with no foot- or handrails for kids to climb. Don't put furniture or decorations close by the fence that kids could use to climb over the fence. Gates should be self-closing and self-latching. Keep tempting pool toys out of the pool. Consider buying a pool alarm and/or cover, but know that these devices haven't been proven to reduce the risk of drowning.
- Bring a cordless phone or your cell phone outside when your kids are playing in or near water.
- Teach your kids to follow all rules at pools, parks, and water parks.

Ironically, small children can be hazards *themselves* in pools! Don't allow your toddler to swim if she has diarrhea. For example, the parasite *Cryptosporidium* can be released into the pool by children with leaky diapers. If other swimmers ingest it, they can get a potentially serious illness with diarrhea, vomiting, and dehydration.

If your toddler isn't yet potty trained, dress her in a well-fitting swim diaper.

◦◦

I grew up near the ocean, and I wanted my kids to enjoy the water too. When my kids were toddlers, we took swimming lessons at the

YMCA. Young children have a natural ability to learn to swim, and most toddlers don't yet fear the water. So I wanted my kids to learn to swim when they were very young.

—*Teresa Hubka, DO, a mom of a 14-year-old son and an 8-year-old daughter, an ob-gyn and the medical director of Comprehensive Wellness Care in Chicago, and an associate professor of obstetrics and gynecology and the chairman and residency program director of the department of obstetrics and gynecology at the Midwestern University/Chicago College of Osteopathic Medicine, in Downers Grove, Illinois*

When my kids were toddlers, I enrolled them in swimming lessons at a local swimming school called the Swim-In Zone. Still, when we were in the water, I abided by the arm's length rule: A parent is within arm's length of a child in the water at all times.

Mommy MD Guides-Recommended Product
Speedo Kid's UV Neoprene Swim Vest

The American Academy of Pediatrics recommends putting a life preserver or life jacket on your child anytime she's near a body of water, including lakes, rivers, and streams. Many states require the use of life jackets on boats. It's also good to know your toddler is supported as she's learning to swim in a pool. Life jackets should fit snugly, and remember it's still important to supervise your child even when she's wearing a life vest.

The Speedo Kid's UV Neoprene Swim Vest has full flotation support and is designed to be a good fit while giving your toddler plenty of room to maneuver her arms as she's learning to swim. It also has 50+ UV protection to block UVA and UVB rays. The swim vests come in pink or blue and cost about $20 to $27 each. The medium size fits kids ages two to four who are 33 to 45 pounds, while the large size fits kids ages four to six who are 45 to 60 pounds. You can buy them at **SpeedoUSA.com** and **Amazon.com**.

When to Call Your Doctor

It might be called swimmer's ear, but an infection of the ear canal can happen even if your child hasn't stepped into a pool in months. Any time the skin in the ear canal breaks—from a lot of moisture in the ear, dry skin or eczema, using cotton swabs to clean the ear, or scratching the ear with fingers or foreign objects—it can lead to an infection from bacteria or fungi.

When it happens, it's important to get treatment for your child to prevent the infection from spreading. Call your doctor right away if your child has ear pain with or without a fever, has trouble hearing in one or both ears, or if you see a discharge coming from your child's ear.

Also, we never used inflatable flotation devices. They can get holes in them and lose air. Plus, even if a child has those inflatable devices around her arms, her face can still fall into the water. Instead, I put actual boating life vests on my kids.

—*Eva Mayer, MD, a mom of an eight-year-old daughter and a six-year-old son and a pediatrician with St. Luke's Pediatrics Associates, in Bethlehem, PA*

One of my greatest fears when my children were toddlers was drowning. Studies have shown that swimming lessons don't decrease the likelihood of drowning, especially in families with swimming pools. It is recommended to have a fence around the pool as well as someone watching children when they're in the water.

My children took swimming lessons, but like any skill, if you don't practice it, you lose it. Experts recommend maintaining a routine of practicing swimming to benefit from the lessons taken, and the kids will be thrilled and feel rewarded once they master their new skills.

—*Aline T. Tanios, MD, a mom of nine- and three-year-old daughters and a seven-year-old son and a pediatric hospitalist at Arkansas Children's Hospital, in Little Rock*

My husband really likes swimming, and he signed our daughters up for swimming lessons. It's important for kids to learn how to swim, especially if you live in an area where there are a lot of backyard pools. More children die of drowning in backyard pools than from handguns at home.

A friend of mine put her child in one of those classes where they learn to swim in a week. Apparently, there's a lot of crying involved. That didn't seem necessary to me.

—*Kate Tulenko, MD, MPH*

When my younger daughter was 18 months old and my older daughter was 5½, I took them to a fabulous swimming instructor. Shortly after we arrived, the instructor sent me into her house.

"I've got this," she said.

I have no idea how she did it, but a half hour later, the instructor had both girls in the pool swimming. Early education on pool safety is vital, especially when you live in an area with lots of swimming pools. My older daughter was delayed in learning due to her physical disability. This instructor worked miracles, and my daughters didn't have the harsh experience of being thrown into the pool.

—*Eva Ritvo, MD*

I really can't stress enough how critical it is to keep your eyes—even your hands—on your toddler in the water. Once, my husband and I were in a pool with our older daughter. She was standing between us, and still she slipped under the water. We were talking, and it took us a few seconds to realize what had happened. After that, my husband and I had an agreement that anytime the kids were in the water, one of us was the designated child watcher.

We have a pool, and on occasion we had pool parties. I always hired a lifeguard. Too often at parties, all of the parents think someone else is watching the kids, and in fact no one is.

—*Susan Wilder, MD, a mom of a 17-year-old daughter and twin 13-year-old girls, a primary care physician, and the founder and CEO of Lifescape Medical Associates, in Scottsdale, AZ*

You really have to up the babyproofing ante with toddlers. We live in Arizona, and so the pool was a big deal. A key to babyproofing with toddlers, who are so clever they can often get around babyproofing devices, is to have several layers of defense. For our pool, for example, we had a fence around the pool, but we also had alarms on all doors and windows, so that a bell chimed if someone opened a window or a door.

We also had a firm rule: For our three children to be in the pool, there had to be at least one adult present for every child under age five. So when my husband was on call and I was alone with my kids, we didn't swim.

Instead, we played a lot in the bathtub! I probably should have bought stock in Mr. Bubble. When my husband was at work, I'd feed my kids dinner, and then we'd go up and take a long bath. It was something my kids enjoyed, and it kept them busy. My kids were happy because even though they weren't in the pool, they still got to play in the water.

—*Lisa Dado, MD*

Toddlers are very susceptible to mollescum, a skin condition that causes wartlike bumps. Mollescum is contagious, and you can catch it by sharing towels and even kickboards.

Pediatricians generally take a wait-and-see approach toward mollescum. But if the condition doesn't go away on its own, a dermatologist can prescribe a treatment.

Also, after your toddler swims, wash her well to remove chlorine from her skin and hair. Chlorine can be very drying.

—*Amy J. Derick, MD*

Keeping Your Toddler and Pets Safe and Happy

Was your dog or cat your baby before your baby was born? No doubt you've worked hard to help everyone to get along. Or maybe you've recently added a new pet to your family, you brave soul!

Here are some ways to keep your toddler and your pets safe and happy.

- Never leave your toddler and a pet together unattended.
- Install a sturdy gate to keep your pet out of the nursery when unsupervised.
- Keep your pet up to date on vaccinations and checked for parasites.
- Provide a comfortable, special area for your pet inside your home, such as a dog crate or a cat bed.
- Move your pet's food and water bowls to a location out of your toddler's reach. The food is a choking hazard, the water is a drowning hazard, and both are unsanitary for your toddler to be playing in.
- Be sure to keep any pet medications, brushes, and leashes away from your toddler.
- Keep your toddler's and pet's toys separate. Don't give your pet plush toys or rattles, or she might be more likely to mistake your toddler's toys for her own.
- If you haven't done so already, consider having your pet spayed or neutered, which might decrease aggression.
- If your dog or cat will tolerate it, encourage your toddler to gently pet your dog or cat by stroking the pet's back and sides but not reaching toward or over her head. Don't allow your toddler to pull at your pet's fur or poke her eyes, or disturb your pet when she is eating, drinking, or sleeping.
- Because your toddler will be touching your pet, keep your dog or cat as clean as possible.
- If your toddler upsets your pet, move your pet to her safe retreat place, such as her crate or bed.
- Keep your indoor pets indoors to minimize exposure to fleas and ticks.
- Don't let your dog or cat run loose in the woods during poison ivy season. It's possible to get a poison ivy rash from touching a pet that has brushed up against the leaves.
- Certainly, keep your toddler far away from the cat's litter box and the dog's poop!

- If there will be times you need to take both your toddler and your pet in the car, come up with a way to keep them separate, such as by confining the pet to a crate or carrier.
- Reward your pet's good behavior around your toddler with treats. And vice versa!

Pets truly can be part of the family. But not an inexpensive part! According to the American Pets Products Association, to own a dog costs about $559 a year, a cat $447, a rabbit $403, and a hamster $216!

But pets do offer many benefits. For one, a recent study found that people who own and walk dogs are 34 percent more likely to get at least 150 minutes of exercise per week, which is precisely the amount experts—and dogs—recommend.

⁓

We have two cats. My younger son doesn't have any chores or responsibilities for our pets yet, but he does know that he needs to be kind and gentle with them. I didn't have to do anything to teach my son that. The cats did! When my son is gentle with them, they will let him play with them and pet them. If he's rough, they run away and hide.

—*Rebecca Reamy, MD*

⁓

One of the first chores our sons had as toddlers was feeding the dog. They can't refill the dog's water bowl because they can't reach the sink. But they can scoop up dog food and put it in the dog's bowl.

I'm pretty sure that each of my sons sampled the dog's food, but they probably found it didn't taste too good. It's not harmful at all, though. It's probably healthier than some food at the grocery store that's marketed to kids!

—*Deborah Gilboa, MD*

⁓

When my daughter was two years old, we got her a Persian cat. She called him Mr. Kitty, and he was her pride and joy. My daughter played with the cat, brushed him, fed him, and helped me fill his water bowl.

She wasn't responsible for him, I was, but I made sure she understood that he was *her* cat.

I believe that my daughter learned a lot about caring for others by taking care of her cat. When other kids came over, my daughter protected her cat, making sure the kids didn't pull his tail. Later she went on to work at a Humane Society. Having that cat really made a difference in her life.

—*Debra Jaliman, MD, a mom of a 20-year-old daughter, a dermatologist in private practice, and an assistant professor of dermatology at Mt. Sinai School of Medicine, in New York City*

We didn't have any pets in our house due to allergies, but my older son loves animals of all sorts and would go up to them without hesitation. We taught him to treat animals with respect, to give them a chance to sniff him and get familiar with him, and to always ask the owner if it was okay to get near a pet. I also made sure my kids knew not to go anywhere with someone with a pet unless they had my permission first.

—*Leena Shrivastava Dev, MD*

RALLIE'S TIP

When my boys were little, they loved our dogs. Sometimes they almost loved them to death! By the time my kids were toddlers, I was more concerned that the boys would hurt the dogs, rather than the other way around. Whenever my kids got too rough with one of our dogs, such as hugging his neck so hard that the dog was in danger of suffocating, I would remind them to be gentle, and I would show them how to give a tender hug that was less like a chokehold.

I wasn't terribly worried that my dogs would bite my children, but I did keep a close eye on the kids and the dogs whenever they were together. I never, ever let my children go anywhere near the dogs when it was doggie dinnertime. I've seen too many kids in the emergency department with dog bites to the face and hands after they had interrupted the family pet while he was eating.

Having an easy-going, loving dog or cat in the family is generally good for kids and their parents. Studies show that children who grow up around pets are less likely to have allergies, and there's plenty of evidence that petting a dog is an excellent stress reliever and mood booster.

Involving children in the care of a pet helps to teach them a lot about responsibility and respect. I think my dogs have taught my children a lot of very important life lessons that they wouldn't have learned otherwise.

∽

One thing that parents with pets might not think about or plan for is what to do when a pet dies. Last fall, our dog Jake was diagnosed with osteosarcoma of the ankle. He was only nine years old. Our vet recommended no intervention because the cancer had likely already spread. It was devastating and heartbreaking. It was a daily struggle not knowing which day would be his last. Some days Jake looked like himself, happy, wagging his tail, and still begging for a walk, even though his body was failing so quickly.

My children adored our dog. Every morning, my daughter would wake up and say, "Jakey"—which was, in fact, her first word—and come downstairs to look for him. My kids always sat beside him, cuddled with him, watched TV with him, and even wanted him to ride in the car to pick up my son from school.

My husband and I didn't know how to approach our dog's illness and death with our children. We sought the advice of our vet and friends, and we searched for help online. Our vet recommended not telling the kids that our dog was sick too early. Many friends told me that I really had to keep it together because the kids would take from the experience what I did. I read on one website, "*Do not* tell your kids that your dog went to a farm." That seemed like a ludicrous thing to say to my kids anyway because there was nowhere else that Jake would have wanted to be than home with us.

My daughter, being a toddler, was a comfort for me to have around. Despite Jake's illness, she always treated him the same way, as if all was well, as if we weren't worried about him.

The night that we knew Jake had to be put down, I had my son sit in my lap. I told him that Jake was very sick. What happened next was unlike anything I had anticipated: My son started violently crying and begging me, "Please let him stay, Mom, please let him stay." It was horrible. If there was anything I could have done to keep that dog with us forever, I would have. He was such a gift to us.

That night after my husband and I got back from the vet, our house was silent. No one wanted to say anything.

"I miss Jake. When is he coming back?" my son asked.

In that moment, my husband and I decided that we could not have that conversation over and over, and we decided that we had to tell our children right away that he had died. I told my son a story about how Jake was walking across a rainbow bridge into Dog Heaven, and he would be watching over our family forever.

For days afterward, my son was concerned that Jake would forget about him. I had to tell him over and over that Jakey would never forget him. I told my son that I had made Jake a new collar with a picture of all of us on his tag to carry with him all the time. We made a Christmas ornament with a picture of Jake in it. We put his stocking up, and we made a photo book of him so that we can look at it. His framed photo is on the end table, and my daughter still points at it and says "Jakey" and then points at his "eyes," "nose," "ears," and "mouth" because he helped her learn those words too. My son's school librarian suggested some books to read. My son read one called *Dog Heaven* quietly and did not say a word about it. I am glad that he did, though, because it gave me a way to frame this sadness for him.

Losing a pet is really hard. I think knowing your belief system about what happens after death is a challenge for all adults. Knowing how to frame it for a child in a way that is palatable and not completely devastating is a serious challenge. Facing our dog's death was one of the hardest things that I've had to do as a mom.

Our family got a new puppy a week after Jake passed away. His name is "Chewy," aka Chewbacca. My children love him. My daughter feels utterly comfortable around him, despite his wild puppy antics. I credit Jake with teaching her to love animals this way at such a young age.

—*Sigrid Payne DaVeiga, MD, a mom of a six-year-old son and a two-year-old daughter and a pediatric allergist with the Children's Hospital of Philadelphia, in Pennsylvania*

Preventing and Treating Cuts and Scrapes and Bumps and Bruises

When you're a toddler, bumps and bruises and cuts and scrapes are a way of life. Luckily, when you're two feet tall, the ground isn't that far away, and most bumps and bruises and cuts and scrapes can be healed with a kiss. And a Hello Kitty or Spiderman Band-Aid.

Often when a child gets a minor bump or bruise, two simple strategies will get you through. First, remain calm. This will help your toddler remain calm too. Second, come up with a distraction. When my kids were toddlers, I would grab an ice pack or a Popsicle to put on the injury. They put the wrapped Popsicle on their skin, and then once they felt better, they ate the Popsicle.

—*Amy Baxter, MD, a mom of 14- and 12-year-old sons and a 9-year-old daughter; the CEO of Buzzy4Shots.com; and the director of emergency research, Scottish Rite, of the Children's Healthcare of Atlanta, in Georgia*

I always keep a few washcloths on hand that are a dark color, such as maroon or navy. When a child is bleeding, using this washcloth will help to camouflage the blood and assuage their fears.

When my kids were toddlers, I explained to them that bleeding is how our bodies clean out wounds. It helps remove the dirt and germs from our cuts. Then I explained that the scab is your own natural bandage.

—*Jennifer Hanes, DO*

When my boys get cuts, I clean them well with soap and water. Then I apply a wound healing prescription gel called Biafine. I put Band-Aids on cuts to keep the gel close to the skin. Most clean wounds don't need to be treated with antibiotics.

I don't use antibiotic creams such as Neosporin because there's a risk of an allergic reaction.

—*Amy J. Derick, MD*

Band-Aids

"With six kids, we've had plenty of bumps and bruises," says Susan Besser, MD, a mom of six grown children, ages 27, 25, 23, 21, 20, and 18, a grandmom of two, a family physician, and the medical director of Doctors Express-Memphis, in Tennessee. "When my toddlers fell, I was careful how I reacted. If I panicked and made a big deal out of it, they would too. But on the other hand, if I was calm, they'd likely stay calm too. If you look at your toddler and say, 'Oopsie!' he will likely look at you like you've lost your mind and go right back to playing. For toddlers' cuts and scrapes that break the skin, I find Band-Aids are a mom's best friend.

"Of course, if your toddler falls and there's a stunned silence followed by that long inhale and then the piercing scream, then you do what you have to do to make it all better."

You can buy Band-Aids at variety stores for around $3 a box. Visit **BAND-AID.COM** for more information.

RALLIE'S TIP

Toddlers get more than their share of bumps and bruises. Generally kids will continue on without the need for any pain medication. I think it's fine to use ibuprofen (Motrin) or acetaminophen (Tylenol) when it's really necessary. The use of all drugs, including over-the-counter medications, carries a small but very real risk, and moms and dads must weigh the risks and benefits of using these drugs before giving them to their children.

But which medication should you choose? While both acetaminophen and ibuprofen can alleviate aches and pains effectively, ibuprofen has the added benefit of reducing inflammation in body tissues, which might make it a better choice for conditions that involve swelling, such as a really painful bruise or a bump. Because ibuprofen is administered every six to eight hours, compared to every four to six hours with acetaminophen, it might be a better choice to use at bedtime.

While most parents don't want to see their children suffer in any way, it's important to remember that aches and pains can play important roles in healing. In some cases, experiencing a bit of discomfort informs us and reminds us that our bodies are in need of rest and healing. If you've strained a muscle, the discomfort will remind you to rest the muscle and avoid overexerting it so that it can properly heal. Children experiencing pain from a serious bruise or a strain might not need to run and play as much as usual; they might need to rest more so that their bodies can heal.

I generally didn't get too excited about the bumps and bruises my toddlers sustained, as long as their heads weren't involved. When my middle son was two, he fell and hit his head really hard on our hardwood floor. Within minutes, he had developed an impressive goose egg on his forehead, and although he wasn't showing any signs of a serious head injury, I was fully prepared to bundle him up and take him to the emergency department for further evaluation. My husband, an emer-

When to Call Your Doctor

A kid on the move means more falls, and that sometimes leads to cuts, scrapes, bumps, and bruises.

A cut needs stitches and requires a trip to the doctor if it's gaping or split open, if it's on the body and longer than half an inch, or if it's on the face and longer than a quarter of an inch. Call your doctor if a wound looks infected: red, tender, and producing pus.

An injury needs immediate medical attention if a puncture wound or serious cut is sustained, if the cut is deep enough that you can see bone or tendons, or if there's skin loss greater than 10 percent (a child's palm represents 1 percent of his body). Immediate medical attention is also required if you can't stop the bleeding after applying direct pressure for 10 minutes, or if you aren't able to clean dirt from the wound.

Also alert your doctor if a cut, scrape, bump, or bruise doesn't heal within 10 days or if it looks as if it's getting worse in any way.

If an injury results in major bleeding that can't be stopped, call 911 right away.

gency physician, examined our son thoroughly and told me that he wouldn't recommend doing a CT scan. Instead, we just watched our son very closely for the next two days, looking for any changes in his behavior. We didn't give him any type of pain-relieving medicine, because if he was experiencing any significant pain, we wanted to know about it. (Give Tylenol—not Motrin—for head bumps, though, to reduce the risk of bleeding in the brain.) After my son's initial pain of whacking his head had subsided, he completely forgot about his injury, even though he had a big shiner on his forehead.

❧

My kids have had plenty of bumps and bruises, and my younger son also had a really bad fall. He's a climber, and one day he climbed up onto the back of one of our living room chairs. He lost his balance, and he fell to the floor, landing directly on the top of his head. I was concerned about his head, and I was even more concerned about his neck.

I raced over to my son. He let out a cry, and I could see him moving his arms and legs—both good signs. He was really dazed, though, so my husband and I agreed that we should take him to the hospital to get checked out. My son didn't fight my husband at all as he got him into his car seat, which is unusual, so that concerned me. It was very scary.

I took my son to the emergency department where I work, and he was evaluated by one of my colleagues. As so often happens when I am at work with my patients, by the time we got to the hospital and were seen 45 minutes after my son's fall, he was acting perfectly fine. This was very encouraging.

My colleague and I discussed whether or not my son should have an X-ray or CT scan. One problem with X-rays and CT scans is that an active child like my son would need to be sedated, which brings with it a whole new set of risks. Also, studies have shown that X-rays and CT scans can increase a child's risk of cancer, which to me far outweighed the concerns I had over my son's head at that point. We opted not to do the X-ray or CT scan, and my son was fine.

—*Rebecca Reamy, MD*

Chapter 9
Preventing and Treating Common Conditions

Your Toddler's Development
During your child's toddlerhood, it's pretty inevitable that he'll get his fair share—or more—of colds, ear infections, and stomach bugs. A toddler's immune system is still developing, and toddlers tend to play in close proximity to other toddlers. They also put toys and their fingers into their mouths, spreading germs all along the way.

How common is the common cold in children? Toddlers catch an average of seven colds a year.

Better stock up on OJ and chicken soup!

Along the same lines, earaches are terribly common in toddlers. Most children will have at least one ear infection by their third birthday. Some children will have many more.

Even less fun, the Centers for Disease Control and Prevention estimates that each year 1 out of every 15 Americans gets norovirus, a stomach bug.

Taking Care of You
Should your toddler share his germs with you, and you come down with his cold or stomach bug, make sure to treat yourself with the same kindness you'd treat anyone else in your family who was sick. You deserve some TLC too!

Justification for a Celebration
The end of cold-and-flu season should be a national holiday!

Preventing and Treating Earaches

What causes pesky, painful earaches? A structure called the Eustachian tube connects the middle ear with the back of the nose. When all is well, this tube lets fluid drain out of the middle ear. When bacteria or viruses infect the lining of the tube, the tube gets swollen and fills with mucus. This prevents the ear from draining properly. Then bacteria can grow in the pooled fluid, increasing pressure behind the eardrum and causing pain.

Acute ear infections usually clear up in a week or two. But sometimes ear infections linger longer and become chronic. In any event, you'll want to help heal your toddler as soon as possible.

The one time my daughter had an ear infection, I put a few drops of olive oil in her ear with an eye dropper. It helps with the pain by helping to balance out the pressure difference between the inner and outer ear. Of course, you don't want to do this if your child has tubes in his ears, if the eardrum is ruptured, or if you see any fluid coming out of your toddler's ear. In Europe, they very rarely prescribe antibiotics for ear infections. They just treat the symptoms of fever and pain.

—Kate Tulenko, MD, MPH, *a mom of four- and one-year-old girls, the author of* Insourced: How Importing Jobs Impacts the Healthcare Crisis Here and Abroad, *and a pediatrician and global health specialist with IntraHealth, in Washington, DC*

I try to avoid giving my kids antibiotics as much as possible. For ear infections, doctors often prescribe antibiotics not for the ear infection but to prevent meningitis, which is a far more serious illness. Thankfully, we now have a vaccine to protect against meningitis, so the need to take antibiotics for ear infections isn't so great anymore. This is especially true once children reach the age of two years.

—Jennifer Hanes, DO, *a mom of a six-year-old daughter and a three-year-old son, an emergency physician, a certified forensic physician, and the founder of Empowered Medicine, PLLC, in Austin, TX*

When to Call Your Doctor

Your child will likely experience the most earaches due to ear infections between six months and two years old. Keep in mind that ear infections tend to crop up on the third day of a cold.

Because it's difficult to know when your child's ears hurt before he's old enough to tell you, pay attention to the way your child acts when you know he has an earache. When the same patterns reappear in the future when he has a cold, make a doctor's appointment.

In the meantime, call your doctor right away—night or day—if your child has the following symptoms.

- Your child appears to be very sick or the earache is severe.
- An earache doesn't go away two hours after your child takes ibuprofen (Motrin).
- There's pink or red swelling on the skin behind your child's ear.
- Your child's neck is so stiff he can't touch his chin to his chest.
- A sharp object such as a pencil or stick was inserted into the ear canal.
- Your child has an earache and has a condition that causes a weakened immune system, such as sickle cell disease or HIV, or your child is on chemotherapy, chronic steroids, or has had an organ transplant.
- Your child's fever is higher than 103°F two hours after treating him for a fever.

If your child has an earache or there's pus draining from the ear without the symptoms listed above, call your doctor during normal business hours.

When my daughter used to pull on her ears, I'd look into her ears with an otoscope. You can buy otoscopes for home use pretty inexpensively.

I generally wouldn't recommend them for moms, but if a child gets a lot of ear infections, it might not be a bad idea to get one. Take it to your pediatrician and ask her to show you how to use it properly and what to look for.

—*Lisa Campanella-Coppo, MD, a mom of a three-year-old daughter, an emergency physician, and the emergency department director of academic affairs at Monmouth Medical Center, in New Jersey*

When my son was two years old, he started on the not-very-merry-go-round of recurrent ear infections. No sooner did we clear up one infection than he was coming down with the next.

My son's pediatrician wanted to have tubes put into his ears. Instead I gave my son a safe children's nighttime decongestant each night for two months. The goal was to dry out the Eustachian tubes. When those tiny tubes become clogged, fluid in the middle ear starts to build up, and that can lead to ear infections. The decongestant worked, and my son never had ear infections again. (Talk with your toddler's doctor before giving your toddler this or any medication.)

—*Dana S. Simpler, MD, a mom of 25- and 20-year-old girls and a 23-year-old son and a specialist in internal medicine in private practice, in Baltimore, MD*

My youngest kids had more ear infections than my other children. Both of them ended up having to have tubes put in, one at age one and the other at age two. That was my first surgical experience with my kids. Even though I'm a doctor, I'm their mother, and so I was as upset about it as any other mommy would be. But after they got the tubes, they didn't have any more significant ear infections.

—*Susan Besser, MD, a mom of six grown children, ages 27, 25, 23, 21, 20, and 18, a grandmom of two, a family physician, and the medical director of Doctors Express-Memphis, in Tennessee*

My son had nine ear infections in his first year of his life. We made many trips to the emergency room, and then to the pharmacy for antibiotics, in the middle of the night.

My son's pediatrician recommended we have tubes put in his ears. This is a surgical procedure, and I was reluctant. If a child has three or four ear infections in four months, or five in 12 months, though, that's too many.

On the way home from the surgery, my son said, "Mommy, that doctor made my ears too loud!" He hadn't been hearing well because of all of the fluid in his ears. At that moment, I knew that we had made the right decision. After my son had the tubes put in, he was like a new boy.

—*Eva Mayer, MD, a mom of an eight-year-old daughter and a six-year-old son and a pediatrician with St. Luke's Pediatrics Associates, in Bethlehem, PA*

My older daughter had chronic ear infections. When she was 14 months old, we had tubes put in her ears. My husband was very reluctant to have it done because it requires invasive surgery, but it was the best thing we ever did for her.

She did still get ear infections, but not the chronic pain. And she was still congested all of the time. I talked with her doctor, who did X-rays. We found out later that she also had infected adenoids. They were removed, and the surgeon said they were the largest adenoids that she had ever removed from a person! She called them "human sushi."

—*Kristie McNealy, MD, a mom of nine- and six-year-old daughters and four-year-old and 22-month-old sons and a blogger at KristieMcNealy.com, in Denver, CO*

Preventing and Treating Colds

Experts say that 80 percent of infectious diseases are spread through touch. Short of carrying a sign that says "Stop touching me!" the best thing to do is to wash your hands frequently, and encourage your toddler to do the same. It's a great idea to get into routines, such as washing your hands right when you get home, or rinsing with antibacterial sanitizer when you get into your car. Wash for at least 20 seconds, and then dry your hands thoroughly so germs don't stick to your wet hands like glue.

Even toddlers are capable of washing their hands, with supervision. But how about blowing their noses? Most kids can't master that skill until about kindergarten. But don't let that keep you from chasing after your toddler with a tissue!

Could your child's "cold" really be the flu? If your child has two or more of the following symptoms, it might be. Place a call to your child's doctor right away.

- Fever
- Aches
- Chills
- Tiredness
- Sudden onset of symptoms

If, despite your best efforts, your child gets a cold, just gut it out. The average cold lasts 7 to 10 days. Hopefully, he doesn't share it with you!

⁓

The key to preventing sore throats, and also colds, is hand washing. Covering a cough and sneezing into your arm or elbow rather than your hands help also.

—Marra S. Francis, MD, a mom of eight-, seven-, and five-year-old daughters and a gynecologist, in San Antonio, TX

⁓

I keep colds away by taking probiotics and giving them to my daughters. A really good study found that taking probiotics daily during winter can cut the number of colds in half.

I buy a probiotics powder, and I stir the recommended dose into my girls' milk each day. Any brand seems to be fine. Since I started doing this, we've really noticed a decrease in the number of colds we catch. But you have to be consistent and take it every day.

—Kate Tulenko, MD, MPH

⁓

When my boys were toddlers, I gave them vitamin C and probiotics supplements to boost their immunity and to ward off colds.

I also fed my boys the most wholesome and nutritious foods I could buy, including plenty of fresh fruits and vegetables. It's sad that our food today is not as nourishing as it used to be. Plus, we're inundated with far more toxins, and our bodies aren't sure how to deal with them. Because of this, we need to try to eat the freshest, least processed foods that we can.

—*Cathie Lippman, MD, a mom of 31- and 29-year-old sons and a physician who specializes in environmental and preventive medicine at the Lippman Center for Optimal Health, in Beverly Hills, CA*

∽◦

My two older sons share a bedroom. When one of my sons gets a cold and the weather outside is mild, sometimes I crack open the window in his bedroom to make the room a bit cooler and more comfortable for him to sleep and breathe. Then I snuggle the sick child under his covers. I take my other son into another room to sleep. The goal is for everyone to get as much sleep as possible.

—*Amy Thompson, MD, a mom of five- and three- and two-year-old sons and an ob-gyn at the University of Cincinnati College of Medicine, in Ohio*

∽◦

With multiple kids, colds spread like the plague. What should last three to five days with one kid can last a month with three kids. When one of my kids gets sick, I take them all to the doctor, trying to nip it in the bud.

Sadly, as a working physician who's never expected to get sick and cancel appointments with patients, having a sick kid at home is tough. For me, prevention is key. We wash our hands often, eat well especially in winter, and avoid other runny-nosed kids.

When all else fails and my toddlers have colds, I put saline spray in their noses to ease the congestion. The problem is, they don't really want you to do that. Once they're able to spray it themselves, it gets much easier.

—*Brooke A. Jackson, MD, a mom of 4½-year-old twin girls and a 2½-year-old son, a dermatologist, and the founder and medical director of the Skin Wellness Center of Chicago, in Illinois*

When children are older than one year old, honey is a great treatment for coughs. It's been shown to be more effective than the over-the-counter cough syrups. When you give your child honey, you don't have to worry about medication interactions or the time since the last dose.

My children love taking a teaspoon of honey for a scratchy throat or to help quiet a cough.

—*Jennifer Hanes, DO*

When to Call Your Doctor

Colds are caused by viruses and need to run their course, so the best treatment is often just to wait it out.

However, colds can lead to other illnesses that require antibiotics, so it's best to call the doctor if your child has any of the following symptoms.

- A fever of 103°F or higher or a fever of 101°F that continues longer than a day
- A cough with an abundance of mucus
- Shortness of breath
- Feeling tired or lethargic
- Unable to keep food down or isn't drinking enough liquids
- A headache that gets worse or the aching spreads to the face or throat
- Drooling or problems swallowing
- Chest pain or stomach pain
- Swollen glands in the neck
- An earache

The following situations also warrant a call to the pediatrician.

- Your child's symptoms get worse after three days.
- The symptoms last longer than a week and happen every year at the same time, which might suggest seasonal allergies.
- Your toddler is wheezing, which could mean she has asthma.

When my children have a very bad cold and can't sleep, I have to admit I sometimes give them an age- and weight-appropriate dose of Benadryl (diphenhydramine). I never gave them cold medicine because that isn't recommended for toddlers and young children.

Benadryl is a single-ingredient medication, and theoretically it helps to ease their congestion. Talk with your pediatrician about the right dose.

—*Eva Mayer, MD*

Other than the occasional cold, my son was healthy during his toddler years. Saline washes helped the most with the nasal congestion. I use

Mommy MD Guides-Recommended Product
Boogie Wipes

"One product that I think is a must-have for moms is Boogie Wipes," says Tanya Douglas Holland, MD, a mom of a two-year-old daughter, a women's health advocate, and a consultant in medical affairs to a pharmaceutical company, in Atlanta, GA.

"Especially in winter, kids pick up viruses, and wiping their little noses with tissues can really dry their skin. Boogie Wipes contain saline, which helps to protect the mucous membranes. Plus, the wipes smell good, which makes it easier to wipe my daughter's nose."

Parents might spend more time wiping their toddlers' noses than doing just about anything else during cold season. While a plain tissue is often greeted with a grimace, your little ones might not run away when you come at them with a Boogie Wipe, saline wipes that are very gentle, help to dissolve mucus, and come in a kid-friendly grape scent, fresh scent, menthol scent, or unscented.

They're available at Target, Toys R Us, Walgreens, and Walmart, or you can buy them at **BOOGIEWIPES.COM**. A pack of 30 wipes costs $3.79.

a commercial preparation for my nasal washes. It has a nozzle with a button for easy application. I use it about twice daily with my sons when they have colds and congestion.

—*Bola Oyeyipo-Ajumobi, MD, a mom of four- and one-year-old sons, a family physician in private practice, and the owner of SlimyBookWorm.com, in Highland, CA*

My older son has a cold right now! To ease his congestion, I run a humidifier in his room at night. It's very important to increase the humidity in the air. I also spray saline up his nose, and then I use a nasal aspirator to suction out the mucus from his nose.

When my son has a cold, I put Little Cold's Baby Rub by Little Remedies on his chest. I don't use Vicks VapoRub, which is made for adults. I'm not sure how much the baby rub helps ease congestion, but it does seem to have soothing properties.

Most of all, when my sons have colds, I give them extra hugs.

—*Deborah Kulick, MD, a mom of two-year-old and eight-month-old sons, a child and adolescent psychiatrist at the Everett Teen Health Center, and an instructor in psychiatry at Harvard Medical School and the Cambridge Health Alliance, in Boston, MA*

Toddlers are very resilient, and sometimes they can be quite sick and not really behave like there's anything wrong. It's important to keep a close eye on toddlers and watch for clues that something might not be right.

When my daughter was a toddler, she had a cold that progressed to a sinus infection, and she had a high fever. I took her to the hospital, and she was admitted. Even being that sick and needing an IV, my daughter was still joking and playing around. Thank goodness, she got better quickly, and all was fine. The lesson is to keep a close eye on toddlers and watch for clues that they might be sicker than they appear to be.

—*Dina Strachan, MD, a mom of a six-year-old daughter, a dermatologist and director of Aglow Dermatology, and an assistant clinical professor in the department of dermatology at New York University, in New York City*

When my younger kids were toddlers, my older ones were in school, and they were always bringing home colds to share with the rest of us. I didn't do much at all to treat their colds, other than chase them around with tissues. Those were the days before cushy, soft Kleenex, and my kids hated those scratchy tissues. So mostly I just let them be. As long as my kids were playing and seemed happy despite their colds, I didn't worry about it.

I really think it's important for moms to realize that kids don't need all those cold and flu medicines. Most of the time, you're just treating yourself so you'll feel better, not the kids. (Kids really don't care that much. They just play on.) Also those medicines are not harmless. Studies show that lots of babies are treated in emergency departments for overdosing on common over-the-counter cold medicines.

—*Susan Besser, MD*

RALLIE'S TIP

I always encourage parents to remember that the signs and symptoms of the common cold are caused by the body's immune system, rather than by the virus that is responsible for the cold. The immune system triggers fever, cough, and runny nose to help fight the infection and heal the body. When we give children over-the-counter cold medications to suppress a cough, reduce a fever, or "dry up" a runny nose, we're actually impeding and interfering with the immune system's ability to overcome the infection and heal the body. In the long run, we might end up prolonging the infection and delaying healing by giving over-the-counter cold medications.

Coughing, for example, is a natural, helpful reaction designed to clear the lungs and airways of disease-causing organisms, mucus, and debris. When we completely suppress coughing in children suffering from colds, we're actually encouraging mucus to accumulate in the lungs and other parts of the respiratory tract. Ultimately, this could result in a worsening of the child's condition and might even lead to pneumonia. It's generally acceptable to suppress a dry, hacking cough that keeps a child awake at night, but loose coughs that result in the expulsion of mucus from the lungs are beneficial and generally don't need to be suppressed.

Likewise, fever can help the body heal. An elevated body temperature helps "pasteurize" the blood, killing invading germs or at least creating an inhospitable environment for them so that they're not able to reproduce.

My mother grew up in Scotland, and she's made all of her children firm believers in the medicinal powers of tea. When my sons started coming down with colds, they knew it was time for tea.

Warm tea is particularly beneficial for children and adults suffering from the common cold because of its antibacterial and antiviral properties. Tea has been shown to enhance the protective powers of the immune system by increasing the body's production of interferon, a substance known to play a key role in protecting the body against infection.

When researchers at Harvard Medical Center asked subjects to drink five cups of black tea each day for four weeks, they found that the volunteers' blood cells contained five times more interferon than before they began drinking tea. The scientists attributed the immune-boosting property to a natural chemical called L-theanine, which is found in green, black, and oolong tea. The researchers expressed their hope that eventually, L-theanine will be used in drugs that bolster the body's defenses against a number of illnesses and infections.

Adding a spoonful of honey to tea improves the taste, and it also boosts the healing properties. Honey has been shown to have wonderful anti-inflammatory and antimicrobial properties, and it's a good source of energy for a healing body. Honey should never be given to infants younger than one year, but it's fine for toddlers.

Preventing and Treating Allergies

If you or your toddler's father has allergies, it doesn't mean he is doomed to getting them too. But it does make it more likely.

Millions of kids have allergies. An allergy is an overreaction of the immune system to a substance that's harmless to most people. It's an immune system gone amok. People can be allergic to just about anything, but the most common nonfood allergens are dust mites, pollen, mold, pet dander, cockroaches, medicines, insect venom, and chemicals. Signs and symptoms of allergies include sneezing, stuffy nose, wheezing, coughing, and itchy eyes, nose, or throat.

❧

When a child has a cold or allergies that are associated with a lot of mucus, I'd stop giving them cow's milk to drink. Cow's milk increases mucus production, worsening a child's congestion.
　—Dana S. Simpler, MD

❧

When my younger son was a toddler, he had severe allergies, and he kept getting croup and conjunctivitis. He seemed to be allergic to everything. I ripped all of the wall-to-wall carpeting out of my home. My son's allergies diminished to almost nothing, and he never got conjunctivitis again.
　—-Cathie Lippman, MD

❧

I've been fortunate that my children haven't gotten any overwhelming infections, and I believe this is mainly due to the vaccines they've received following the Centers for Disease Control's guidelines. They did have seasonal allergies, though. When their allergies were flaring up, I gave them an age- and weight-appropriate dose of Children's Benadryl. (Talk with your toddler's doctor before giving your toddler this or any medication.)
　—Aline T. Tanios, MD, a mom of nine- and three-year-old daughters and a seven-year-old son and a pediatric hospitalist at Arkansas Children's Hospital, in Little Rock

❧

Kids have so many runny noses and colds that sometimes it can be hard to distinguish if nasal symptoms are from colds or allergies. Children usually don't develop allergies to seasonal pollens until after the age of two or three years, but many children can have allergies to pet dander and dust mites from an even younger age.
　Signs and symptoms to look out for are itchy eyes and nose, watery eyes, and runny nose. If your child has a lot of ear infections,

it's a good idea to have him checked for nasal allergies. This will help you prevent repeat ear infections. An allergist can provide simple skin testing to tell you whether or not your child has allergies.

—Sigrid Payne DaVeiga, MD, a mom of a six-year-old son and a two-year-old daughter and a pediatric allergist with the Children's Hospital of Philadelphia, in Pennsylvania

My kids had seasonal allergies. I addressed the problem by cleaning up their environment. I removed as many carpets as possible in our home and replaced them with washable floors. I removed as many fabric curtains as reasonable and replaced them with washable blinds. I covered the mattresses and pillowcases with allergy covers. I kept pets out of the bedrooms. (No exceptions!) I also kept the furnace filters clean.

Then we cleaned up our diet. I bought organic foods, avoided

Mommy MD Guides-Recommended Product
Dr. Hana's Nasopure 2 Squirts

The Nasopure nasal wash system gently cleans the inside of the nose. It doesn't flood the sinuses, but the patented design encourages the sinuses to drain naturally. Hana R. Solomon, MD, a mom who raised four children, a grandmom of three, a board-certified pediatrician, the president of BeWell Health, LLC, and the author of *Clearing the Air One Nose at a Time: Caring for Your Personal Filter*, in Columbia, MO, developed a special bottle that makes it easy for kids and adults to wash the nose comfortably. She even has advice on her website for encouraging your toddlers to start using the system on their own.

You can get everything you need for two children or for your child and you in Dr. Hana's Nasopure 2 Squirts kit. It includes two four-ounce bottles (BPA free), 10 buffered salt packets, instructions, and a reusable tote bag for $20. You can buy the kit at NASOPURE.COM or at health food stores.

processed artificial foods, and tried to rotate foods. Back then not many people believed that there was a relationship between foods and allergies and asthma, but now it is proven. Allergies to fish, nuts, milk, pork, and other foods are well known.

In addition to cleaning our home environment and cleaning up our diet, I also would wash my children's noses. I understood that allergy and asthma episodes always began with a snotty nose, so washing it made sense. Now we know that rinsing with the correct solution will remove 80 percent of the allergens! Cleaning the environment and the diet and the nose helps decrease the toxic load on the body.

—*Hana R. Solomon, MD, a mom who raised four children, a grandmom of three, a board-certified pediatrician, the president of BeWell Health, LLC, and the author of* Clearing the Air One Nose at a Time: Caring for Your Personal Filter, *in Columbia, MO*

My youngest child had allergies and asthma and was admitted to the hospital with pneumonia each year of his life until age five. It was a scary time. I could manage him at home to a point, and then he would need to be admitted to the hospital to be treated for dehydration or to receive steroids.

It was really important to me to find out what my child was allergic to and then avoid that trigger as much as possible. As he grew older, his allergies did improve, and he got fewer infections. I would say that many children have reactions to foods, pets, and chemicals in our environment, and we don't even know what they are! If you know a good allergist, that is a blessing. When a child with allergies is exposed to viruses on top of the allergies, the child can quickly develop a serious illness.

I tried to make sure all my kids were sleeping well, were eating a well-balanced diet, and had a minimum of stress. I acted quickly when I noticed they were congested from a cold to help prevent complications. We had a steam shower, and I would put the kids in swimsuits so we could sit together in the steam room. I would try to rinse their noses with saline, but that was more challenging.

—Laura M. Rosch, DO, a mom of a 12-year-old daughter and 7-year-old boy-girl twins, a board-certified internist who works at Central DuPage Hospital Convenient Care Centers in Winfield, IL, and an instructor in the department of family medicine at the Midwestern University/Chicago College of Osteopathic Medicine, in Downers Grove, IL

Preventing and Treating Sore Throats

Far too often, the first sign of a cold is a scratchy, painful throat. One of the best ways to prevent a sore throat is to prevent a cold. And we all know how that works out. Fortunately, there are a number of ways to ease a sore throat.

૭⁄○

It can be difficult to know if a toddler has a sore throat. They don't always understand the concept of "throat." Sometimes a child will say his neck hurts or point into his mouth. Those are signs I watch my daughter for when she's sick.

—Jennifer Bacani McKenney, MD, a mom of a one-year-old daughter and a family physician, in Fredonia, KS

૭⁄○

Sore throats are tricky in toddlers because until they can speak better, they can't tell you that their throats hurt.

One thing to watch out for is if your toddler is drooling a lot more than usual. This could be a sign of a sore throat, but I've found it more often to be a sign of a condition called hand, foot, and mouth disease, caused by the Coxsackie virus. It causes painful ulcers in the back of a child's mouth.

For either a sore throat or an infection with the Coxsackie virus, I'd give my sons Popsicles to eat and cold water to drink. Otherwise, all they need is time. Antibiotics won't treat these viruses, and they just have to run their course. The exception is strep, of course, but that's less common in this age group.

—Leena Shrivastava Dev, MD, a mom of 15- and 11-year-old sons, a general pediatrician, and an advocate for child safety, in Philadelphia, PA

Your child will need an antibiotic if strep throat is causing his sore throat, so it's important to go to the pediatrician and have his throat swabbed and tested if he has any of the following symptoms, which tend to come on suddenly.

- A fever that climbs to its highest on the second day
- A sore, red throat that might have white spots
- Headache, nausea, chills, or an overall feeling of sickness
- A loss of appetite or if your child says food tastes funny
- Swollen glands in the neck
- Trouble swallowing
- A rash

Also take your child to the doctor if he's already being treated for strep throat but isn't feeling better after 48 hours.

When my sons had sore throats, I would give them a homeopathic remedy, such as Sambucus or some form of elderberry or Oscillococcinum, whichever I had on hand at the time. Homeopathic remedies are gentle, safe, very diluted substances that you can buy over the counter at health food stores and online. I also gave them more vitamin C.

—*Cathie Lippman, MD*

There's really not much to do to prevent sore throats. If kids go to day care, they're going to get colds and sore throats.

When my kids have sore throats, I try to ease their symptoms. Back home in Pakistan, we avoid cool foods and beverages when we have sore throats or colds. So we don't eat ice cream or drink ice water. We also avoid sour foods and beverages such as fruit and juices. Instead, to soothe a cold or sore throat, we give warm foods and beverages, such as hot tea or room temperature water.

When a child has a sore throat, it's important to keep him hydrated. Try to give him food to keep his energy up, but not so much that he vomits or gets diarrhea.

I also treat my toddlers' sore throats with over-the-counter pain medication such as acetaminophen (Tylenol) or ibuprofen (Motrin), as recommended for age and weight. When you have sick kids, you can never have too much help. (Talk with your toddler's doctor before giving your toddler this or any medication.)

—*Sadaf T. Bhutta, MD, a mom of a six-year-old daughter and four-year-old triplets and an assistant professor and the fellowship director of pediatric radiology at the University of Arkansas for Medical Sciences and Arkansas Children's Hospital, both in Little Rock*

RALLIE'S TIP

My sons all had sore throats as toddlers, usually as a result of a cold. Infection with a cold virus is one of the most common causes of sore throat, although it can be caused by a bacterial infection, such as streptococcus, or strep. Sore throats can also be the result of sinus drainage related to allergies or breathing dry air through the mouth, and a very small percentage of toddlers might have a sore throat caused by something lodged in the throat or esophagus, such as a coin or a small part from a toy.

As long as my toddlers were breathing well, able to swallow normally, and not too sick to eat or drink well, I tried not to medicate them with prescription drugs or over-the-counter medicines. I kept a close eye on them until the illness had run its course. In the meantime, I'd offer them foods like chicken noodle soup and applesauce, which are easy to swallow, and plenty of liquids to drink. Sometimes they'd enjoy crushed ice or fruit popsicles, which helped keep their throats moist and cool and eased their discomfort. I'd also make them a warm "tea" of honey and lemon, which is very soothing to inflamed tissues.

If my boys didn't feel better in a day or two, or if they developed any other symptoms, such as an earache, a stomachache, swollen neck glands, or a rash, I'd take them to the pediatrician. With that said, I might have felt more comfortable taking this kind of watch-and-wait route because of my medical training. It's important to remember that a sore throat is merely a symptom of an underlying condition, and it can be really difficult to determine exactly what the underlying condition is without the help of a physician. Even physicians can't always make the diagnosis without performing a test or two, such as a throat swab and culture or a blood test.

Although it's far more common for young children to have a sore throat caused by a cold than by a strep infection, toddlers can get strep throat, and it's very important for them to be diagnosed and treated properly. Children with strep infections who don't receive treatment with antibiotics are at risk for developing rheumatic fever, which is an inflammatory illness that can lead to serious consequences, including permanent damage to the heart.

Whenever I had any doubt about the cause of a sore throat in one of my toddlers, we'd make a trip to the doctor's office. Usually we'd leave the clinic with nothing more than negative test results and the doctor's reassurance, but I always felt better knowing that my boys were going to be just fine. To me, the peace of mind was well worth the minor hassle of going to see the doctor.

Preventing and Treating Constipation

Nine out of 10 children don't eat enough fiber, which helps to keep stools soft and easier to pass. Plus, toddlers are often so busy playing they don't want to stop to poop. The longer they wait, the harder the poop gets, and the harder it is to poop. Also, sometimes if a toddler is going through a phase of emotional stress, his intestines might get upset, resulting in constipation, or diarrhea. So is it any wonder that children get constipated? Luckily, there are some easy ways to get things moving again.

⤚⤚

Preventing constipation is all about hydration! I don't keep soda in the house though. My kids only drink soda on "special occasions." Fresh fruit juices, milk, and water make up my daughters' fluid intake each day.
  —Marra S. Francis, MD

⤚⤚

I've been fortunate that my daughter eats and poops like a champ. I think it's helpful that I give her diluted juice to drink. In fact, if she drinks too much juice or eats too much fruit, she gets diarrhea.

—*Jennifer Bacani McKenney, MD*

When my younger daughter was a toddler, she became very constipated for a while. I tried giving her Miralax. It was effective, but my daughter could tell when we mixed it into her drinks!

—*Cheri Wiggins, MD, a mom of six- and three-year-old daughters, a specialist in physical medicine and rehabilitation at St. Luke's Magic Valley, and the cofounder of the Mommy Doctors Bakery (makers of Milkin' Cookies), in Twin Falls, ID*

Both of my kids had issues on and off with constipation. At one point, my older son was in so much pain that I thought he might have had an intestinal obstruction. My husband and I took him to the emergency department. It was poop, and after an enema and a dose of Miralax, my son felt better.

When to Call Your Doctor

It's best to take care of constipation early, before it becomes a major problem, so call your doctor if your child is going several days without a bowel movement; has dry, hard stools; complains of stomach cramps and seems bloated in the abdomen; has a waning appetite; is trying to hold in a bowel movement because of pain; or is leaking liquid or soft stools into his underwear.

It's especially important to call your pediatrician if:

- Your child has been constipated for three weeks or longer.
- Your child doesn't want to engage in normal activities because of constipation.
- Your child can't push the stool out during a bowel movement.
- Stool or liquid is leaking from the anus.
- There are small tears in the skin around the anus.
- Your child develops hemorrhoids.

We keep Miralax in our cupboard. My kids call it their "poop sugar."
—*Carrie Brown, MD, a mom of eight- and six-year-old sons and a general pediatrician who treats medically complex children and specializes in palliative care at Arkansas Children's Hospital, in Little Rock*

When my son was a toddler, he had a bit of a problem with constipation. It hurt him to go to the bathroom, so he became afraid to go.

Mommy MD Guides-Recommended Product
Natural Calm

Rallie's Tip: For kids who struggle with chronic constipation, a fiber-rich diet is critical. It's also important for kids to drink plenty of water, eat plenty of fruits and vegetables, and get plenty of regular exercise to prevent constipation.

But for the occasional bout of constipation, you might want to use a natural remedy to get things moving. Magnesium is an excellent remedy for occasional constipation. It also soothes and relaxes the gastrointestinal tract. This is why so many over-the-counter constipation remedies include magnesium, such as Milk of Magnesia, magnesium citrate, and various antacids.

One of the best natural remedies I've found is Natural Calm. It's a tart-tasting liquid that offers 240 milligrams of magnesium per capful, a safe and effective dose for youngsters. Children younger than age eight years should take only half a capful, 120 milligrams of magnesium, per day. It helps soothe and relax the GI tract and promote normal elimination. You don't want to go overboard and give your kids too much magnesium, as it can cause diarrhea.

Millions of people suffer from symptoms that can result from lack of magnesium, including stress, fatigue, inability to sleep, muscle tension, and headaches.

You can buy an eight-ounce container of Natural Calm in raspberry-lemon flavor for $13.77 at **VITACOST.COM**.

He eats a high-fiber diet, but sometimes that isn't enough. I gave my son some of my company's Milkin' Cookies to eat. Cheri Wiggins, MD, and I created them to help increase a nursing mother's milk supply, but because they are also high in fiber, they helped to ease my son's constipation. You can buy Milkin' Cookies at Milkin-Cookies.com for about $21 for a two-week supply. I prefer not to use medicines, but sometimes I had to give my son a bit of Miralax. You buy it over the counter. I experimented a bit, beginning at the age- and weight-recommended dose and then decreasing it from there. I found that just ¼ teaspoon mixed into my son's milk or a little bit of juice was enough to soften his stools so it didn't hurt for him to go to the bathroom.

—*Lennox McNeary, MD, a mom of a three-year-old son, a specialist in physical medicine and rehabilitation at Carilion Clinic, and a cofounder of the Mommy Doctors Bakery (makers of Milkin' Cookies), in Roanoke, VA*

To keep my older daughter pooping regularly, I would give her lots of water on a daily basis. However, when my daughter turned two, she became more of a picky eater. Her fiber intake dropped, which led to her not having a bowel movement for three to four days. I started to give her four ounces of either apple or prune juice every day. Once I started this, she didn't have any problems with constipation.

I am still struggling to this day to get my daughter to eat her veggies and get more fiber in her diet. I have resorted to making fresh smoothies for her at home. I add vegetables to the blender along with yogurt or a probiotic (such as Florastor or Culturelle). It works like a charm. My daughter loves the smoothies, and we are both happy!

—*Jeannette Gonzalez Simon, MD, a mom of three- and one-year-old daughters and a pediatric gastroenterologist in private practice, in Staten Island, NY*

One of my triplets has autism. GI disturbances, such as constipation and diarrhea, are common among children with autism. My son has struggled with them all of his life, swinging from one to the other. If I

Mommy MD Guides–Recommended Product
Sunsweet Essence Orange-Flavored Prunes

"When my children were toddlers, they sometimes had issues with constipation. Of all things, they loved to eat Sunsweet Essence Orange-Flavored Prunes," says Eva Mayer, MD, a mom of an eight-year-old daughter and a six-year-old son and a pediatrician with St. Luke's Pediatrics Associates, in Bethlehem, PA.

"I used to cut the prunes into quarters so they were small and safer to eat. They were like plump, juicy raisins. My kids would eat those prunes for a snack, and it helped a lot with the constipation."

When you're looking for a nutritious, sweet snack that's portable, prunes are a great pick. They're full of antioxidants, fiber, and nutrients such as potassium, magnesium, calcium, and vitamin B_6. They sure beat those so-called fruit snacks that are packed with more sugar than fruit. But if your child is on the picky side and turns his nose up to the fruit, we have you covered. Sunsweet now has orange-flavored prunes that make such a tasty snack you'll hear no complaints from the little one. Other flavors include cherry and lemon. A seven-ounce bag costs $2.35. If you can't find them in your supermarket, you can buy them at SUNSWEET.COM.

treat his constipation, then he ends up with diarrhea. If I treat the diarrhea, he becomes constipated.

I talked with my son's pediatrician about this, and he referred my son to a pediatric gastroenterologist. We're still trying to fix the problem. The take-home message is that not everything is perfect. You have to deal with parenting challenges as best you can. I try to take it one day at a time.

—*Sadaf T. Bhutta, MD*

Preventing and Treating Nausea and Vomiting

Stomach bugs seem to make the rounds every winter. Because stomach bugs are usually caused by viruses, not bacteria, antibiotics won't help. Only time will heal.

The best prevention is to wash your hands, and your toddler's hands, frequently, especially after using the bathroom and before touching food. It's incredible to think that one out of every three people leaves a public bathroom without washing his or her hands, according to the Centers for Disease Control and Prevention (CDC). Yuck.

Stomach viruses can become serious. For example, according to the CDC, infection with the norovirus causes around 18,500 kids under age five to be hospitalized each year. If your child is vomiting, keep a close eye on him and, most important, get fluids into him, even in tiny amounts, to prevent dehydration.

Few things are more painful to watch than a little one vomiting. Probably the only good thing we can say is it's often caused by stomach bugs that usually last for only 24 hours.

⤳⤺

I'm very big on hand sanitizer to prevent illnesses like stomach bugs. I have a bottle of sanitizer in every room of my house, plus in my diaper bag and purse. We sanitize all of the time. Even my one-year-old knows to rub her hands together when we squirt sanitizer gel on her hands.

—*Kate Tulenko, MD, MPH*

⤳⤺

When my kids have nausea or vomiting, I immediately put them on a very light diet. When they were little, they used to love to eat plain bread if they were sick. Once they were starting to feel better, I might put a tiny bit of butter on it to flavor it. A scrambled egg is another bland food to try when a child is sick.

—*Eva Mayer, MD*

⤳⤺

My older son had gastroenteritis, commonly called the stomach flu, on his first birthday. It was awful. He vomited everything up, and he was so lethargic he just wanted to lie on the floor. I knew that he had to get some fluid in him or he'd become dehydrated. So I gave him tiny amounts, around 1 teaspoon, of water or Pedialyte every five minutes with an eye dropper.

It's so hard when children are vomiting because they get hungry and ask for food, but as an adult, you know that they'll throw up anything they eat. My general rule was that once a child had gone three hours without throwing up, he could eat a bit of food, such as plain bread or Cheerios.

—*Leena Shrivastava Dev, MD*

೨∽

It's so awful to watch a baby or toddler vomit. There's not much you can do besides just get through it.

When my kids had stomach viruses, I was very glad that our washing machine has a sanitizing cycle! I would wash their sheets, pillowcases, pajamas, and clothes in hot water to kill all of the germs.

—*Cheri Wiggins, MD*

೨∽

So far my sons haven't gotten any stomach bugs. Only my husband and I have caught them!

My one son is very gaggy with food smells, though. They make him gag and almost vomit.

"He's not going into medicine," my husband jokes. "I don't think he's doctor material."

—*Amy Thompson, MD*

Mommy MD Guides-Recommended Product
Pedialyte and Pedialyte Freezer Pops

"One of the hardest things during my kids' toddler years was when they were sick. Even as a physician, it's hard to see your own children not feeling well," says Eva Mayer, MD, a mom of an eight-year-old daughter and a six-year-old son and a pediatrician with St. Luke's Pediatrics Associates, in Bethlehem, PA.

"To be prepared for times when my kids had diarrhea or were nauseated, I always kept Pedialyte products on hand," says Dr. Mayer. "I especially loved Pedialyte Freezer Pops. I still keep some in my freezer. I give them to my kids if their bellies hurt."

Pedialyte Pops are better than regular Popsicles because the sugar in regular Popsicles can worsen an upset stomach or diarrhea. Pedialyte's formula is specifically designed with the right balance of sugar and electrolytes to promote fluid absorption during diarrhea and vomiting so that your child can feel better fast.

"Pedialyte can taste slightly salty because it replaces the vital minerals and nutrients (such as sodium) lost during diarrhea and vomiting," says Dr. Mayer.

Dehydration can make your child feel worse. If you give your child Pedialyte when he's vomiting or suffering from diarrhea, you'll feel better knowing that you're helping him replace the minerals and nutrients he's lost. Pedialyte comes in fruit, strawberry, grape, and bubble gum flavors for older children and unflavored for infants. If your toddler is reluctant to drink, try Pedialyte freezer pops in grape, cherry, blue raspberry, and orange flavors. You can find Pedialyte at drugstores, where it costs about $6 for 34 ounces or 16 freezer pops. Visit **PEDIALYTE.COM** for more information.

Rallie's Tip

Fortunately, all of my sons now enjoy good gastrointestinal health, but when they were younger, they had their fair share of GI issues.

At one time or another, my sons all suffered from an upset stomach or a bout of gastroenteritis and the nausea and vomiting that came with it. One of my favorite remedies for these conditions is an herb called slippery elm. The bark of the slippery elm is extremely mucilaginous, which allows it to coat, soothe, and protect the lining of the GI tract. Mucilage is a long chain of sugars, known as polysaccharides, that becomes a gooey, slippery substance when combined with water. This mucilage helps soothe the digestive tract. Slippery elm is also rich in nutrients, and it's easy to digest, making it an excellent food for kids when they're suffering from digestive discomfort and are unable to tolerate or digest many other foods.

Slippery elm bark is typically dried and ground and can be used to make a tea or a gruel. It's sold in bulk, and it's also available in capsules. Slippery elm bark is very safe and effective for toddlers. According to legend, soldiers in George Washington's army at Valley Forge ate slippery elm bark to sustain themselves and to survive the grueling winter.

Another natural remedy I gave my toddlers when they had belly-aches was peppermint tea. Peppermint has been shown to have antispas-modic properties because it acts locally on smooth muscles in the gastrointestinal tract. This property allows the tea to relax the upper and lower GI tract and ease cramps and discomfort. Peppermint tea is an excellent way to administer peppermint to toddlers. It's as tasty as it is effective!

Preventing and Treating Skin Problems and Rashes

Skin problems and rashes are very common in toddlers, and they're tricky to diagnose and to treat. They can be caused by so many things, including an illness, exposure to an irritant, or an emotional upset. Sometimes the best treatment for a rash is patience.

◦◦◦

My motto for self-limited conditions, such as viral rashes, is "less is more." Let these things be, and with a tincture of time they should resolve. If a rash itches, a little topical antihistamine or cortisone used as directed by a physician might help, but otherwise, let Mother Nature heal!

—*Mona Gohara, MD, a mom of five- and three-year-old sons, a dermatologist in private practice, an assistant clinical professor in the department of dermatology at Yale University, and a cofounder of K&J Sunprotective Clothing, in Danbury, CT*

◦◦◦

When my toddlers get bug bites, I apply a topical, over-the-counter steroid cream such as cortisone, and that usually reduces inflammation and itch.

—*Amy J. Derick, MD, a mom of three-year-old and 19-month-old sons who's expecting another baby and a dermatologist in private practice at Derick Dermatology, in Barrington, IL*

◦◦◦

One of my sons has eczema, mainly on the extensor surfaces of his body, such as the bend of his elbows and on his knees. Our

When to Call Your Doctor

Unless it's a run-of-the-mill diaper rash that you can easily treat with an over-the-counter diaper rash cream, call your doctor any time your child's skin looks red, irritated, and painful, because it could be a sign of an allergy or a serious infection.

It's especially important for you to call your doctor if your child's rash is accompanied by a fever or illness or if areas of the skin are filled with pus. Another red flag that requires a call to the doctor is a rash that begins making the rounds in your family.

pediatrician recommended minimizing bathing, so we give our son a bath only every third night. When I do bathe him, rather than washing his skin directly, I wash his hair and let the soap run down his body.

—*Amy Thompson, MD*

One of my twins has severe eczema. We discovered it's caused by her food allergies. Researchers are developing a desensitization program of sublingual medicine that holds promise for the treatment of eczema.

—*Susan Wilder, MD, a mom of a 17-year-old daughter and twin 13-year-old girls, a primary care physician, and the founder and CEO of Lifescape Medical Associates, in Scottsdale, AZ*

Many children suffer from eczema, which can be related to allergies. My son had eczema as an infant, and it still flares up from time to time. The most important thing to remember is that this condition is typically caused by excessive dryness of the skin and in some cases irritation by allergens, such as grass pollen or ragweed pollen.

It's important to keep your toddler's skin clean and well moisturized by using mild soaps without fragrances or perfumes and avoiding any agent that has alcohol listed as an ingredient. Usually, bathing your child regularly, patting his skin dry following the bath, and applying a thick moisturizer, such as Vaseline or

Eucerin Cream, to the entire body can be enough to prevent eczema from worsening.

—*Sigrid Payne DaVeiga, MD*

My daughter is 2½, and I have been fortunate that she's been a pretty healthy toddler. In the wintertime, her biggest challenge is dry lips. I've increased her fluid intake to help keep her skin moist. Plus, I apply Boudreaux's Baby Kisses Lip Balm and Vaseline throughout the day to her lips. This has helped significantly.

—*Tanya Douglas Holland, MD*

Mommy MD Guides-Recommended Product
Eucerin Cream

"Our daughter continued to have very dry skin and some patches of eczema during her toddler years," says Melody Derrick, MD, a mom of a two-year-old daughter who's expecting another baby and a family physician in private practice with Cadence Physician Group, in Winfield, IL.

"We used Eucerin Cream with Alpha-Hydroxy. This helped with the dry skin and eczema.

"As an added bonus, Eucerin also helped my daughter with keratosis pilaris," Dr. Derrick notes. "This is a common, benign condition characterized by bumps on the backs of the arms.

"I had to convince my husband that I was using the lotion to help with the health of our daughter's skin. He thought that I was just putting lotion on her to make her smell good or give her soft, pretty skin!"

Eucerin offers a variety of skin products, including Aquaphor Baby Healing Ointment. This product helps soothe and protect skin that's irritated because of eczema, diaper rash, drooling, minor burns, or abrasions, and it's safe to use anywhere on baby's skin.

A three-ounce tube of Aquaphor Baby Healing Ointment costs around $8 and can be found at supermarkets and drugstores. Visit **EUCERINUS.COM** for more information.

Treating Fever

In healthy toddlers, a mild to moderate fever is your friend. When your toddler is sick, his body temperature rises, most likely to fight the germs that cause infection and to make his body a less comfy place for them to be. The fever itself isn't an illness, but rather a symptom.

If your toddler is playing comfortably, is eating and drinking, is alert and smiling, *and* has a temperature lower than 102°F, you might not even want to treat it. Let the fever run its course. If your child is younger than three years old and has a fever of 102.2°F, call your child's doctor for advice. (Talk with your toddler's doctor before giving your toddler any medication.)

∽◦∾

When my boys have a fever, I allow them to have an age- and weight-appropriate dose of acetaminophen (Tylenol) or Motrin (ibuprofen). I buy the infant formula, rather than the children's version, because I don't want my babysitter to have to think too hard. It is easier to dose than trying to calculate the difference with the children's pain reliever.

—*Sharon Boyce, MD, a mom of three- and one-year-old sons and a family physician at DayOne Family Healthcare Clinic, in Battle Creek, MI*

∽◦∾

I was so lucky that my kids have always been very healthy. However, I'm a big believer in acetaminophen (Tylenol) and ibuprofen (Motrin) for symptom relief. It you have a fever or aren't feeling well, and you know what's causing it, and it's nothing that requires more serious medical attention, I think it's okay to give toddlers an age- and weight-appropriate dose of acetaminophen or ibuprofen so they'll feel better.

—*Siobhan Dolan, MD, MPH, a mom of 16- and 13-year-old daughters and an 11-year-old son, a consultant to the March of Dimes, and an associate professor of obstetrics and gynecology and women's health at Albert Einstein College of Medicine/Montefiore Medical Center, in Bronx, NY*

∽◦∾

I'm not a believer in pushing drugs. I think sometimes when doctors prescribe medication for kids' colds, they're really treating Mommy.

I never gave my kids medicine just because it tastes good. That's a really bad behavior to get into. If they had a fever of 101°F or higher and they looked sick, I'd give them an age- and weight-appropriate dose of acetaminophen (Tylenol). That was before they sold kids' ibuprofen (Motrin). Both work well for fever. If a child has a fever and also muscle aches, I'd give him ibuprofen, which has an anti-inflammatory effect. But if a child has a sensitive stomach, I'd give him Tylenol because ibuprofen can irritate the stomach.

—*Susan Besser, MD*

When my older son is sick, I try to stay ahead of the fever. That means, if his temperature is 100°F or higher, I give him medication to make sure it doesn't keep climbing.

When to Call Your Doctor

There's usually no need to worry if your child has a fever but is still eating and drinking, has a normal skin color, is interested in playing, smiles, is alert, and looks healthy once his temperature comes down. But be sure to call your doctor if your child has a fever and:

- Recently received immunizations
- Is younger than two years old and has a fever longer than 24 to 48 hours or is older than two years old and has a fever longer than 48 to 72 hours
- Has a fever of 103°F that doesn't go down when treated with acetaminophen (Tylenol) or ibuprofen (Motrin)
- Has a sore throat, earache, cough, or other symptoms
- Has developed a rash or bruises
- Is having pain during urination or frequent urination
- Has been getting fevers for a week or longer
- Has a heart problem, diabetes, or another illness
- Has lowered immunity due to steroid therapy, an organ transplant, cancer, or another serious medical condition
- Recently traveled to a third-world country

The most important thing is to determine what is causing the fever. This might of course require a call or visit to your pediatrician. If my son has a fever, and I know it's caused by a virus, I will give him an age- and weight-appropriate dose of ibuprofen (Motrin), but not more than three times a day.

Even though my son is two, I still use a rectal thermometer to check his temperature. I worry about other types of thermometers giving me an accurate reading. Vicks makes one that has a safeguard so it can only go in so far, and I put a water-soluble lubricant on it before I insert it.

—*Deborah Kulick, MD*

When my sons got a fever, I didn't give them any medicine if they were still playing and in good spirits. If they looked and acted sick, I'd give them an age- and weight-appropriate dose of acetaminophen (Tylenol) or ibuprofen (Motrin).

I had to abide by the day care's rule of keeping them out of school until they were fever free for 24 hours. That wasn't a problem because if they weren't feeling well, I'd want them to be home anyway.

—*Leena Shrivastava Dev, MD*

RALLIE'S TIP

Like all toddlers, my boys got fevers from time to time. Rather than immediately giving them a fever-reducing medication, I'd try to wait out the fever for a while, because I wanted to know what was causing it. In the vast majority of cases, fever is a result of some type of infection, and it's important to pinpoint the source of infection if at all possible, because the type of infection determines the best treatment.

If, for example, one of my children had a bacterial infection that resulted in strep throat, I knew he was going to need antibiotics. If he just had a viral infection that resulted in the common cold, on the other hand, I knew that antibiotics wouldn't be effective. Fever-reducing medications also reduce pain, and pain helps you pinpoint the source of infection. If moms give their toddlers acetaminophen or ibuprofen at the first sign of a fever, it makes it far more difficult to determine the site of the toddler's pain and the source of his infection.

Fevers also help the body overcome the infection. A low-grade fever is the body's way of "pasteurizing" the blood. Infection-causing viruses and bacteria invade the body at its normal temperature of roughly 98.6°F. The child's normal body temperature is one that is favorable for the organisms to set up housekeeping and to multiply, thus causing infection. The immune system reacts to this microbial invasion by elevating the body temperature. An elevated temperature is far less hospitable for the organisms and causes them to die. A slightly elevated body temperature also speeds biochemical reactions, so that the body can deliver nutrients and components of the immune system to the site of infection more rapidly. It also allows wastes and toxins to be removed more rapidly from the site of infection.

Additionally, fever generally slows children down and encourages them to rest or sleep. That's just what the body needs when trying to overcome an infection. Children with fevers should be allowed to stay home from day care so that they can sleep a little longer in the morning, take a nap, and avoid the physical and mental rigors of preschool. Rest and sleep are critical to healing. As an extra bonus, staying home from preschool will help prevent the spread of the illness.

Even a low-grade fever increases thirst, and drinking extra fluids is helpful to the body as well. Offer children plenty of fluids regularly while they're suffering from a cold. If the child is eating well, water is usually the best fluid to offer, but juice, Pedialyte, and sports drinks are also acceptable, especially if they're diluted with water.

If your toddler has a high fever and you know what's causing it, you might give him an age- and weight-appropriate dose of acetaminophen (Tylenol) or ibuprofen (Motrin). But which one? Some scientific studies suggest that acetaminophen and ibuprofen alleviate fever equally well when given at the age-appropriate doses. But at least one study suggests that ibuprofen reduces fever faster and longer.

Preventing and Treating Other Common Conditions

Besides colds and allergies, rashes and sore throats, children get a myriad of other common conditions.

As much as I knew about human development and health, when my own children got sick, it was as if I didn't remember a thing. Often my husband would ask, "Did you think about this?" or "How about such and such?"

The takeaway message is that moms, even moms who are physicians, can't think of everything all of the time. It's important to have other people with whom to bounce ideas off and with whom to talk things through.

—*Cathie Lippman, MD*

∾

My sons tend to get croupy coughs that wake us all up in the middle of the night. It sounds like we have a seal in our house! The first time it happened, I was afraid it was a condition called epiglottitis, which is a bacterial infection that children get that causes a condition similar to laryngitis in adults, only worse because it can be life threatening. I took my son to the doctor to rule that out.

Now that I can recognize the croupy cough, when one of my sons gets it, I wrap him in a blanket and take him downstairs to the kitchen. Then I open the freezer door and let him breathe in the cool air.

—*Amy Thompson, MD*

∾

My son got sick a lot as a toddler. It was so very stressful for me. A few times, he got croup. When that happened, I wasn't a doctor anymore. I was a very scared mother.

My son would wake up in the middle of the night having great difficulty breathing. It's so super scary. Hard as it was, I knew it was critical that I stayed calm, to help my son stay calm. The more upset my son was, the harder it was for him to breathe. I bundled him up in fleece blankets and took him out in the cool, even cold, night air for 10 minutes. That helped him to breathe, and thank goodness I never had to take him to the emergency department.

—*Eva Mayer, MD*

RALLIE'S TIP

My oldest son had pinkeye when he was a toddler, and the experience was something I never wanted to go through again. His swollen, itchy, goopy eyes made him miserable, especially when he woke up in the morning and his eyelids were stuck together, and he couldn't go to day care for an entire week. His eyes stayed red and watery for several days, even after I took him to the pediatrician and started him on antibiotic eye drops.

Pinkeye, or conjunctivitis, can be caused by an infection of the eyes with a bacteria or a virus, and it can also be related to allergies. Only bacterial conjunctivitis requires treatment with antibiotics, but some cases of viral conjunctivitis require treatment with antiviral medications. Of course, it's hard to know the cause of the infection when it first appears. If your toddler goes to day care or is normally around other children, it's probably a good idea to take him to the doctor pronto at the first sign of pinkeye, because it can be contagious.

In most cases, pinkeye isn't serious, but occasionally an infection of a child's eye can have serious consequences, so it's always worth the time

Mommy MD Guides-Recommended Product
FeverAll Suppositories

"One of the best-kept secrets is that acetaminophen comes in a suppository," says Jennifer Hanes, DO, a mom of a six-year-old daughter and a three-year-old son, an emergency physician, a certified forensic physician, and the founder of Empowered Medicine, PLLC, in Austin, TX. "With a suppository, it becomes possible to help a sick child feel better from a fever even when his tummy is upset."

Suppositories are a great option for when oral acetaminophen won't go or stay down. Parents will know their child received the exact dosage of acetaminophen required for their age every time.

FeverAll sells acetaminophen suppositories in infants', children's, and junior strength at drugstores. For children up to age three, use the infants' strength of 80 milligrams unless otherwise instructed by your doctor. FeverAll Infants' Strength is the only acetaminophen suppository approved for infants as young as six months. FeverAll costs approximately $7 for a pack of six. For more information on FeverAll, visit FEVERALL.COM.

and effort required to see a pediatrician. One of the best ways to keep pinkeye from spreading like wildfire through your home is to make sure everyone's washing their hands frequently with lots of soap and water and a little elbow grease. Washing sheets and blankets is also helpful.

The hardest part of treating my son's pinkeye was getting the eye drops into his eyes. I gave him a very long and detailed explanation of why the eye drops had to go into the eyes, and then I spent even more time cajoling, bargaining, and bribing. He wasn't buying it.

Fortunately, I grew up on a farm, and I've had years of experience catching and detaining young farm animals. This comes in very handy as a parent. I finally gave up on trying to get my son to cooperate. I just placed his wriggly little body firmly between my knees, held his head snuggly against my chest with one hand, and squirted the drops into his eyes with the other. It was over in about 20 seconds, and after he realized that the eye drops didn't hurt a bit, he cooperated from then on.

? When to Call Your Doctor

A common condition that parents might be unfamiliar with is pinkeye, which is also called conjunctivitis. Some types of pinkeye will go away on their own, but others need to be treated, so it's best to check with your child's doctor if your child's eye is pink or red, especially if he's complaining that it feels like there's sand in his eye. If your child has a fever and increasing swelling, redness, and tenderness around the eye and on the lids, be sure to call your doctor immediately because it might mean the infection is spreading.

In some cases, what might look like pinkeye is really another eye condition. Have your child checked by a doctor if he has any of the following symptoms.

- Severe eye pain
- Poor eyesight
- Sensitivity to light
- Pinkeye continues for longer than a week untreated or longer than two or three days after treatment

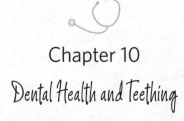

Chapter 10
Dental Health and Teething

YOUR TODDLER'S DEVELOPMENT

Most toddlers have at least four baby teeth by the time they're a year old. Then they generally have all 20 baby teeth by the time they're two. But like so many things, there's a wide range of normal. Some kids don't have all of their baby teeth until they're 3½.

Sometimes people call teeth pearly whites, and you should care for your toddler's teeth as if they are as precious as pearls. Tooth decay affects children in the United States more than any other chronic infectious disease. Not taking care of your toddler's teeth can lead to decay. That decay in turn can cause pain and infections that might lead to problems in eating, speaking, playing, and learning.

Tooth decay and other dental diseases are preventable. By investing just a few minutes a day to brush and floss your toddler's teeth and by taking her to regular dental checkups, you can care for her baby teeth and protect her beautiful smile.

The tooth fairy likely won't start to make visits to your house until your child is five or six years old. That gives you plenty of time to ask your friends who have older kids about the tooth fairy's going rate.

TAKING CARE OF YOU

When was *your* last dental appointment? If it's been more than six months, schedule one today.

JUSTIFICATION FOR A CELEBRATION

Your toddler's first trip to the dentist is a great reason to celebrate.

Choosing a Dentist

Do you want to take your child to a dentist, or to a pediatric dentist? Pediatric dentists are the pediatricians for dentistry. They have to complete two to three years of specialized training following dental school. They treat infants up to teens, including kids with special health needs.

This choice might not be entirely yours to make. There might not be a pediatric dentist in your area, or this type of specialist might not be covered by your insurance. It's a good idea to first check with your dental insurance company, if you have one, to see what's covered.

∽

Having a pediatric dentist or a regular dentist who is kid friendly makes all the difference. Our dentist and her entire staff were wonderful with kids! It was important that I could schedule all of our appointments around the same time, and they were willing to work with me on that.

—*Marra S. Francis, MD, a mom of eight-, seven-, and five-year-old daughters and a gynecologist, in San Antonio, TX*

∽

We live in a very small town. There's only one pediatric dentist, and so that's where my husband takes our girls. I'm very glad that he takes them because I'm afraid of the dentist!

The pediatric dentist really does a great job with kids, and my girls love to go there. Just the other day, my older daughter asked, "When can I go to the dentist again?"

—*Cheri Wiggins, MD, a mom of six- and three-year-old daughters, a specialist in physical medicine and rehabilitation at St. Luke's Magic Valley, and the cofounder of the Mommy Doctors Bakery (makers of Milkin' Cookies), in Twin Falls, ID*

∽

We live in a small town, so we don't have the luxury of a pediatric dentist. The closest regular dentist is 45 minutes away!

That's the dentist my husband and I go to, and I think there's value in taking our daughter there. Our daughter will see us go there too, and it will be more like a family event than if she was going to her own pediatric dentist. We'll also save time and gas by taking everyone to the dentist at once.

—Jennifer Bacani McKenney, MD, a mom of a one-year-old daughter and a family physician, in Fredonia, KS

⟜⟝

When I was looking for a dentist, I asked my family and friends where they take their kids. I started taking my boys to the dentist when they were 2½ years old.

In the end, I chose a pediatric dentist for my sons. Certainly, you don't have to take kids to a pediatric dentist, but they *know* kids. They know how to cajole kids and get them through the visit. Our pediatric dentist is so patient and amazing. You don't want to take your kids to an old-school dentist who's going to strap them down and make it an awful experience!

—Heather Orman-Lubell, MD, a mom of 11- and 7-year-old sons and a pediatrician in private practice at Yardley Pediatrics of St. Christopher's Hospital for Children, in Pennsylvania

RALLIE'S TIP

I took all of my boys to the dentist when they were toddlers. I had heard great things about a pediatric dentist in our town, and she definitely lived up to her reputation. She had a kid-friendly waiting room with a playhouse and lots of toys, and my boys always looked forward to going to her office. She was very kind and incredibly patient, and she had lots of really neat tricks to keep my sons entertained while she was examining their mouths. She gave them cool sunglasses to wear and headphones so they could listen to music while they were sitting in the exam chair. Afterward, she always took time to answer my questions and teach me what I needed to know to keep my boys' teeth healthy. The only bad thing about visiting her office was that my children didn't want to leave!

I don't think it's absolutely necessary to take children to a pediatric dentist, but it is important to find a dentist that you and your toddler feel safe and comfortable with. Those early visits will help determine how comfortable your child feels visiting the dentist and having dental work for years to come.

Going to the Dentist

Dentists recommend taking your child to the dentist when her first tooth appears or at least by her first birthday. If that ship has sailed, it's a great idea to make an appointment as soon as you can and return for a visit every six months.

I took each of my girls to the dentist for the first time when they were two years old. I made sure that they got to see me have my exam first, and then I let them sit or recline on top of me in the chair while they got their exams.

    —*Marra S. Francis, MD*

Thankfully, I've never had a problem taking my kids to the dentist. I started to take my kids to the dentist when they were two years old. I call our dentist the "tooth doctor." Before we go, I explain to my kids that the tooth doctor will look at, clean, and count their teeth. It's important to prepare kids and to explain things on a level that they can understand. This way there are no surprises.

    —*Sadaf T. Bhutta, MD, a mom of a six-year-old daughter and four-year-old triplets and an assistant professor and the fellowship director of pediatric radiology at the University of Arkansas for Medical Sciences and Arkansas Children's Hospital, both in Little Rock*

The earlier you start taking your kids to the dentist, the better. My sons go to my family dentist, and they started sitting on my lap watching what the dentist did to me when they were six months old. By the time my sons could talk, they were asking for a turn. We started doing very brief exams and applying fluoride every six months, which is what's recommended from the time they get teeth, but certainly by age two years.

My oldest son's molars came through without any enamel. He has needed extensive dental work, but he still thinks of the dentist as his friend. My youngest has had no dental issues at all.

    —*Carrie Brown, MD, a mom of eight- and six-year-old sons and a general pediatrician who treats medically complex children and*

specializes in palliative care at Arkansas Children's Hospital, in
Little Rock

❧

I took my daughter with me to the dentist for my regular appointment, and then I scheduled a separate appointment for her with a pediatric dentist. The first appointment for her was really just to look at all of the instruments and get used to the dentist looking in her mouth. She got a kick out of it. Also, my daughter's preschool class took a trip to the dentist's office, which was a huge help.

— *Jeannette Gonzalez Simon, MD, a mom of three- and one-year-old daughters and a pediatric gastroenterologist in private practice, in Staten Island, NY*

❧

I took my kids to the dentist for the first time. My son was very intrigued by the dentist. I found that buying a book about going to the dentist was very helpful. I also told my son that the dentist would give him a brand-new toothbrush after the visit was over. My son loves gifts, so the thought of a new toothbrush was more than enough to get him excited about dental hygiene!

— *Shilpa Amin-Shah, MD, a mom of a two-year-old son and a one-year-old daughter and an emergency physician at Emergency Medical Associates, in Livingston, NJ*

❧

My younger son had a hard time at the dentist's office initially because he didn't like the taste of the toothpaste the dentist used. So we bring our familiar toothpaste from home whenever we visit the dentist.

— *Heather Orman-Lubell, MD*

❧

The best way to smooth the path for toddlers visiting the doctor or dentist is to choose the doctor or dentist wisely! Health care professionals who know how to connect with small children are precious gems. Community networks and parent grapevines can help you find someone who uses state-of-the-art professional techniques and is skillful at negotiating with toddlers. Then the problems with fears and reluctance are likely to be minimized. In

When to Call Your Dentist

The American Academy of Pediatric Dentistry recommends taking your child to a pediatric dentist around the time her first tooth makes an appearance, which tends to be when she's between six months and one year old. Having dental checkups early in life means your child is less likely to have dental problems in the future. When it comes to finding a dentist for your child, pediatric dentists are good choices because they have had two to three years of additional training in the treatment of infants, children, and adolescents, and they tend to have offices that are specially designed for kids.

addition, if the parent gives some kind of breezy, brief, and matter-of-fact description of what it's like to see the dentist and to say, "Ahhhh" while the dentist looks at the teeth, then children will know what to expect.

Little children are naturally likely to cry and wail if they have a dental procedure. I don't believe it is helpful to give youngsters under the age of four much advance explanation of the procedure until the moment it's about to happen. If parents are calm and soothing throughout the entire experience, the toddler usually follows along and forgets the unpleasantness. As with many matters, if the parent is very anxious about the toddler's potential reaction, this might serve as a self-fulfilling prophecy.

—*Elizabeth Berger, MD, a mom of a 29-year-old son and a 27-year-old daughter, a child psychiatrist, and the author of* Raising Kids with Character, *in New York City*

Caring for Teeth and Gums

Whoever said, "An ounce of prevention is worth a pound of cure" might well have been talking about going to the dentist. A regular checkup is often covered by dental insurance, or costs about $150 out of pocket. But a filling costs up to $300!

Brushing your toddler's teeth is probably not your favorite thing to do, nor hers. But it's crucial. Dentists say that children aren't ready to brush their own teeth until they're around seven years old. It's not until that age that children can move the bristles of a toothbrush at a 45-degree angle to get between the tooth and the gumline, where the plaque likes to party. So you've got quite a long way to go!

Interestingly, one in five Americans admits to not brushing their teeth twice a day! Nevertheless, you should brush your toddler's teeth twice a day. It's a great idea to give her a chance to brush too, but then make sure you give it a go-over.

Ideally, you should brush your toddler's teeth for two minutes. You could set an egg timer, count to 120, or buy a toothbrush that has a timer built in.

If you, or someone you know, can't afford to take the kids to the dentist, check into the American Dental Association's Give Kids a Smile Day. It provides free checkups for children in low-income families.

⚬⚬⚬

When my kids were toddlers, we lived in a home with well water, so it didn't have any fluoride. I had to give my kids those awful-tasting fluoride supplements. I got them the chewable tablets, which taste a little bit better than the liquid. I crumbled them up into yogurt or applesauce.

—*Eva Mayer, MD, a mom of an eight-year-old daughter and a six-year-old son and a pediatrician with St. Luke's Pediatrics Associates, in Bethlehem, PA*

⚬⚬⚬

Since my daughter's teeth came in, I've brushed her teeth and gums with a finger brush. She loves it! Right now it's a game for my daughter because she tries to bite the brush, so we have to be quick and efficient. We'll probably be switching to a toddler toothbrush soon because she's getting a lot quicker at biting, and she's getting more teeth!

—*Jennifer Bacani McKenney, MD*

When my kids were toddlers and I brushed their teeth, we would practice saying the vowels in a long AAAA-EEE-IIII-OOOO-UUUU. The various mouth shapes for the letters helped me reach all of their teeth and tongue. Plus, my kids learned their vowels quickly!

—*Jennifer Hanes, DO, a mom of a six-year-old daughter and a three-year-old son, an emergency physician, a certified forensic physician, and the founder of Empowered Medicine, PLLC, in Austin, TX*

My older son used to hate every minute of brushing his teeth. But then he started to sing the alphabet song while he brushes his teeth, and he loves it. Now I have a new challenge: getting him out of the bathroom to move on to the next activity.

Luckily, my younger son just follows what his big brother does. So already, he's happy to brush his teeth.

—*Sharon Boyce, MD, a mom of three- and one-year-old sons and a family physician at DayOne Family Healthcare Clinic, in Battle Creek, MI*

I started to brush my sons' teeth as soon as their teeth came in. It's so much easier to brush a baby's teeth than a toddler's. With a baby, you just brush the teeth and gums with gauze and water, and babies are generally tolerant of that. But some toddlers really don't like having their teeth brushed. You have to do it. It's not a choice.

I brush my sons' teeth twice a day even if it's a struggle. I give them positive feedback afterward, like a big hug. I want them to learn that brushing their teeth is quick, it's over, and now you get a hug from Mom.

—*Heather Orman-Lubell, MD*

Mommy MD Guides-Recommended Product
Tom's of Maine Toothpaste

You'll find two types of toothpaste for kids: those that contain fluoride and those that don't. Before your child is able to spit, it's important to brush her teeth with baby toothpaste that doesn't contain fluoride to avoid fluoride poisoning if swallowed. Too much fluoride while your child's teeth are developing can cause problems with her tooth enamel. (However, it's important to make sure your child is getting some fluoride, which is in public drinking water in most areas of the United States.)

If you're using toothpaste with fluoride, the American Academy of Pediatric Dentistry recommends putting a smear of toothpaste on the brush for children under age two. After age two, use just a pea-size amount and tell your child to spit after brushing.

Tom's of Maine sells both fluoride-free and fluoride toothpaste for kids, and the company's products are made with natural ingredients. The fluoride-free toothpaste comes in strawberry, and the fluoride toothpaste comes in strawberry and orange mango. Both cost $3.99 a tube at **WWW.TOMSOF MAINESTORE.COM**. You can also find the toothpaste at **DRUG STORE.COM**, **AMAZON.COM**, CVS, and Walgreens.

None of my kids have particularly liked having their teeth brushed. With my three oldest, it was pretty much a fit to be had each night until they were around 2½ years old. I brushed their teeth each night before bed. Morning brushings were rather hit-or-miss.

With my younger son, I came up with a new approach. I buy two identical toothbrushes, and I brush with one and give him the other one to play with.

—*Kristie McNealy, MD, a mom of nine- and six-year-old daughters and four-year-old and 22-month-old sons and a blogger at KristieMcNealy.com, in Denver, CO*

Each morning, my kids brush their teeth at the same time my husband and I do. That's helpful because they see us brushing, so they want to brush too.

At night, because my kids go to bed earlier than I do, they brush their teeth earlier than I do. It's part of their bedtime routine. They drink some milk, brush their teeth, read a book, and then go to sleep.

To make this easier, I have two sets of toothbrushes for my kids: one set in my bathroom for the mornings and another set in their bathroom for evenings.

—*Shilpa Amin-Shah, MD*

I let my daughter eat candy on occasion, but I stress to her that if you're going to eat candy, you must brush your teeth extra carefully to take care of them. I let my daughter watch me brush and floss my teeth so that she'll want to do it too. You have to be careful with kids having floss because it's a choking hazard.

I'm a little nervous that I let my daughter use my adult toothpaste sometimes, and I fear she might have brown spots from the fluoride when her adult teeth come in. (This is another tip that I somehow missed being told as a Dr. Mom.) Babies and toddlers should only use fluoride-free toothpaste.

—*Lisa Campanella-Coppo, MD, a mom of a three-year-old daughter, an emergency physician, and the emergency department director of academic affairs at Monmouth Medical Center, in New Jersey*

I brushed my toddlers' teeth, took them to the dentist, and fed them a very healthy diet, and they never had any cavities. If they had needed to have fillings, I would have made sure the dentist used porcelain or ceramic fillings, not metal ones.

I had all of the metal fillings removed from my mouth and replaced with porcelain or ceramic. I am grateful that I did this because we find heavy metal toxicity in children who themselves do not have metal fillings, but whose mothers do.

—*Cathie Lippman, MD, a mom of 31- and 29-year-old sons and a physician who specializes in environmental and preventive medicine at the Lippman Center for Optimal Health, in Beverly Hills, CA*

RALLIE'S TIP

Making sure that toddlers drink fluoridated water can dramatically reduce the risk of tooth decay. Dentists are finding that young children today are at high risk for developing cavities because many parents give their kids only bottled water to drink, and many brands of bottled water don't contain any fluoride at all. While making sure that toddlers get a tiny bit of fluoride is important, too much of a good thing is definitely bad. Too much fluoride can lead to dental fluorosis, a developmental disturbance of the tooth enamel caused by excessive exposure to high concentrations of the mineral during tooth development. The risk of fluoride overexposure occurs between the ages of three months and eight years. In its mild forms, fluorosis often appears as faint white streaks or specks in the tooth enamel. In more severe cases, the teeth develop brown marks or other discolorations and the surface of the enamel can be pitted or rough and hard to clean. Unfortunately, the changes are generally permanent.

When my sons were toddlers, we used fluoridated toothpaste because our water supply didn't have added fluoride. My youngest son obviously didn't rinse well, and he must have swallowed more toothpaste than he spit out. I was so upset with myself when his permanent teeth came in and I noticed that he had some bright white spots on his two front teeth! Now that he's a teenager and his teeth are fully emerged, the white spots are barely noticeable. Still, I learned a very important lesson that I pass on to my patients whenever I get the chance. Fluoride is nothing to mess around with. Kids who live in areas that don't have access to a fluoridated water supply should be given water with added fluoride, or they should take the exact dose of a fluoride supplement prescribed by their pediatrician, family doctor, or dentist. Kids who don't get enough fluoride are at risk for tooth decay, and kids who get a bit too much fluoride are at risk of having discolored permanent teeth. Neither is a good option!

Easing Teething Pain

It's pretty impossible to think that pointy, hard teeth pushing through soft, tender gums wouldn't hurt. Yet amazingly, older children who are getting their permanent teeth and teens getting wisdom teeth often report it doesn't hurt a bit. But if your toddler is having teething pain, there are ways to help.

However, skip the over-the-counter teething gels containing benzocaine. In breaking news, the Food and Drug Administration recently warned against using products containing benzocaine, the main ingredient in some over-the-counter teething liquids and gels. Benzocaine is associated with a rare but serious condition called methemoglobinemia, which greatly reduces the amount of oxygen carried through the bloodstream. In the most severe cases, this condition can be life threatening. The symptoms come on suddenly, and they can happen after the first use. Symptoms include shortness of breath, dizziness, fatigue, and rapid heart rate.

The FDA says products containing benzocaine should never be given to children younger than two years old. (Talk with your toddler's doctor before giving her any medications.)

༄

When my daughter was around one year old, she pulled on her ears a lot. I looked in her ears every five minutes, but I didn't see any signs of an ear infection.

? **When to Call Your Dentist**

? **When to Call Your Dentist**

The dreaded teething process usually starts sometime between ages four months and seven months, but some children don't start teething until they're older than one. By age two, toddlers usually have their first 20 teeth.

A child who's teething typically has pain and might be quite restless and fussy. When normal soothing techniques such as cold teething rings and over-the-counter pain relievers aren't working, call your dentist or doctor. Although teething might increase your child's temperature slightly, it doesn't cause a high fever, so call your doctor if your child has a fever because it might be a sign of an illness.

I learned later that ear pain can actually be referred pain from teething! So an age- and weight-appropriate dose of acetaminophen (Tylenol) or ibuprofen (Motrin) might have eased her pain.

—*Lisa Campanella-Coppo, MD*

Before my sons were a year old, I'd usually give them acetaminophen (Tylenol) only for teething pain. But after a year, I'm more likely to give ibuprofen (Motrin) because it has anti-inflammatory properties in addition to pain relief.

—*Sharon Boyce, MD*

A frozen Lender's mini bagel is a cool "teething ring" that is also a nutritious treat. This can get messy if you let it thaw all the way, though.

I also gave my toddlers acetaminophen (Tylenol) before naptime and bedtime when they were teething.

—*Marra S. Francis, MD*

For my older son's teething pain, we gave him a lot of cold things that he could chew on, such as teething rings. My son's favorite was a cloth puppy with rubber feet that each had a different texture. As long as we kept that puppy cold, my son was okay.

My second child never really seemed bothered by his teeth. We never knew they were coming until we could see them.

—*Carrie Brown, MD*

∽

After my kids got their first few teeth, I don't think the rest of the teeth hurt too much coming in. You'd think it would hurt, but my kids didn't seem to mind. If they ever did complain of pain, some acetaminophen (Tylenol) would take care of it.

—*Sadaf T. Bhutta, MD*

RALLIE'S TIP

When a child is experiencing teething pain, the pain doesn't serve any great purpose. In fact, the pain might interfere with eating, so it makes good sense to give a child a dose of acetaminophen (Tylenol) or ibuprofen (Motrin) to ease this type of discomfort.

How do you know which medicine to use? While both acetaminophen and ibuprofen alleviate aches and pains effectively, ibuprofen has the added benefit of reducing inflammation in body tissues, which might make it a better choice for teething pain, which involves swelling of the gums. Because ibuprofen is administered every six to eight hours, compared to every four to six hours with acetaminophen, it might also be a better choice to use at bedtime.

When my boys were teething, I always offered them cold teething rings to chew on. The cold temperature and the counterpressure offered by teething rings are pretty effective in numbing minor pain. If those didn't work and my boys were too miserable to eat, I would give them ibuprofen. Fortunately, teething pain generally doesn't last long, so I didn't have to keep them on the medicine for more than a day or two.

Putting Nonfood Items in Mouth

At one year old, many children still put things into their mouths. Your job: Keep-away!

Ironically, pacifiers get a bad rap for a lot of reasons, but I found that because my daughter liked to have her pacifier in her mouth, it prevented her from putting other nonfood items into her mouth. By the time my daughter gave up her pacifier at age 2½, she wasn't so apt to put nonfood items into her mouth anymore.

—*Jennifer Hanes, DO*

My daughter still puts everything into her mouth. Everything gets explored. The biggest challenge is the dog's and cat's food. We can't put it up high so my daughter can't reach it, because then the pets wouldn't be able to eat.

At this age, my daughter knows she's not *supposed* to eat pet food. She'll go over to the pet's bowl, casually look over at me, I say, "No," and then she usually puts it into her mouth anyway. It's become like a game to her. But this phase should quickly pass. For now, we just continue to tell her "No," and we ask her to give the food in her hand to the dog or cat so that she knows it's for them and not her.

—*Jennifer Bacani McKenney, MD*

When to Call Your Doctor

It's typical for babies to put everything in their mouths—and sometimes ingest things that they shouldn't. But if your child is eating nonfood items after age two, call your doctor right away. It could point to an eating disorder called pica, in which a child eats things that will make you cringe, such as dirt, hair, paper, paint chips, feces, pencil erasers, strings, light bulb pieces, needles, cigarette butts, plaster, or burnt matches.

Pica is most common in children with developmental delays, and it can be dangerous and life threatening. Pica can lead to infection, gastrointestinal issues, lead poisoning, and other health problems, plus kids with the disorder can cause serious damage to their teeth.

When my children were toddlers, I worried a great deal about them putting nonfood items into their mouths, not because they might get sick, but because they might choke. I've seen so many children come to the hospital after swallowing things that they shouldn't have.

This is especially challenging when there's a wide age gap between children. It's difficult, for example, to keep my son's Legos away from my younger daughter. My son is a huge Lego fan, and he plays with his Legos all of the time. I am very consistent about telling my daughter not to put things into her mouth. And my son tries his hardest to quickly pick up any small parts that fall on the floor.

—*Aline T. Tanios, MD, a mom of nine- and three-year-old daughters and a seven-year-old son and a pediatric hospitalist at Arkansas Children's Hospital, in Little Rock*

❧

My older daughter didn't put much that wasn't food into her mouth. *Oh, this is so great,* I remember thinking.

Then my younger daughter was born. She put everything into her mouth. I've had to watch her carefully all of the time because of this and carefully consider what toys we got her. As my daughter got older, I explained to her the dangers of putting things into her mouth because she might choke. But it didn't help much.

Even now at three, my daughter still puts things into her mouth. We got the girls a Marble Run toy this past Christmas, and two days later I caught her with a marble in her mouth!

—*Cheri Wiggins, MD*

RALLIE'S TIP

My youngest son was especially curious and adventurous, and he would try to eat just about anything he could fit in his mouth until he was around three years old. Even at the age of four, he would still eat the dog's kibble if I didn't keep it out of his reach! I had to grow eyes in the back of my head and keep a constant watch on him to make sure that he didn't choke. Whenever I would take one of these nonfood items away from him, I'd remind him that it was "Yucky!" and not to be eaten.

If your toddler seems determined to munch on nonfood items, it's a good idea to discuss this issue with your pediatrician. In some cases, craving nonfood items can be a sign of a nutritional deficiency, and your doctor can check for that. It's wise to take your toddler to a pediatric dentist as well. The dentist can check to make sure that there's not a problem with her teeth that might cause her to want to chew on hard items.

Weaning Your Toddler from the Pacifier or Thumb

Dentists agree that using a pacifier or sucking a thumb isn't generally a problem, unless it goes on for a long period of time. Most children give up these habits on their own, but if your child is still using a paci or sucking a thumb at age three, it's a good idea to talk with your dentist or doctor. In extreme cases, your child might need to be fitted for a mouth appliance to correct any teeth problems.

∽

I believe there's a window of time, when a baby is around six months old, when it's easiest to wean him from a pacifier. Unfortunately, with my second child, I completely missed that window.

By the time my son was three years old, he had amassed a huge pacifier collection. He was able to dictate what color paci he wanted to use each day. My husband and I tried to take the pacifiers away, but our son would cry, and we'd give in.

In hindsight, we should have taken them away a lot sooner, cold turkey. I think my husband and I were the ones more addicted to the pacis, and how they soothed our son. If we had taken them all away at once, he'd have cried and gotten over it much more quickly.

—*Victoria McEvoy, MD, a mom who raised four children; a grandmom of six-, four-, and two-year-old grandsons; an assistant professor of pediatrics at Harvard Medical School; the medical director and chief of pediatrics at Mass General West Medical Group; and the author of* 24/7 Baby Doctor, *in Boston, MA*

I was always so happy that my daughter took to a pacifier, instead of sucking her thumb! You can't take a toddler's thumb away!

As my daughter neared her third birthday, I explained to her that her third birthday was the time to give up her nook. She very rationally accepted that, and on her birthday, she gave it up, cold turkey.

—*Christy Valentine, MD, a mom of a six-year-old daughter, a specialist in pediatrics and internal medicine, and the founder of the Valentine Medical Center, in Gretna, LA*

When I was in residency, a patient asked me how to get her pre-schooler to stop using a pacifier! At that moment, I resolved I wasn't going to have a four-year-old with a pacifier in his mouth. So that very day, I went home and had my son, who was a bit younger than one, quit the paci cold turkey. I was also concerned that at this age, my son could drop his pacifier, pick it up, and pop it back into his mouth, with-out me even seeing it to stop him to clean it first.

"You're not going to be a preschooler with a pacifier," I explained. My son resisted a bit, but not too much, and I held firm. Unfortunately (or maybe fortunately), when he turned one, he had a stomach bug, so I gave him the pacifier back to comfort him. But he had already forgot-ten about it and didn't know what to do with it!

—*Leena Shrivastava Dev, MD, a mom of 15- and 11-year-old sons, a general pediatrician, and an advocate for child safety, in Philadelphia, PA*

When my daughter was 2½ and I was pregnant with her brother, I really wanted her to give up her pacifier. It was around Christmas time, so we wrapped up her pacifier and left it with the milk and cookies for Santa on Christmas Eve. I explained to my daughter that Santa would take the pacifier and give it to a baby on Christmas.

In return, Santa left a gift for my daughter in the pacifier's place. It was a small stuffed animal that filled in nicely for the pacifier. My daughter cuddled with that stuffed animal instead of asking for her pacifier.

—*Jennifer Hanes, DO*

Only one of my children ever wanted a pacifier. But he didn't want to ever give it up! About two months before my son's third birthday, my husband and I told him that when he turned three, he'd be a big boy, and big boys don't use pacifiers. We made it into a game.

"What happens when you're three?" we'd ask.

"No more paci!" our son would exclaim.

On our son's birthday, he woke up with the pacifier in his mouth. When he came downstairs, we asked him, "What happens when you're three?"

"No more paci!" he yelled and whipped the pacifier triumphantly out of his mouth. We grabbed the paci, cheered, and that was the end of that. When my son asked for his pacifier at bedtime that night, we reminded him he was a big boy, and he believed it.

—Amy Baxter, MD, a mom of 14- and 12-year-old sons and a 9-year-old daughter; the CEO of Buzzy4Shots.com; and the director of emergency research, Scottish Rite, of the Children's Healthcare of Atlanta, in Georgia

Toddlers sometimes hang on to their pacifiers or to thumb-sucking—along with the soft items that are stroked along with the sucking, such as a twirled lock of their own hair, a blanket or bit of rag, or a stuffed toy—long beyond the time when their mothers feel that these habits are cute and sanitary. Impatience with these patterns is not really necessary however. These habits represent a transition from total dependency on the mother as the source of all comfort to the children's independent capacity to comfort themselves. Toddlers will relinquish these things on their own, with time, and there is no need to hurry the process along.

If the dentist states that the child's thumb-sucking is bad for the teeth, naturally there should be some active negotiation with the child about phasing out this habit and replacing it with another one that doesn't damage teeth. Otherwise, parents can make a tactful suggestion that the toddler might try leaving the pacifier or tattered blankie at home one day and see how it goes.

—Elizabeth Berger, MD

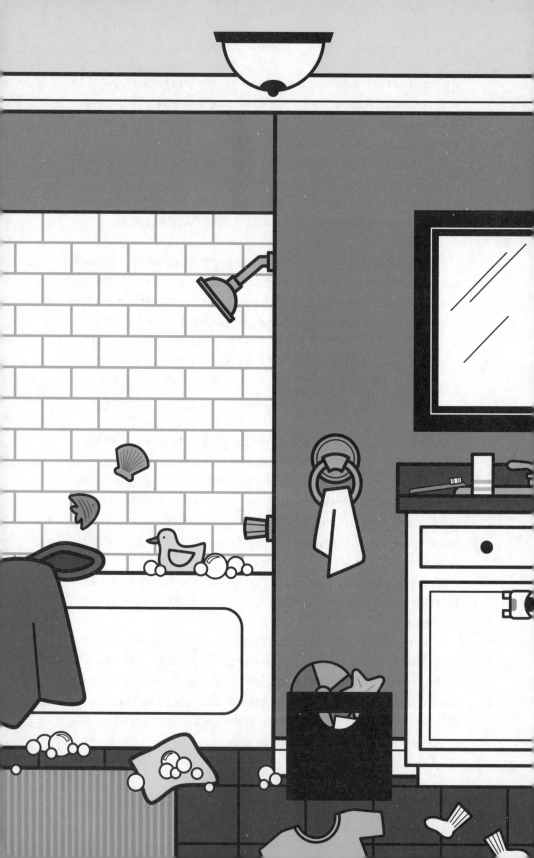

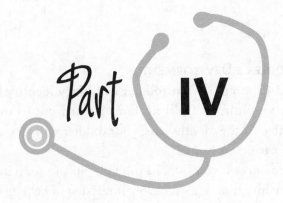

Part IV

BATHING AND GROOMING

Chapter 11
Bathing Safely

YOUR TODDLER'S DEVELOPMENT

By around 15 months, your toddler can likely identify his own reflection in a mirror. He'll no longer reach out to touch the "other" baby. As the months pass, your toddler will take a greater interest in caring for himself.

By around two years old, he might be able to wash his hands, if you show him how. He's probably interested in helping to bathe himself too. But it'll still be a while before you can delegate that task to him. And it'll definitely be a while before your child can be left in the tub unattended.

TAKING CARE OF YOU

By now you've given your toddler approximately 1,000 baths! Treat yourself to a bubble bath—or better yet, a spa day!

JUSTIFICATION FOR A CELEBRATION

When the time comes that your toddler doesn't cry or fuss while having his hair washed or his nails clipped, that'll be a great day!

Making Bathtime Safe and Fun

Bathtime can be a wonderful time to connect with your toddler. He's a totally captive audience, and you're sitting there at eye level. What a wonderful time to talk about the day and dream about the future. Enjoy these fun, quiet moments together.

ᴗ

Sometimes bathtime used to be a challenge with my daughter. She didn't want to stop playing to take a bath. Plus, she knew that after bathtime came bedtime!

My daughter loves music, and she enjoys watching *Sid the Science Kid*. On that show, they sing a catchy song, "It's rug time!" I modified that to "It's bathtime!" That makes my daughter giggle, and she's more willing to come take a bath. I try to make things fun for her.

—*Tanya Douglas Holland, MD, a mom of a two-year-old daughter, a women's health advocate, and a consultant in medical affairs to a pharmaceutical company, in Atlanta, GA*

ᴗ

I worried a great deal about drowning when my toddlers were in the bathtub. I was hyper vigilant, watching each one of them every second. This is especially important if there are older children in the tub too. They cannot be responsible for their younger siblings in the water. It only takes an instant for a toddler playing in a slippery tub to slide underwater.

—*Aline T. Tanios, MD, a mom of nine- and three-year-old daughters and a seven-year-old son and a pediatric hospitalist at Arkansas Children's Hospital, in Little Rock*

ᴗ

I gave my sons baths together for a really long time because it was so convenient and easy. Plus, it was safer because I knew where everyone was! You can never leave a toddler unattended in any water, even the tub.

Now my sons take showers, but occasionally they still take baths. I put a nonstick mat on the floor of the tub to prevent them from slipping.

—*Heather Orman-Lubell, MD, a mom of 11- and 7-year-old sons and a pediatrician in private practice at Yardley Pediatrics of St. Christopher's Hospital for Children, in Pennsylvania*

My son loves bathtime, and he's usually a step ahead of me, running to the tub when it's time for a bath. He's a happy camper when he's in the tub. As my son has become more mobile, bathtime has become more fun for him and more terrifying for me. I have a nonskid mat on the bottom of the tub, and we have a "bottoms down" rule. If his bottom doesn't stay down, he has to get out of the tub. To keep him from trying to turn on the real faucet, I bought a Flow 'N' Fill Spout. An unexpected bonus is that it keeps him from trying to pour water on the floor too.

—*Lennox McNeary, MD, a mom of a three-year-old son, a specialist in physical medicine and rehabilitation at Carilion Clinic, and a cofounder of the Mommy Doctors Bakery (makers of Milkin' Cookies), in Roanoke, VA*

I used to give my kids baths together, but I don't anymore. My son likes to play in the tub, and that often involves throwing bubbles into the air, which all too often would wind up in my daughter's eyes. To eliminate this problem, I give my daughter a bath first. Then while my husband or nanny puts her to bed, I give my son a bath. This gives him time to play in the tub. It also gives me nice one-on-one time with each of them.

—*Shilpa Amin-Shah, MD, a mom of a two-year-old son and a one-year-old daughter and an emergency physician at Emergency Medical Associates, in Livingston, NJ*

For my sons, I don't use bubble bath with fragrance. I don't use tear-free shampoo because that has fragrance in it too. I use fragrance-free products, such as California Baby. Also, I don't let my sons stay and play in the bathtub for too long. I get them in and out in five minutes, and then I apply moisturizer to their skin.

—*Amy J. Derick, MD, a mom of three-year-old and 19-month-old sons who's expecting another baby and a dermatologist in private practice at Derick Dermatology, in Barrington, IL*

∽

A child's skin is thinner than an adult's, and their skin-surface-to-body-volume ratio is much larger than ours. So their bodies have greater exposure to dangerous chemicals. You have to choose bath products very carefully. I knew I didn't need to use a lot of soap for my son, and the only places that really got dirty were his face (which I don't use soap for anyway), hands, scalp (he was quite the sweater and he actually smelled in the summer months!), feet, and diaper area. I bought a bottle of Burt's Bees Shampoo & Wash, and I never used more than a dollop the size of a quarter for his hair and body, so that one bottle lasted a really long time.

Another thing is that I never use a Q-tip to clean the inside of the ear canal (where it's pitch black and you can't see!). If you can't see, inserting a Q-tip is guaranteed to puncture something, like the eardrum. But always clean the *outside* of the ear canal, which is where earwax will sit as soon as the body extrudes it. Those folds are called the auricular folds, and it's perfectly safe to clean there. Another tip is to use a warm, wet jumbo cotton ball to clean the ear; it's simply too big to insert into the ear canal, but you can get it into those tiny ear grooves perfectly!

One thing I do use a Q-tip for is to clean my son's belly button. It's amazing how much dirt gets trapped there. I do it about once every week or so.

—*Cheryl Wu, MD, a mom of a four-year-old son, a pediatrician at LaGuardia Place Pediatrics in New York City, and a pediatric emergency physician at the Joseph M. Sanzari Children's Hospital of Hackensack University Medical Center, in New Jersey*

My daughter loves to take a bath. I think she'd stay in the tub forever if she could.

At this age, she's so small, it's practically like swimming. When I tell my daughter that it's time for her bath, she goes running up to the bathroom. I have to watch her very carefully because she wouldn't hesitate to hop right into the tub.

I know the exact spot between the hot and cold marks to set the faucet handle so that the water temperature is safe. I check it anyway with my hand before I let my daughter get in the bathtub. I fill the tub with water only up to my daughter's belly button. I sit right there next to the tub, of course, the entire time she's taking her bath. I bring my phone into the bathroom with me in case it rings.

We have a bunch of bathtub toys, but I only let my daughter play with a few of them at a time. I like to rotate them so she can have a variety, and I want to make sure there is enough room for her in the tub.

—*Rachel S. Rohde, MD, a mom of a one-year-old daughter, an assistant professor of orthopaedic surgery at the Oakland University William Beaumont School of Medicine, and an orthopaedic upper-extremity surgeon with Michigan Orthopaedic Institute, P.C., in Southfield, MI*

Keeping Bath Toys and Tub Clean

"Rubber Duckie, you're the one . . ." Yes, you make bathtime so much fun, right up until you start squirting out more black mildew than water. Eew. One would think the bathtub and bath toys would be self-cleaning (like the cat!), but oddly enough they're not.

My daughter has a lot of bath toys. After she's done in the tub, I rinse the toys off. I also rinse the tub out well. I worry about my daughter getting the chemicals from soaps and cleaners into her mouth.

—*Jennifer Bacani McKenney, MD, a mom of a one-year-old daughter and a family physician, in Fredonia, KS*

I wash our bathtub and tub toys each week with a bleach solution. The toys and the tub are often moist, providing the perfect environment for germs to grow. It's important to wash away any molds on toys that might cause skin infections in kids.

—*Aline T. Tanios, MD*

○○○

My son loves to play with old cups in the tub, so those just go right in the dishwasher. Foam letters go in a mesh bag in the washing machine. My favorite purchase was a set of tub crayons and paints. They're made of soap, so I can convince myself that we're actually cleaning him and the tub at the same time.

—*Lennox McNeary, MD*

○○○

I'm generally not fanatical about cleaning. In small doses, germs aren't such a bad thing. I love it that my daughter plays outside in the garden and even touches worms. I teach her not to eat dirt (or the worms), and I teach her about washing her hands. However, I draw the line on mold in tub toys! If I see that black mold inside a tub toy, I throw it away.

—*Lisa Campanella-Coppo, MD, a mom of a three-year-old daughter, an emergency physician, and the emergency department director of academic affairs at Monmouth Medical Center, in New Jersey*

RALLIE'S TIP

When my two youngest sons were toddlers, I was amazed at how quickly their toys took over the bathtub. They loved to drag their favorite toys into the tub at bathtime, and of course I had to leave the toys there afterward until they were dry. Because you can stack only so many toys on the sides of the tub, my husband and I were constantly tripping over boats, cars, and rubber snakes.

I finally bought a small plastic laundry basket to use as a bathtub toy container, and I would toss all the toys into the basket when the boys were finished with their baths. Then I would spray the toys and the tub with a little bleach water that I kept in the bathroom before rinsing everything under the shower. I'd leave the basket full of toys in the tub to drain and dry out overnight.

When it was time for me to get ready for work the next morning, I could just lift the mostly dry laundry basket full of toys out of the tub and take a shower without worrying that I was going to trip over a rubber duckie and kill myself.

Washing and Detangling Hair

Some things become easier as your child gets older. Washing his hair might not be one of them. Take heart in the fact that this stage won't last forever. Someday you'll be tearing your hair out about how long your teens spend fixing and fretting about their hair!

My daughter is unusual in that she loves to have her hair washed and combed. Perhaps it's because she's only one year old. She loves bathtime, and we always give her a good head massage with each washing.

My daughter has a lot of hair, and every morning it stands straight up. I have her watch me brush my hair, and then I hand her the brush. My daughter holds it up to her head in an attempt to brush her hair, and then I take it and gently brush her hair. I show her the finished product in the mirror, and she always laughs.

—*Jennifer Bacani McKenney, MD*

I wash my sons' hair every day. One son has straight hair, and one son has curly hair. I use California Baby Super Sensitive Shampoo on them.

To keep things simple, I use the same hair care products, such as detangler, on my sons that I use on myself.

—*Amy J. Derick, MD*

⁓⁓

I found that goggles are a great solution for the fear of hair washing. My children loved to put on goggles in the bathtub and explore their world. When my kids were wearing the goggles, they no longer feared having their hair rinsed.

—*Jennifer Hanes, DO, a mom of a six-year-old daughter and a three-year-old son, an emergency physician, a certified forensic physician, and the founder of Empowered Medicine, PLLC, in Austin, TX*

⁓⁓

Washing and detangling my girls' hair has been quite a challenge. My younger daughter has baby fine hair, so I rinse it with water every night but I only shampoo it about once a week. That cuts down on the battles. Now that my older daughter is six years old, I'm teaching her how to wash her own hair.

—*Cheri Wiggins, MD, a mom of six- and three-year-old daughters, a specialist in physical medicine and rehabilitation at St. Luke's Magic Valley, and the cofounder of the Mommy Doctors Bakery (makers of Milkin' Cookies), in Twin Falls, ID*

⁓⁓

One day, my older son put Children's VapoRub in his hair! He sees his dad put styling products in his hair, so he was imitating that. Fortunately, the VapoRub washed right out. That's a good lesson in the importance of keeping these sorts of things out of a child's reach!

—*Deborah Kulick, MD, a mom of two-year-old and eight-month-old sons, a child and adolescent psychiatrist at the Everett Teen Health Center, and an instructor in psychiatry at Harvard Medical School and the Cambridge Health Alliance, in Boston, MA*

⁓⁓

Although my son loves to take a bath, he hates to have his hair washed, especially if he gets soap in his eyes. When it's time to rinse his hair, I tilt his head way back and tell him to look up at the ceiling and close his eyes. Then I use a cup to carefully pour warm water over his head.

—*Lennox McNeary, MD*

Having Your Toddler's Hair Cut

Your experience having your toddler's hair cut can change with the wind. One haircut might be a fun, pleasant experience; the next one could be a nightmare. It pays to do some research ahead of time to find a salon that specializes in kids' cuts, or to find a stylist who has a knack for cutting kids' hair, or at least one who's fast.

~○~

My daughter has really pretty hair and a lot of it. I haven't had it cut yet. I sweep it off her face and put a bow in it to hold her hair back. We've been putting bows in her hair since she was just a few months old, so she's used to them by now and doesn't pull them out. She rarely goes out without something cute in her hair!

—*Jennifer Bacani McKenney, MD*

~○~

Having my girls' hair cut hasn't been too bad. We're not very fashionable people, so we all go together to an inexpensive hair cut chain in our town. It's fun, quick, and cheap, and my kids get a lollipop at the end to boot.

—*Cheri Wiggins, MD*

~○~

We live within walking distance of a neighborhood barber. It's like going back in time to the 1950s. We usually go there as a family, and I'm usually the only woman there.

All of my sons had their first haircuts there. It gets easier with each son because they watch their dad and their older brothers have their hair cut too.

—*Amy Thompson, MD, a mom of five- and three- and two-year-old sons and an ob-gyn at the University of Cincinnati College of Medicine, in Ohio*

I cut my kids' hair myself. I bought a pair of trauma shears; they're special scissors we use at the hospital. The way they're designed, they cut hair and clothing but not skin. You can find them online by searching for "trauma shears."

My kids' haircuts might not have looked great. But they also didn't cost the $30 the salon charged!

—*Jennifer Hanes, DO*

∽

I barely have time to get my own hair cut every few months, let alone take my son to have his hair cut every few weeks! To save time

MomMy TIME: Changing Your Hairstyle

Most nights you might be up to your elbows in bath bubbles getting your toddler's hair clean, but wouldn't it be nice to get some much-needed pampering while updating your own tresses?

One Marist Poll found that more than half of Americans haven't changed their hairstyle in the past couple of years, and as many as 29 percent haven't gotten a new look in more than 10 years.

Making a change can be fun, and you'll be doing yourself a favor if you choose a simple style that doesn't take much work in the mornings. Try one of the following chic cuts.

- **Long layers:** They add volume to one-length hair and frame your face.
- **A bob:** Make it straight or wavy, and keep in mind that it looks best when it's slightly longer in the front.
- **A pixie cut:** If you're daring enough to go super short, taking care of your hair doesn't get any easier.
- **Bangs:** They're a surefire way to look younger, but remember that they need trimming every three weeks, so you might want to ask how to trim them on your own in between salon visits.
- **Color:** Highlights add depth and dimension to your style, or go for an overall color to cover up pesky gray.

and emotional energy, I usually cut my son's hair myself. I put a towel on the den floor, turn on the TV to a special show, and then trim as much as he'll let me do in one sitting. Last year I decided that I'd take him for a professional haircut before we went to visit our families at Christmas. It didn't go well, and the haircut was awful. Now I'm back to doing it myself. His haircuts aren't perfect, but this method is far less traumatic for him—and for me.

—Lennox McNeary, MD

RALLIE'S TIP

My boys were all bald for what seemed like forever after they were born. I was so happy when they finally got hair that I waited a long time to have it cut by a professional. I trimmed their wispy baby hair until it grew in thick enough for me to botch it up.

My oldest son wanted to be a soldier like his grandfather, so when it was time to get his first real haircut, I told him he was going to get a Marine haircut, and that helped him to be brave.

My youngest two boys didn't have the same military aspirations as toddlers, and I had a little more trouble with them. I considered taking them to a salon that specialized in kids' haircuts, but the closest one was nearly 20 miles from my house. My husband and I decided to take the boys to his barber, because they had already been there a few times and they knew from experience that this particular barber had never hurt their dad or made him cry.

My middle son sat really still from the very first time and seemed to enjoy the experience. My youngest son, who has always been especially wriggly, was determined not to cooperate, and I didn't try to force it. I just asked the barber to do the best he could on a moving target in three minutes or less. As a result, my son didn't have a really good haircut until he was about four years old, but at least he didn't have a terrible experience, and he wasn't traumatized.

Fortunately, the barber was very kind and patient, and he made a game of cutting the boys' hair. He always gave them a sucker while they were sitting in his chair, and I have some really great photos of my boys' sticky, hair-coated fingers and faces!

Trimming Fingernails and Toenails

Young toddlers likely still squiggle and squirm when having their nails cut. Fortunately, as your toddler gets older, he'll start to understand that having one's nails trimmed is a necessary evil, it doesn't take long, and the less he fights, the sooner it'll be over and he can get back to playing. If all else fails, consider bribery.

❦

I keep my toddlers' nails clean and short. Bacteria can hide under dirty nails. Uncut nails can result in inadvertent scratches. One week, I got a little behind schedule on cutting my sons' nails, and both of my sons ended up with scratches on their noses.

—*Amy J. Derick, MD*

❦

When I need to cut my son's nails, I usually give him something to hold in his other hand. I set my expectations low, and I only try to cut the nails on one hand in a sitting. Then I cut the nails on his other hand the next day.

—*Michelle Davis-Dash, MD, a mom of a one-year-old son and a pediatrician, in Baltimore, MD*

❦

When I cut my son's fingernails and toenails, it's the perfect time to work on counting. I count each nail as I go, and I encourage him to count with me, either up from 1 to 10 or down from 10 to 1. The counting serves as a great distraction too.

—*Lennox McNeary, MD*

❦

Trimming toenails and fingernails is a challenge, even with my super easygoing toddler. I usually still try to do it when she's sleeping. But that doesn't always work, so I try to make it into a game. I pretend to clip my nails, and then I sneak in a trim of one of hers. I don't have high expectations: If I get one or two nails trimmed a night, that's good.

—*Jennifer Bacani McKenney, MD*

❦

Ever since my kids were babies, I kept to a schedule of trimming their fingernails and toenails each weekend. I usually sit down on the couch, and my kids all line up to have their nails trimmed. They sometimes lie on their backs on the floor and put their feet on my lap to get their toenails trimmed. It's amazing how fast kids' nails grow!

—*Sadaf T. Bhutta, MD, a mom of a six-year-old daughter and four-year-old triplets and an assistant professor and the fellowship director of pediatric radiology at the University of Arkansas for Medical Sciences and Arkansas Children's Hospital, both in Little Rock*

When my daughter was younger, trimming her nails was such a challenge that I would have to trim them while she was sleeping. Lucky for me, I now have a dainty little girl who always wants her nails painted like Mommy's. We change my daughter's nail polish weekly, and she knows that the only way I will paint her nails is if we trim them first. My daughter waits patiently while I cut her nails, and then she picks the color of quick-dry nail polish she wants. Since we started this, I have not had any problems cutting her nails.

—*Jeannette Gonzalez Simon, MD, a mom of three- and one-year-old daughters and a pediatric gastroenterologist in private practice, in Staten Island, NY*

Chapter 12
Diapering and Dressing

YOUR TODDLER'S DEVELOPMENT

By age two, your toddler is probably able to help to get herself dressed and undressed—quite possibly at inopportune moments. You'll probably need to help her to put on her pants until she's around four. Elastic waistbands help to simplify this for her, and they're especially helpful for potty training.

By around age three years, your toddler can probably put on her coat, though she might not be able to zip it. You might want to start teaching her how to tie her own shoes, though it'll be a while before she masters this skill. You could take the easy way out and buy shoes that fasten with Velcro!

TAKING CARE OF *YOU*

You've been working so hard buying, organizing, and cleaning your child's clothing and shoes for years now. It's a great time to treat yourself to something, such as a new outfit, pair of shoes, or a handbag. We love PonyUP! Kentucky, equestrian fashion with purpose and passion. Their unique, high-quality handbags are made in the United States, and a portion of all profits benefits retired and rescued horses in need. Their hobo handbags are the perfect I-don't-need-a-diaper-bag-anymore size! Check out their catalog at PonyUPKentucky.com.

JUSTIFICATION FOR A CELEBRATION

Your toddler put on her shoes without help? It's gonna be a great day!

Changing a Toddler's Diaper

Babies and toddlers use between 2,000 and 3,000 diapers a year. By now, you are an expert diaper changer. You can probably change your toddler's diaper in the dark, in back of your (parked!) car, in two seconds flat. But toddlers don't make it easy! When you're a toddler with so much to do, who has time for a diaper change? Come to think of it, when you're a *mom* with so much to do, who has time for a diaper change?

❧

Lawyers are fond of saying, "Never ask a question you don't already know the answer to."

With toddlers, I amend that to, "Never ask a question that could back you into a corner." So, for example, when I needed to change my toddler's diaper, I'd never ask, "Can I change your diaper?" Of course the answer to that question would be "No!"

Instead I tried to always ask questions that would generate the response I wanted. In this case, I'd ask something like, "Would you like me to change your diaper now, or in five minutes after you finish coloring that part of your picture?"

—*Cathy Marshall, MD, a mom of 28-, 14-, and 11-year-old daughters and a pediatrician in private practice, in Encino, CA*

❧

Changing a toddler's diaper can be difficult. My mother-in-law told me to change my toddlers' diapers on the floor. This way they can't roll off a changing table and get hurt.

To distract my son when I'm changing his diaper, I usually give him a toy to hold. I often enlist my older boys to entertain my youngest son when I change his diaper. My older son does remarkably well with that!

—*Amy Thompson, MD, a mom of five- and three- and two-year-old sons and an ob-gyn at the University of Cincinnati College of Medicine, in Ohio*

❧

It's challenging to change my toddler's diaper, especially when she has a diaper rash. Then she's extra fussy and wriggly. I feel bad because I know that it hurts to wipe her. When my daughter has a rash, we are extra careful to clean her gently.

Every time my daughter is on the changing table, I hand her something to play with like a toy or book. That way she's distracted, and we can maybe even do a little learning at the same time.

—Jennifer Bacani McKenney, MD, a mom of a one-year-old daughter and a family physician, in Fredonia, KS

⌐∽⌐

The key to changing a toddler's diaper is speed. My son was born prematurely, so I learned how to change his diaper when he was still in an isolette. I had to put my hands through portholes and maneuver around tubes and wires to change a diaper that was smaller than the palm of my hand. By the time my son was a toddler, I could change his diaper superfast, even while he still had his pajamas on, in the dark. With my eyes closed. (It's one of my hidden talents!)

—Lennox McNeary, MD, a mom of a three-year-old son, a specialist in physical medicine and rehabilitation at Carilion Clinic, and a cofounder of the Mommy Doctors Bakery (makers of Milkin' Cookies), in Roanoke, VA

Mommy MD Guides-Recommended Product
Pampers Cruisers

Rallie's Tip: Pampers were my favorite brand of diapers when my kids were babies and toddlers. The cheaper brands just weren't the same. They leaked, and they were scratchy. Instead of saving money buying cheaper diapers, I usually ended up wasting the money I had spent on them. I'm perfectly happy to buy generic versions of some items, but it just didn't pay to scrimp on diapers.

A toddler on the move can't be encumbered by a bulky, restrictive diaper. Pampers Cruisers have a three-way fit that allows for optimal movement while keeping the diaper leak free for up to 12 hours. A 27-pack of size 4 Cruisers costs around $10 at drugstores, supermarkets, and discount stores. Visit **PAMPERS.COM** for more information.

I've used cloth diapers for my younger three children. When they became toddlers, though, I had to simplify my system because toddlers don't want to lie still long enough to change a cloth diaper. When they were babies, I loved flat diapers, and I would experiment with different folds, pins, and Snappis. I swore by covers with Velcro closures. For an impatient toddler, I gave up on my "favorite" diaper folds, and I switched to a cover with snaps, because it makes it a little harder for a toddler to take it off.

—*Kristie McNealy, MD, a mom of nine- and six-year-old daughters and four-year-old and 22-month-old sons and a blogger at KristieMcNealy.com, in Denver, CO*

Preventing and Treating Diaper Rash

Diaper rash is more common in babies younger than a year old than in toddlers, but toddlers still can get diaper rashes. Parents of toddlers, having by now changed approximately 6,324 diapers, sometimes don't change their toddler's diaper as frequently, which can lead to a painful diaper rash.

∽

I used cloth diapers for my son, so I was lucky to have very little personal experience with treating diaper rash. When we used disposables on vacation, my son did develop a little diaper rash. At work, we use Calmoseptine on our adult patients with skin irritation. It works wonders on tiny tushies too.

—*Lennox McNeary, MD*

∽

The most important way to prevent diaper rash is to change diapers frequently. Of course, by the time a child is a toddler, parents are tired of changing diapers and want to stretch out the time between diaper changes.

My older son has been out of diapers since he was 2½, and I change my younger son's diapers frequently to minimize or prevent diaper rashes.

—*Amy J. Derick, MD, a mom of three-year-old and 19-month-old sons who's expecting another baby and a dermatologist in private practice at Derick Dermatology, in Barrington, IL*

Thankfully, we did not struggle with diaper rash too much, and I'm sure that's partially due to genetics and partially due to luck. When I changed my sons' diapers, I used hypoallergenic wipes when the kids went poop, but I only used warm water on a washcloth when they went pee. I also lubricated with Vaseline with each diaper change to help give the skin an extra barrier.

—*Mona Gohara, MD, a mom of five- and three-year-old sons, a dermatologist in private practice, an assistant clinical professor in the department of dermatology at Yale University, and a cofounder of K&J Sunprotective Clothing, in Danbury, CT*

My kids didn't have a lot of problems with diaper rash. I think that's because after every bath I slathered them up with Vaseline. It created a nice barrier between their skin and the diaper.

Diaper rash creams are great for helping diaper rash heal. But sometimes they can dry out the skin, which isn't as good as protecting healthy skin.

When I treat babies with diaper rashes, I recommend the moms put Maalox or Mylanta on their kids' diaper rashes caused by diarrhea. Simply moisten a cotton ball with the liquid and dab it on. It

Mommy MD Guides-Recommended Product

Triple Paste

"My daughter used to be very prone to diaper rash. I discovered Triple Paste, and that's now my go-to cream," says Shilpa Amin-Shah, MD, a mom of a two-year-old son and a one-year-old daughter and an emergency physician at Emergency Medical Associates, in Livingston, NJ.

When your toddler's behind is looking rosy more often than not, try soothing it with Triple Paste. It's a prescription-strength diaper rash cream that's gentle enough to use every day.

Two ounces cost around $9, and you can buy it at drugstores. For more information, visit TRIPLEPASTE.COM.

neutralizes the acid from the diarrhea. Make sure you label the bottle *only* for external use so there is no accidental diaper contamination the next time an adult has heartburn.

—*Jennifer Hanes, DO, a mom of a six-year-old daughter and a three-year-old son, an emergency physician, a certified forensic physician, and the founder of Empowered Medicine, PLLC, in Austin, TX*

I try to change my daughter's diapers very often to prevent rashes. I see a connection when I give my daughter a lot of fruit. I think the acidity of the fruit or fruit juice causes her to get a rash, so we are careful about how much fruit or juice she gets in a day. We also use Pampers Sensitive wipes.

When my daughter gets a diaper rash, I put Boudreaux's Butt Paste on it to keep it from getting worse. If her bottom is especially tender, we'll often wipe her gently and then put her right into the bath.

Boudreaux's Butt Paste treats diaper rash and chafed skin and protects your toddler's skin from diaper rash by sealing out moisture. It's available at drugstores and costs $3.85 for a two-ounce tube. For more information, visit ButtPaste.com.

—*Jennifer Bacani McKenney, MD*

When my daughter gets a diaper rash, I stop using wipes because they sting. Instead, I wipe her skin with a washcloth soaked in warm water and then put her diaper on.

If we're going to be home, I actually let her roam free sans diaper. The open air helps to dry out and heal the diaper rash.

—*Shilpa Amin-Shah, MD, a mom of a two-year-old son and a one-year-old daughter and an emergency physician at Emergency Medical Associates, in Livingston, NJ*

Buying Clothing

It's amazing how quickly babies outgrow those tiny zero-to-three-month clothes, three-to-six-month clothes, and then six-to-nine-month clothes. Toddlers' growth slows, though, and so you'll get to spend a lot more time with your child's one year, 2T, and 3T clothes. That's less work for you, and it puts a whole lot less strain on the pocketbook too.

❧

When my daughter was a toddler, she was very into pink, so much so that if she wore another color, people who know her well would comment on it, "Wow, no pink today?" I actually got some criticism from other mothers about it. I chose to ignore them. My daughter is happy; let her wear all the pink she wants!

—*Dina Strachan, MD, a mom of a six-year-old daughter, a dermatologist and director of Aglow Dermatology, and an assistant clinical professor in the department of dermatology at New York University, in New York City*

❧

I'm not a clothes person, so my goal is to dress my kids comfortably. Even for day care, I dressed my kids in soft, comfortable clothing, such as clothes made from cotton. Even though my younger girls are twins, I didn't dress them alike. I take a very low-stress approach to dressing, and I just bought them easy-to-wear clothing.

—*Susan Wilder, MD, a mom of a 17-year-old daughter and twin 13-year-old girls, a primary care physician, and the founder and CEO of Lifescape Medical Associates, in Scottsdale, AZ*

❧

My daughter's cousins are 5½ and 2 years old, so we've been fortunate to receive a lot of their outgrown clothing. My daughter is starting to catch up with the two-year-old in clothing size, though.

I buy a lot of clothing at Target and Marshall's. I buy my daughter's clothing on sale, a year or two ahead. It's hard to pay $25 for a dress that I know she'll outgrow in a month!

—*Rachel S. Rohde, MD, a mom of a one-year-old daughter, an assistant professor of orthopaedic surgery at the Oakland University William Beaumont School of Medicine, and an orthopaedic upper-extremity surgeon with Michigan Orthopaedic Institute, P.C., in Southfield, MI*

On my daughter's first day of preschool, I dressed her in comfortable clothing—jeans and a T-shirt. Turns out the other parents dressed *their* kids in $800 French dresses bought on Madison Avenue! I overheard another parent comment on my daughter's clothing, "I can't believe someone sent her daughter to school in *those* clothes."

I continued to dress my daughter in comfortable clothes so that she could paint and play. Her clothes were still expensive NYC clothes. They were purchased in a boutique but were not over the top.

—Debra Jaliman, MD, a mom of a 20-year-old daughter, a dermatologist in private practice, and an assistant professor of dermatology at Mt. Sinai School of Medicine, in New York City

When my twins were toddlers, I was ridiculous about clothing. I dressed them alike like doll babies in all-matching clothes. I was *that* twins' mom. I loved to dress my kids in their fancy church clothes and take their pictures.

Of course, my kids had comfortable play clothes too. I bought a lot of them at Target and the Gap. I also went to consignment stores, and I found a lot of great deals there. We have a local twins club that has a consignment sale. I could even find matching, inexpensive, gently used outfits there! I sold some of my twins' clothes on consignment too, so I could feed my obsession with matching clothes! I could only do that for so long, so I enjoyed it while it lasted.

—Ann Contrucci, MD, a mom of 13-year-old boy-girl twins who works as a pediatric emergency physician, in Atlanta, GA

Getting Your Toddler Dressed

Before your child turned a year old, she was probably helping you to help her get dressed. For example, she'd probably hold her arm out to help put on her shirt. Sometime between 13 and 20 months, your toddler will probably figure out how to take off her own clothes. This is helpful at home, not so helpful at the grocery store. It could make for some funny stories to share with her friends when she's a teenager. When your toddler is around 20 months old, she'll probably be able to put on loose-fitting clothing herself. She might not be able to dress herself completely until she's around three years old.

⁓

I think the key to the toddler years is giving toddlers choices with limits. For example, I'd never send my toddler to his closet to pick out an outfit! Instead I get out two shirts, and I ask him, "Do you want to wear this shirt or that shirt?" Toddlers are all about autonomy. That's wonderful, but if you give them too many choices, they will drive you bananas.

> —*Deborah Gilboa, MD, a mom of nine-, seven-, five-, and three-year-old sons, a parenting speaker whose advice is found at AskDoctorG.com, and a family physician with Squirrel Hill Health Center, in Pittsburgh, PA*

⁓

When my daughters were toddlers, they had strong opinions about everything, including what they wanted to wear. I was careful to use language that was nonadversarial to them. I also gave them choices.

"Would you like to wear this outfit, or that one?" I'd ask. That way they got to choose, but either way, they were wearing something acceptable to me.

> —*Cathy Marshall, MD*

⁓

People by nature like choices, and toddlers are no exception. Whenever possible, I gave my toddlers choices on how they wanted to get dressed.

"Would you like to put your shirt on first or your pants?" I'd ask, for example. Whichever my toddler chose, I was happy.

> —*Dana S. Simpler, MD, a mom of 25- and 20-year-old girls and a 23-year-old son and a specialist in internal medicine in private practice, in Baltimore, MD*

⁓

One of the biggest challenges I have with my toddlers is their desire to be independent. For example, they don't want to get dressed in the morning. They want to be off doing something else.

Just this morning, I was trying to get my younger son dressed.

He had his toothbrush in one hand, and he did not want to let that toothbrush go. I tried to explain to him that it was very difficult to take his pajamas off and put his T-shirt on while he was holding onto that toothbrush. This good logic got me nowhere. I had to take the toothbrush out of my son's hand, set it down, quickly swap out the pjs for the shirt, and then give him the toothbrush back.

The good thing is that I know this phase won't last forever. My older son already is able to understand logic like this. He would

When to Call Your Doctor

Children start being able to dress and undress themselves around age three, progressing to being able to dress without help at around age four. However, your child will master a developmental skill like dressing at her own pace, so don't be worried if your child is taking longer.

Instead, consider all of the signs of a developmental delay. Call your doctor if your child has any of the following signs by age three or four.

- Won't dress, use the toilet, or sleep on her own
- Doesn't throw a ball overhead
- Can't jump in place
- Isn't able to ride a tricycle
- Doesn't hold a crayon between thumb and fingers
- Isn't scribbling or copying a circle
- Can't stack four blocks
- Doesn't want to play interactive games
- Doesn't interact with other children
- Doesn't engage in fantasy play
- Clings and cries when separating from parents
- Won't respond to people who aren't family members
- Doesn't show self-control when she's upset
- Isn't talking in sentences with more than three words
- Doesn't use the words "me" and "you" properly

simply move the toothbrush to his other hand or put it down until we are done.

—*Sharon Boyce, MD, a mom of three- and one-year-old sons and a family physician at DayOne Family Healthcare Clinic, in Battle Creek, MI*

ೋ

My daughter is learning how to dress herself. She can put on her socks, but she still needs help with her pants and shirt. Sometimes, my daughter tries to play the cutesy card to get me to help her get dressed. But at this age, I'm really starting to encourage her to dress herself.

"You can do it! I know you can!" I tell my daughter to encourage her to try to dress herself.

Getting my daughter undressed for her bath can be a bigger struggle. She knows all too well that after bath comes bed! To make getting undressed fun, I positioned the clothes hamper in a corner. When I take my daughter's clothes off, I make a big to-do out of having her toss the clothes into the hamper like she's shooting a basket.

"Swish! Two points!"

—*Tanya Douglas Holland, MD, a mom of a two-year-old daughter, a women's health advocate, and a consultant in medical affairs to a pharmaceutical company, in Atlanta, GA*

Washing and Organizing Clothes

With a toddler who's trying to feed herself, doing arts and crafts, playing outside, and potty training (with an accident here and there), you might be considering buying stock in Procter & Gamble. Toddlers generate a lot of laundry.

Here's some good news: In a few years, your child will have the ability to match up socks and the desire to help out around the house. These are great tasks to delegate!

If you're still washing your toddler's clothes separately with baby detergent, you might want to give your family's soap a try now. Wash one item of your toddler's clothes in your regular laundry detergent. Pajamas are a great bet because they're easy to remember. Let your toddler wear those for a few nights and watch her for a skin reaction. If her skin turns red or develops a rash, keep using the baby detergent. If not, you can wash everyone's clothes together now, saving both money and time.

～◌～

With kids, the laundry just never ends. I feel like I'm constantly doing laundry. Especially when my kids were toddlers, and especially when they were potty training, I did at least a load of laundry each day to keep up with it.
—*Ann Contrucci, MD*

～◌～

I try to maintain our simple approach to clothing. Once someone gave one of my daughters a dress that was dry-clean only.

Are you kidding me? I thought.

If it's not machine washable, it's not worth it.

For washing clothes, I buy products that are fragrance free and hypoallergenic. I feel there are too many chemicals in our environment that are potentially harmful. I never use air fresheners or petroleum-based sprays either. I think they are poison.
—*Susan Wilder, MD*

Mommy MD Guides-Recommended Product
All Free Clear

"My kids have sensitive skin, so I launder my entire family's clothing in All Free Clear," says Amy J. Derick, MD, a mom of three-year-old and 19-month-old sons who's expecting another baby and a dermatologist in private practice at Derick Dermatology, in Barrington, IL. "I don't use any dryer sheets or fabric softener. These products can be irritating to dry or sensitive skin."

All Free Clear doesn't contain perfumes or dyes, is hypoallergenic, and shouldn't irritate skin. You can buy a 50-ounce container of All Free Clear, which will last 32 loads, at supermarkets and Target, Walmart, and Kmart for about $8. Visit **ALL-LAUNDRY. COM/FREECLEAR** for more information and coupons.

My secret weapon against dirt and germs is bleach. And my favorite, surprising, tip is that I buy my kids as much white clothing as I can. It sounds counterintuitive, but I can bleach white clothes, but not colored ones.

I also use a bleach solution to clean other areas of my house, such as my kitchen countertops. I think people sometimes think that bleach isn't safe. But actually it's very safe, safer in fact than some products that are marketed as "natural." Bleach is also inexpensive.

—*Jennifer Hanes, DO*

Once my son was old enough to find his own clothes in drawers, the drawers turned to chaos in seconds. I bought a sweater hanger that attaches to the bar in my son's closet with Velcro. It has five cubbies, so I use one for short-sleeved T-shirts, one for long-sleeved T-shirts, one for shorts, one for sweaters, and one for swimsuits. I find this makes it easier to see what he has, and it keeps things neater.

—*Lennox McNeary, MD*

Buying and Organizing Shoes

It's important to buy properly fitting shoes for your child. The bones and cartilage in a child's foot aren't fully developed until age five. While the foot is developing, the cartilage can be affected by badly fitting shoes.

Does your young toddler have flat feet? That's because babies' feet don't have arches. When a child is around two years old, the arches in her foot start to develop.

Toddlers who are just learning to walk need all the help they can get. Consider buying shoes with bendable rubber soles that grip the floor and also let your toddler "feel" the ground beneath her feet. Steer clear of open-toed shoes and backless ones, which can be tripping hazards. Toddlers need the support of shoes that surround the entire foot.

By 27 months, your toddler can probably take off her own shoes. Good luck trying to get her to put them back on the right feet!

My cousin gave my daughter a pair of Faded Glory boots from Walmart that came with one of the best inventions ever. The soles of the shoes are made of a transparent material under the toe. If I peek at the bottom of my daughter's boots, I can tell if the boots fit her or not. I can't believe no one ever thought of doing that before!

—*Jennifer Bacani McKenney, MD*

I keep a shoe rack at our back door. From a very early age, my son learned to to plop down on the floor, take his shoes off, and put them on the rack as soon as we came inside. Now I've even trained him to put my shoes on the shoe shelf. Success!

—*Lennox McNeary, MD*

To keep our family's shoes and boots tidy and to prevent them from getting lost, I put a large canvas bin right inside our front door. We put all of our shoes and boots in that bin.

This works very well because we pretty much always know where our shoes are, so we're not searching for them when we're getting ready to go somewhere. Plus, even my toddler can walk around the house, gather up any stray shoes, and toss them into the bin.

—*Rebecca Reamy, MD, a mom of seven- and two-year-old sons and a pediatrician in emergency medicine at Children's Healthcare of Atlanta, in Georgia*

By the time my kids reach adult size, shoes are going to make us broke. I buy my kids new shoes seasonally, at least twice a year. Even though my sons are triplets, they all wear different shoe sizes, so they can't share shoes.

I have a no-shoe-wearing policy in my home. I started it when my kids were babies because I didn't like the idea of them crawling around on the floor where we had walked with our shoes on. When we get home, we all take our shoes off in the mudroom. I bought an inexpensive basket for each member of our family, and then I labeled the baskets with our names. I keep the baskets in the same location. This way, even before my kids could read their names, they knew which shoe basket was theirs. Everyone knows to put their shoes into their basket, and then everyone knows where to find their shoes!

—*Sadaf T. Bhutta, MD, a mom of a six-year-old daughter and four-year-old triplets and an assistant professor and the fellowship director of pediatric radiology at the University of Arkansas for Medical Sciences and Arkansas Children's Hospital, both in Little Rock*

Anytime it crosses my mind that my sons have outgrown their shoes, I check, usually by taking my boys to a shoe store to have their feet measured. My husband believes that the shoe store's answer will always be, "Yes, they need new shoes." But actually that didn't always happen. I think the key is that you have to find a reputable shoe store!

When my sons were younger, I bought them each several different pairs of shoes, to match with different outfits. Once my sons were toddlers, I streamlined this so each boy has a pair of tennis shoes to wear with everything and a pair of sandals for summer.

I pass shoes down from son to son, unless the shoes are in really deplorable condition. Then I throw them out.

—*Amy Thompson, MD*

I try not to take my toddler into shoe stores—at least grown-up shoe stores—because she'll always find the five-inch heels, try them on, and admire herself in the mirror. Other people in the store find it adorable. Meanwhile, I'm chasing after my daughter, picking up her little shoes and socks that she has flung off.

To avoid this scenario, I measure my daughter's feet at home, and I either order her shoes online or make sure we take a family trip to the shoe store so Daddy can keep my daughter entertained while I actually buy her shoes.

—*Jeannette Gonzalez Simon, MD, a mom of three- and one-year-old daughters and a pediatric gastroenterologist in private practice, in Staten Island, NY*

Mommy MD Guides-Recommended Product
Stride Rite Shoes

Fitting kids' shoes can be stressful. To make this task easier, Stride Rite's toddler shoes now come with removable insoles that show you where your child's toes should hit so you know when you need to replace them. What a simple, wonderful idea.

You can buy Stride Rite's shoes in Stride Rite stores and at STRIDERITE.COM.

RALLIE'S TIP

My two youngest sons were toddlers at the same time, so we usually had a lot of little shoes scattered around the house. On those rare occasions when I was on top of my housework, I kept all of the boys' shoes in a basket in their room. I kept the basket on the floor right next to their dresser, instead of in their closet. That way, my boys wouldn't have to open the closet door to put their shoes away. They could just toss them into the basket whenever I could talk them into helping me clean up. When it was time to get dressed, they could pull matching shoes out of the basket and bring them to me so we could put them on.

I love baskets, because it's really easy to throw things in them without any special sorting or stacking, and unlike drawers, you can see what's in a basket at a glance. I'm probably trying to make excuses for my lack of organizational skills, but I really believe that using baskets helped my toddlers be more independent, and it engaged them in a few problem-solving tasks. In the case of their shoes, they could put their shoes "away" and get them out of the basket when they were ready to wear them with little or no help from me or my husband. When they found one of their shoes in the basket, they'd have to solve the brainteaser of finding the matching shoe to make a pair. As toddlers, they weren't ready to open heavy dresser drawers or closet doors, but they could easily rummage through a basket on the floor.

I kept a plastic bag in my laundry room for all the shoes and clothes that my sons couldn't wear anymore. As soon as I found that they had outgrown a shirt or a pair of shoes, I'd carry those items into the laundry room and put them in the bag. When the bag was full, I'd toss it in the car and drop it off at the Goodwill store or the Salvation Army on my way to work. This system helped me keep the clutter in my boys' room to a minimum, and it also helped cut down the number of face-offs my boys and I had when they insisted on wearing a shirt or a pair of shoes that simply did not fit. Even better, most of the clothes and shoes that my boys outgrew were still in good shape, and I was happy knowing that some other toddler could put them to good use.

Keeping Your Toddler Warm in Winter and Cool in Summer

Toddlers are full of lots of things—fun and mischief come to mind—but common sense isn't one of them! It's critical that parents watch out for temperature, to make sure toddlers are warm enough in the winter and cool enough in the summer.

Toddlers develop hypothermia faster than older children and adults. Plus, if their clothing gets wet—such as when playing in the snow—their body temperature will drop quickly. In the wintertime, if the wind chill is 32°F or higher, it's probably okay to play outside, as long as your child is dressed in layers, with a hat and mittens. If the wind chill dips between 13°F and 31°F, play outside very cautiously. If the wind chill drops to below 13°F, it's not safe to play outside. Bring everyone inside to warm up with a cup of cocoa!

Because you can take off only so many layers, it can be harder to keep kids cool in summer than warm in winter. Once you've dressed your toddler in lightweight clothing, be sure to cool her from the inside out with plenty of cool water to drink. If you're playing actively outside, such as playing tag, have her drink five ounces—10 big gulps—every hour or so.

∽◦

I believe with toddlers you have to choose your battles wisely. My older son never wants to wear his coat. Rather than arguing, I dress him in warm clothes, such as sweaters and turtlenecks. When we go out, I bring his coat along. As long as I get a great parking spot close to our destination, I don't fight him. Fortunately, we've had a very mild winter!

—*Amy Thompson, MD*

❦

My son loves to play outside in the cold, and he never seems to get chilled. When he was a toddler, he never wanted to wear his coat. I took a bunch of his favorite warm baby blankets, and I had them made into a patch coat. My son loved that coat, and he wore it quite willingly until he outgrew it.

—*Teresa Hubka, DO, a mom of a 14-year-old son and an 8-year-old daughter, an ob-gyn and the medical director of Comprehensive Wellness Care in Chicago, and an associate professor of obstetrics and gynecology and the chairman and residency program director of the department of obstetrics and gynecology at the Midwestern University/Chicago College of Osteopathic Medicine, in Downers Grove, Illinois*

? When to Call Your Doctor

Frostbite happens when your child's skin, usually on the fingers and toes, becomes frozen from being out in the cold too long. If you notice your child's fingers, toes, ears, lips, or nose become pale, gray, and blistered and if your child complains that her skin is burning or feels numb, bring her inside at once.

The American Academy of Pediatrics says to soak a child's hands or feet in warm water (instead of hot water) or place washcloths soaked in warm water on her nose, ears, or lips without rubbing the frozen areas. After a few minutes, dry the areas, put warm clothing and blankets on your child, and give her something warm to drink. If the numbness doesn't go away after a few minutes, call your doctor.

Keeping my son warm in winter has been a challenge. He doesn't believe in wearing jackets, and he often pitches a fit if I try to put his jacket on before we go outside. So I don't fight it. I ask if he wants to wear his jacket or carry it. If he chooses to carry it, I let him know it's available anytime he wants to wear it. If the temperature is in the single digits, though, I pull rank and make him wear it.

My son also didn't like to wear a hat, but our nanny bought him a really cool one. He'll wear that one without complaint.

—*Lennox McNeary, MD*

In the wintertime, I always layer my daughter's outfits. I will usually put an extra onesie under my daughter's clothes. I don't snap it; I just put it on her for an extra layer of warmth.

My daughter doesn't mind wearing coats and hats. If I put a hat on her, she'll wear it all day, inside and outside the house.

To organize all of my daughter's little hats and mittens, I have baskets on her dresser. This way I don't have to match anything up; I just throw them into the baskets.

—*Jennifer Bacani McKenney, MD*

One of the easiest ways I find to keep my son warm in winter is to dress him in long-sleeved onesies. They are also great for in-between seasons: I put a long-sleeved onesie under a short-sleeved T-shirt, and it's easy to pull off the T-shirt when the day warms up.

—*Michelle Davis-Dash, MD, a mom of a one-year-old son and a pediatrician, in Baltimore, MD*

My daughter loves to wear sandals. This is great in summer, not so great in winter. I try to be flexible and let her wear sandals when possible. But on cold days, I have to say, "No, we're not going to wear sandals today. Maybe another day!"

—*Tanya Douglas Holland, MD*

My daughter is little enough that she can run around the house in summer with only her diaper on. But when we go outside in summer,

When to Call Your Doctor

When your child is active in very hot temperatures and she becomes dehydrated, she's at risk for heatstroke. When that happens, a child's brain isn't able to control her body temperature, and she needs immediate medical attention.

Call 911 if your child has the following signs or symptoms.
- A fever of 105°F or higher after exercising in the heat
- Sweating stops and your child's skin is hot, dry, and flushed
- Dizziness
- Nausea
- Stomach cramps
- Rapid breathing

After calling 911, undress your child and place her in a cool bath. (Be sure the water is cool, not cold.) Massage her arms, legs, and body to help with circulation.

I make sure to keep her covered, or in the shade. I take her for a lot of walks in the stroller, and I put the stroller shade up so the sun stays off of her.

—*Jennifer Bacani McKenney, MD*

We have a small blow-up pool we keep in our backyard, and when it's hot, I take my son for a dunk in the pool. We empty the pool and hang it on a hook on a wall when not in use.

Also, I always keep glasses of water nearby. I encourage my son to take a drink very often. Kids are so interested in playing that they can forget to drink and get overheated. I also like to have lots of fresh fruit around for him. That's a good way to keep him well hydrated.

—*Lennox McNeary, MD*

Chapter 13
Potty Training

YOUR TODDLER'S DEVELOPMENT

As your toddler approaches his second birthday, you're probably thinking about potty training. Truth be told, you've probably been *thinking* about it for quite a while, but now you can realistically start it.

Many children are ready to be toilet trained after their second birthday. Boys tend to be ready slightly later than girls. A good time to start is when your toddler is past the "no" stage of toddlerhood and into the "parent pleasing" stage, where he wants to please you and be like you. This often happens when a child is between 18 and 24 months.

TAKING CARE OF YOU

An all-too-common "symptom" of motherhood is urinary incontinence. If you've been having a problem with leaking, such as when you lift something or laugh, cough, or sneeze, talk with your doctor about it. Physicians can offer a variety of ways to help. For example, your doctor might suggest reducing caffeine or prescribe medication. She might suggest wearing a pessary, which is a device inserted into the vagina that puts pressure on the urethra. In some cases, surgery might resolve the problem.

JUSTIFICATION FOR A CELEBRATION

No more diapers! Less money spent on diapers = more money for much more fun things!

Timing Potty Training Right

Ask 62 doctors when the right time is to potty train, and you'll get 62 different answers. We know; we did! You're the expert on your toddler, and you will know when the time is right for your toddler, for you, and for your family to potty train. Whenever you begin, it's comforting to know that it really doesn't matter in the grand scheme of things when your toddler started—and finished—potty training.

Here are a few signs of readiness to watch for.

- Your toddler's bowel movements occur on a fairly regular basis and a predictable schedule.
- Your toddler's diaper stays dry for at least two hours at a time during the day or is dry after naps.
- He can—and will—follow simple instructions.
- He shows an interest in using the potty.
- He gives you clues that he knows that he has to "go."
- Your toddler can walk to the bathroom and can pull his pants down.

My son is 2½, and we just started potty training. He's at the point now that he tells me when he peed in his diaper and asks for a diaper change. He doesn't like the way the wet diaper feels against his skin, so we thought this was the perfect opportunity to start potty training.

—*Shilpa Amin-Shah, MD, a mom of a two-year-old son and a one-year-old daughter and an emergency physician at Emergency Medical Associates, in Livingston, NJ*

It's a shame: I think a lot of parents feel pressured to potty train their kids because of preschool and day care rules. The parents in turn pressure the toddlers to potty train before they are ready. This is traumatic for everyone involved.

I waited to really work on potty training until my daughter was three. At that age, she was much more aware of when she needed to use the potty. That helped a lot.

—*Christy Valentine, MD, a mom of a six-year-old daughter, a specialist in pediatrics and internal medicine, and the founder of the Valentine Medical Center, in Gretna, LA*

I think the biggest mistake parents make with potty training is that they start before the kids are ready. This is frustrating for everyone, and it makes the process take three times as long.

I found that if I waited until my sons had the words to tell me if they were dry or if they had to go, potty training was a pretty easy process. But if you start too early, before your toddler can express those things to you, the parents are being trained, not the kids. The parents are going through the motions, but the kids aren't actually learning.

It's also important to begin potty training at a time that's good for you. If you have a really crazy schedule and aren't going to be home much, that's not the time to begin. On the other hand, if you have a week off from work and your toddler seems ready, that might be a great time.

—*Heather Orman-Lubell, MD, a mom of 11- and 7-year-old sons and a pediatrician in private practice at Yardley Pediatrics of St. Christopher's Hospital for Children, in Pennsylvania*

Potty training is a huge rite of passage and also a major milestone. One of the most important things I found is that the parent has to be ready for it, perhaps even more than the toddler. Talk with friends who have kids, your pediatrician, and even your own parents to get yourself prepared.

Then when you're ready, talk with your toddler about it. It helps to watch videos and read books to get excited about it. Make it into a family project by going together to buy the potty. Then when your toddler is ready to start using the potty, encourage him by saying things like, "Big boys use the potty. You're becoming a big boy!"

—*Eva Ritvo, MD, a mom of 21- and 16-year-old daughters, a psychiatrist, and a coauthor of* The Beauty Prescription, *in Miami Beach, FL*

My four kids have all potty trained at different ages. It's been all over the map. Generally, I haul out the potty when they're 18 months old. I let them sit on it and get used to it being there. No pressure at all! I start to talk about actually using the potty and potty training once they start to show an interest in it.

My youngest son will probably be the earliest one potty trained. The problem is he doesn't want to go in the bathroom. He just finds a spot on the floor! When I hear the little unsnapping sound of his pants, I come running!

—*Kristie McNealy, MD, a mom of nine- and six-year-old daughters and four-year-old and 22-month-old sons and a blogger at KristieMcNealy.com, in Denver, CO*

༄

Potty training my twins went really well. I admit part of this might have been luck. I believe potty training is all about the toddler's control. The toddler will be ready when he's ready.

I was very relaxed about potty training, not in a hurry at all. When my twins were twoish, I bought a potty seat. My twins liked to sit on it with their clothes on.

"This is where you can go pee and poopy," I'd casually say. But I never pushed.

One day when my daughter was almost 2½, she announced, "I want to wear big-girl panties." So we all went to Target to buy them. When we got home, my daughter put them on, and that was pretty much it. She potty trained herself.

At Target, my son had expressed interest in the Buzz Lightyear underwear, so I bought some for him. Two days after his twin sister, he told me he wanted to wear them. That was it; I pretty much did nothing. Potty training was up to them, no stress, no problems. I think it's another one of those issues where if parents will just stay calm and not get in a power struggle, it will happen with little difficulty. I was confident they would not go to college (or even elementary school) not potty trained!

—*Ann Contrucci, MD, a mom of 13-year-old boy-girl twins who works as a pediatric emergency physician, in Atlanta, GA*

There's a wide range of normal in the age that kids potty train. My kids are close in age, and my son potty trained a little later than usual, and my daughter a little earlier, so I potty trained them at the same time.

My son just didn't want to potty train. I tried to reward him with M&M's, and I put Cheerios in the potty as targets, but nothing worked.

My daughter, on the other hand, would take a book into the bathroom and sit on the potty and read! Pretty soon, my son was wondering, *What's the big deal? What am I missing?* So he started to do it too.

—*Antoinette Cheney, DO, a mom of a seven-year-old son and a six-year-old daughter and a family physician with Rocky Vista University College of Osteopathic Medicine, in Parker, CO*

Tricks and Techniques

Toddlers take many different roads to potty training—some short and some that will have *you* asking, "Are we there yet?"

I bought my daughter a Dora the Explorer potty chair. I put it in the bathroom for her to look at and to get used to having it around.

My daughter likes to pretend everything is a hat, and the potty chair is no exception. Of course, right now it's brand-new and perfectly clean!

—*Rachel S. Rohde, MD, a mom of a one-year-old daughter, an assistant professor of orthopaedic surgery at the Oakland University William Beaumont School of Medicine, and an orthopaedic upper-extremity surgeon with Michigan Orthopaedic Institute, P.C., in Southfield, MI*

We just started my son potty training. We have good days and bad days. My son is starting to get the whole idea of potty training.

We take our son to the bathroom every hour or so to sit for a couple of minutes. We don't force him; he decides how long he wants to stay there. When our son goes on the potty, we reward him with an M&M.

—*Shilpa Amin-Shah, MD*

When my toddlers were potty training, I took them to the bathroom every hour or two, and I gave them rewards just for participating. In time, they *will* be successful, and they'll go on the potty. At this point, you just want to keep them in the game. I would give my toddlers a small sticker just for trying. Sometimes I gave them glow-in-the-dark stars to put on their bedroom ceilings. This gave them a very visual sign of how well they were doing.

—*Cathy Marshall, MD, a mom of 28-, 14-, and 11-year-old daughters and a pediatrician in private practice, in Encino, CA*

Certainly, you don't want to punish your child when he's toilet training. You want him to think of going on the potty as a happy experience. It's easy to get frustrated, though, and kids pick up on that right away.

One thing that worked for my kids was rewarding them with M&M's. I gave one M&M if they peed on the potty and two M&M's if they pooped on the potty.

—*Eva Mayer, MD, a mom of an eight-year-old daughter and a six-year-old son and a pediatrician with St. Luke's Pediatrics Associates, in Bethlehem, PA*

Mommy MD Guides-Recommended Product
Potty Tots

By the third potty accident of the morning, who doesn't wish for some help in the potty training department? Wish granted. For $19.95, you can buy a potty training kit from Potty Tots for a girl or a boy that includes a story book, animated DVD with songs and music videos, an illustrated potty chart, and even a toilet bowl game. If you don't want the whole kit, Potty Tots offers potty charts for $4.95 each and books and DVDs for $5.95 each that teach kids the six steps of potty training. Here's a cool feature: Your child can choose the "potty tot" character he likes best, from aspiring super hero Enrique to Polynesian dancer Leilani.

You can find them at **POTTYTOTS.COM**.

Although many experts recommend an "all-or-nothing" approach to potty training, I found that a blend worked best for our son. Once my son started potty training, he would begin the day in underwear, and then he let me know when he was ready to change back into a diaper. This gave my son confidence that he was in charge of the process.

As a mom, this strategy was wonderful because I would plan travel or errands in the afternoon when he would be wearing a diaper and thus not have to run to find bathrooms.

—*Jennifer Hanes, DO, a mom of a six-year-old daughter and a three-year-old son, an emergency physician, a certified forensic physician, and the founder of Empowered Medicine, PLLC, in Austin, TX*

My husband and I read a book, *3-Day Potty Training*, by Lora Jensend. After reading the book, we told our son he could no longer wear diapers. Period. Not even at night. At first, my son fussed, but he quickly realized it was easier to go in the potty than to have an accident. He was potty trained in a weekend.

—*Amy J. Derick, MD, a mom of three-year-old and 19-month-old sons who's expecting another baby and a dermatologist in private practice at Derick Dermatology, in Barrington, IL*

My daughter is 2½, so I am still knee-deep in the toddler phase! The biggest challenge (which we are still working through) is her potty training. Early on, she was very nervous about sitting on the regular toilet. I started taking her with me when I go to the bathroom so that she sees Mommy sitting on the "big girl toilet." We also converted her small potty seats to the step stools, which she can use to stand on to wash her hands at the sink. My daughter no longer sits on the potty seats in any of the bathrooms.

Incentivizing my daughter to tell me when she has to go has also been helping. We give her "potty stickers" when she tells us she has to go and when she goes in the "big girl toilet."

—*Tanya Douglas Holland, MD, a mom of a two-year-old daughter, a women's health advocate, and a consultant in medical affairs to a pharmaceutical company, in Atlanta, GA*

Don't be surprised if pooping on the potty comes well after peeing on the potty! For about five months after my son was potty trained, he'd ask for a Pull-Up to go poop. He refused to poop on the potty.

—*Heather Orman-Lubell, MD*

❧

Potty training was tough. I felt a great deal of pressure to potty train my daughter before she started a certain day care. I did one of those potty-train-your-toddler-in-a-weekend routines where I let her run around sans diaper for a weekend. She had peeing down in no time, but all the pressure really slowed things down for bowel movements. It took about a year before she figured out "number two." Needless to say, we did not make the day care deadline!

I believe that like eating and sleeping, you really have to follow your child's lead on potty training. You can't make a kid eat, sleep, or poop if she doesn't want to. If you make eating, sleeping, or pooping into a battle, the kid is likely to "win."

—*Katja Rowell, MD, a mom of a six-year-old daughter, a family practice physician, and a childhood feeding specialist with TheFeedingDoctor.com, in St. Paul, MN*

❧

My two toddlers—a boy and a girl—were close in age. One day I brought home some underpants with colorful unisex stitching.

"Hey guys," I announced, "try these on! Try to keep 'em dry, and I'll bake some cookies!"

My kids had already shown some interest in using the toilet like Mom and Dad, so I guessed that they were ready.

The most powerful motive for all social behavior in children is the desire to be like admired adults. This is certainly true of bathroom habits, and the best way to help toddlers master the use of the toilet is to support the child's natural inclination to do what the big folks do. When moms add their own anxiety to the performance, or make a power struggle out of it, the fun and the child's sense of achievement tend to get lost.

Like all growth, the child's use of the potty has its moments of back and forth. Understanding that forward progress is bound to be a bit uncertain helps parents and toddlers to stay cheerful and optimistic about mishaps that might occur along the way.

—*Elizabeth Berger, MD, a mom of a 29-year-old son and a 27-year-old daughter, a child psychiatrist, and the author of* Raising Kids with Character, *in New York City*

◦◦◦

I always used cloth diapers on my son, so when it was time to start potty training, I bought cloth training pants. I believe that cloth helps toddlers to potty train because they feel it instantly when they're wet. I'll never forget the look of disbelief on my son's face the first time he peed wearing the cloth training pants, and he felt the pee running down his legs! Using cloth training pants made potty training much quicker, and much cheaper too.

I did buy a pack of pull-up diapers to use when our family went away on trips. They were easier for travel. But my son told me he didn't want to wear the "paper" diapers. He wanted to wear the cloth ones.

My nanny tried a trick with my son to get him to pee in the potty that she had seen work with other kids. She put blue food coloring into the toilet, so when my son peed in the toilet, it would "magically" turn the water green. My son didn't buy it.

To help my son learn to go poop on the potty, I gave him a high-fiber diet full of fruits, vegetables, and whole grains. That way it didn't hurt when he went to the bathroom.

—*Lennox McNeary, MD, a mom of a three-year-old son, a specialist in physical medicine and rehabilitation at Carilion Clinic, and a cofounder of the Mommy Doctors Bakery (makers of Milkin' Cookies), in Roanoke, VA*

◦◦◦

Potty training was a challenge. Our daughter seemed to be laid-back and easygoing and learned new skills fairly easily. But potty training was a stop-and-start process that lasted for months.

When my daughter was around two years old, she showed interest in going to the potty, and for about two weeks, she made almost every poop in the potty. My husband and I were excited, and we bought pull-up diapers and encouraged her to keep trying. Then one day, my daughter decided she would *not* go in the potty at all no matter what. So we decided to let it go because she was still young, and we knew that we could try again later.

A few months later, we were on vacation, and so we had more 24/7 continuous time with our daughter to work on the potty training. By the end of the week, she was making almost every pee and poop in the potty. Then when we got home, my daughter totally regressed and showed no interest in going in the "big girl potty." A few months later, when my daughter was 2½ years old, I decided that it was time to potty train. I had another baby on the way, and I was determined not to have two kids in diapers at the same time. We used stickers to reward her when she went on the potty. Basically, it didn't work!

I had this high ideal in my head that you shouldn't motivate kids with food, so I wasn't going to use candy or treats to reward the potty training. Then one night at Grandma's house, Grandma told my daughter that she could have an M&M if she went to the potty. Immediately my daughter went to the potty and did it all on her own! We had a few days off over the holidays and we let her wear big-girl underwear and rewarded her with M&M's. Within a week, my daughter was potty trained. It seemed like it took forever, but I think the key was finding the right thing to motivate her and to use as a reward.

—*Melody Derrick, MD, a mom of a two-year-old daughter who's expecting another baby and a family physician in private practice with Cadence Physician Group, in Winfield, IL*

Coping with Accidents

Accidents happen. A toddler might have a potty accident because he couldn't think ahead to know he was going to have to "go." Or maybe he was having too much fun to stop playing. He might have an accident because he's feeling stressed or upset about something. Or maybe because of a cold, he was sleeping more deeply than usual.

The fact that your toddler has an accident is far less important than how you react to it. Be calm, be quick, and be kind.

Like so much in parenting, it helps in potty training to be positive. You'd never want to punish a child for an accident. Make it a positive experience by *being* positive.

—*Cathy Marshall, MD, a mom of 28-, 14-, and 11-year-old daughters and a pediatrician in private practice, in Encino, CA*

I keep a duffle bag in both of my cars with a change of clothes for both

When to Call Your Doctor

When your toddler first gives up the diaper or pull-up at night, he might wet the bed two or three times a week. That's completely normal. Things will improve, though, until he can go all night without wetting the bed, usually around age five. However, one in four five-year-olds, one in five seven-year-olds, and one in twenty 10-year-olds continue to wet the bed at night while asleep, according to the American Academy of Pediatrics. The majority are boys, particularly those whose fathers had problems with bedwetting when they were kids.

If your child wets the bed, don't worry. It's usually not a sign of any physical or emotional problem unless he consistently has accidents during the day and night. Most of the time, kids will have accidents during the day and at night only occasionally. A call to your doctor is in order, however, if your child has the following signs.

- Has frequent accidents during the day and at night six months to a year after finishing potty training
- Wets the bed even when he's going to the bathroom regularly before bed
- Is straining while urinating, there's a very small urine stream, or there's dribbling after urinating
- Has urine that's cloudy or pink or if there's blood in his underwear
- Has a red rash in the genital area
- Is hiding his underwear so you don't see that he's had an accident

kids, plus extra diapers. This is very handy for accidents! Anytime I take anything from those bags, I replace it right away, so I don't forget.
—*Shilpa Amin-Shah, MD*

My youngest daughter is mostly potty trained, but I still keep a pull-up diaper in my bag. If she really needs to go, and we can't make it to a bathroom in time, I can put the pull-up on her discreetly in the car.
—*Aline T. Tanios, MD, a mom of nine- and three-year-old daughters and a seven-year-old son and a pediatric hospitalist at Arkansas Children's Hospital, in Little Rock*

While a child is potty training, there will be accidents. My advice is to not make a big deal out of nighttime accidents. I just cleaned them up, gave lots of hugs and kisses, and moved on.
—*Heather Orman-Lubell, MD*

My twins potty trained very easily when they were 2½. For nighttime, though, it took a lot longer. My son had some nighttime accidents, and so he wore a pull-up diaper at night for a year or two.

My daughter wore a pull-up diaper at night until she was almost eight years old. In many kids, the ability to stay dry throughout the night is a question of how mature their bladders are. It's not something you can rush or do much about. I just checked my daughter's pull-up, and once it was consistently dry in the morning, I had her wear underwear to bed at night.

We also tried a bed-wetting alarm when she was around seven years old, which gave some good results. Most toddlers will have nighttime wetting until their bladders mature, so it shouldn't raise much concern for parents at that age.

—*Ann Contrucci, MD*

RALLIE'S TIP

As the old saying goes, accidents happen, and that's especially true with toddlers. Whenever my children didn't make it to the bathroom in time,

? When to Call Your Doctor

When bacteria from the bowel end up in the urinary tract, your child's body is normally able to eliminate the bacteria before a urinary tract infection (UTI) can develop. But sometimes the body can't effectively fight the bacteria and your child will get an infection. Girls tend to have more UTIs than boys, but they're usually not serious when they are treated with an antibiotic.

Signs and symptoms of a UTI can be as mild as frequency of urination and urine with an unusual smell, or they can be far more alarming, such as lethargy and a high fever. Some children might have no signs or symptoms at all. Because toddlers aren't very good at communicating how they're feeling, the only signs that they have an infection might be a high fever, poor appetite, and fussiness. Any time your child seems sick and has a high fever for longer than a day without a runny nose or another obvious cause, call your doctor to have her checked for a urinary tract infection.

and even when they didn't try to make it to the bathroom on time, I didn't make a big deal about it, and I never punished them or fussed at them. I just tried to handle the incident very matter-of-factly.

Toddlers learn soon enough that it's uncomfortable and a little embarrassing to have an accident, so I didn't want to do anything to add to their discomfort. When they had an accident at home, it was easy enough to clean up. I'd just help them get into clean clothes and throw the dirty ones in the washer.

As soon as toddlers gain better control over their bodies and learn to better communicate their need to go to the bathroom, they quickly outgrow this stage. If your toddler seems to have trouble making it to the bathroom on time, discuss it with your pediatrician, because it could be a sign of a bowel or bladder issue that requires medical attention.

Keeping the Potty Clean

Cleaning the potty chair isn't the most glamorous part of motherhood, and certainly not the most fun.

⤫

Once you finally get your kids to use the potty, you have a new challenge: getting them to flush to help keep the potty clean. I used a rather silly technique that worked really well for my son. I told my son that there was a poop party, but the only way for the poop to get to the party was to flush. It worked like a charm!

—*Eva Mayer, MD*

⤫

I bought two potty chairs, and I put one in each of our bathrooms. This way I don't have to race my son upstairs to a potty chair if he has to use the bathroom. I keep a container of Clorox Wipes near each potty chair. When my son uses the potty, I put a bit of water into it, dump it into the toilet, and then wipe it out with a Clorox Wipe.

—*Lennox McNeary, MD*

⤫

My kids used a potty seat for about six months. Cleaning it was not my favorite thing to do. As soon as I could, I transitioned my kids to the toilet seats that sit atop the toilet because they are easier to keep clean.

My family is from Pakistan, and in our culture/religion, we clean ourselves with water after using the toilet. We had our house custom built, and we put a handheld bidet shower in each bathroom. Everyone gets their bottoms quickly cleaned and patted dry after using the toilet.

—*Sadaf T. Bhutta, MD, a mom of a six-year-old daughter and four-year-old triplets and an assistant professor and the fellowship director of pediatric radiology at the University of Arkansas for Medical Sciences and Arkansas Children's Hospital, both in Little Rock*

RALLIE'S TIP

I kept the boys' potty chair in the bathroom, right next to the big-boy commode, so that they'd get the hang of going into the bathroom to answer the call of nature. I've never particularly enjoyed cleaning any commode or potty chair, but I'd much rather clean one that is only slightly soiled than one that is really far gone.

After emptying the removable bowl into the toilet, I would spray the potty chair with bleach water and rinse it off under the shower after each use. Once a week or so, I'd put the entire chair into the shower and scrub it with Lysol and a specially designated brush. As soon as my boys were big enough to use the big-boy commode, I got rid of the potty chair. I was really happy to see it go!

Mommy MD Guides-Recommended Product
Bemis Next Step Potty Seat

"For potty training, my husband found a toilet seat for toddlers that fits in the adult toilet lid, and our daughter can pull it into place when she is ready to go," says Melody Derrick, MD, a mom of a two-year-old daughter who's expecting another baby and a family physician in private practice with Cadence Physician Group, in Winfield, IL. "One brand is Bemis Next Step Potty Seat."

The seats cost $40 to $45 at home improvement stores and online retailers such as **AMAZON.COM**.

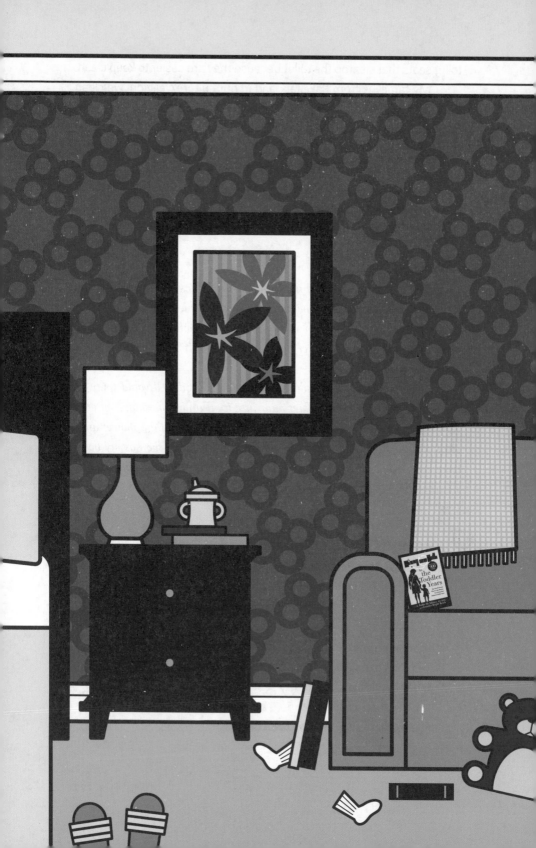

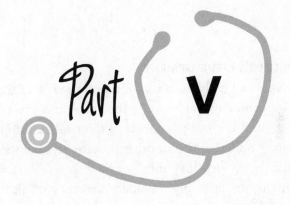

Part V

EMOTIONAL HEALTH AND DISCIPLINE

Chapter 14
Nurturing Relationships

YOUR TODDLER'S DEVELOPMENT

Your one-year-old child has a very interesting view of the world. She's at the center of her world—the sun—and she considers everyone around her in the context of their relationship to her. She, of course, understands that other people exist, but she doesn't really think about what they think or how they feel. If she gives it any thought, she probably concludes that they think the same way that she does!

As time goes on, your toddler will become more aware of herself as separate from other people. By age three, your child will be much less selfish. She'll be more independent, and less dependent on you. Her identity, her sense of self, will be stronger. She'll start to understand that other people have their own ideas and opinions about things. Your toddler will start to form relationships of her own with her family and with friends. It's one of the greatest joys of parenting to watch these bonds develop.

TAKING CARE OF YOU

As moms, we rarely see ourselves as the center of our worlds. Our needs are eclipsed by the needs of our children, our spouses, our friends, our coworkers, other people in line with us at the grocery store, pretty much everyone. Take some time to reclaim the spotlight!

Put yourself in the center of your world and picture a series of concentric circles around you. They sort of look like ripples in a pond after someone has tossed in a stone. First consider which relationships are in the closest circle: your relationships with your spouse and children, perhaps? Now consider which relationships are in the next circle: your relationships with your parents, siblings, and closest friends, maybe? Then consider which relationships are in the farther-away circle: your relationships with other friends and coworkers? Prioritizing relationships will help you to focus on and nurture the relationships that you hold most dear. This will also make it easier when you're faced with choices, such as going to a coworker's sister's wine tasting or watching your toddler's karate practice.

JUSTIFICATION FOR A CELEBRATION
It can be hard to say no. When you say no to something so you can say yes to something more special to you, celebrate your courage!

Taking Care of Yourself
Hello, you! Remember you? It's time to take better care of *you*!

When my kids were toddlers, I took care of myself by getting up super early with a running buddy and training for a marathon in the dark!
>—*Nancy Rappaport, MD, a mom of 22- and 17-year-old
>daughters and a 19-year-old son, an assistant professor of
>psychiatry at Harvard Medical School, an attending child and
>adolescent psychiatrist in the Cambridge, MA, public schools, and
>the author of* The Behavior Code

When my kids were toddlers, I bought the *Don't Sweat the Small Stuff* day calendars. I read those tips religiously each day. It's all too easy to sweat the small stuff when you have toddlers!
>—*Eva Mayer, MD, a mom of an eight-year-old daughter and
>a six-year-old son and a pediatrician with St. Luke's Pediatrics
>Associates, in Bethlehem, PA*

I had several friends I traded child care with. I also had several adult friends who helped out with child care, so I could go folk dancing and play tennis.

—Stuart Jeanne Bramhall, MD, a mom of a 31-year-old daughter and a child and adolescent psychiatrist in New Plymouth, New Zealand

∽

I'm getting much better at saying "no." Life is about choices, and as I get older, I realize more and more that I can't do it all. I've had to say no to some things I really didn't want to say no to. I try to remember that saying no lets me say yes to other things, like spending more time with my children.

—Michelle Paley, MD, PA, a mom of two and a psychiatrist and psychotherapist in private practice, in Miami Beach, FL

MomMy TIME Try Meditating

Once your nights are your own again and you've caught up on your sleep, it's the perfect time to take 10 or 15 minutes in the morning before the kids wake up to do something for you. Here's one idea: meditate.

Meditation is well known for bringing a sense of calm and emotional balance, and it's even helpful for dealing with stress, anxiety, depression, insomnia, pain, and other physical and emotional symptoms.

You can choose from many different ways to meditate. One common way is mindfulness meditation, which is part of Buddhism. To do it, find a quiet place and get into a comfortable position while sitting or lying down. (Some types of meditation can even be done while standing or walking.) Then focus on your breath as it flows in and out of your body, and let thoughts and emotions come and go without judging them.

Another technique uses a mantra, in which you repeatedly say a word or make a sound such as "ohm" quietly or in your head to help you avoid distraction.

With super-active toddlers, I found it so critical to keep my energy level up. For me, the hardest thing about having toddlers was their nonstop energy and constant demands for attention. You just don't have enough hands or energy. It's very hard for adults to keep up. I do my best.

—*Susan Wilder, MD, a mom of a 17-year-old daughter and twin 13-year-old girls, a primary care physician, and the founder and CEO of Lifescape Medical Associates, in Scottsdale, AZ*

My spiritual life is central, so that was always important to me. When my kids were toddlers, it was hard to take time for myself. But I tried to find quiet time where I'd have no TV or phone, and sometimes I'd spend quiet time with like-minded people. That quiet time was helpful for me to ground and center myself.

—*Lauren Feder, MD, a mom of 18- and 14-year-old sons, a nationally recognized physician who specializes in homeopathic medicine, and the author of* Natural Baby and Childcare *and* The Parents' Concise Guide to Childhood Vaccinations, *in Los Angeles, CA*

When my kids were toddlers, it was very difficult to find time for myself. I'm fortunate that my husband can tell when I've had a rough week.

"Do you need some time at the spa?" he'll ask me gently.

Yes! I find that a massage or spa treatment is very energizing.

Also, I have a favorite chair in my home that I love to sit in and read. It's wonderful quiet time.

—*Teresa Hubka, DO, a mom of a 14-year-old son and an 8-year-old daughter, an ob-gyn and the medical director of Comprehensive Wellness Care in Chicago, and an associate professor of obstetrics and gynecology and the chairman and residency program director of the department of obstetrics and gynecology at the Midwestern University/Chicago College of Osteopathic Medicine, in Downers Grove, Illinois*

Me? Who has time for me?

Before I started back to work, I met with a knitting group once a week. Now I try to meet up with friends from church on my day off, or I sometimes go to another knitting group on Sundays.

I like to have hobbies such as knitting, where I do something I enjoy and I also have something tangible at the end. It makes me feel productive. I knit scarves and hats to give as gifts and to donate to people in need.

—*Sharon Boyce, MD, a mom of three- and one-year-old sons and a family physician at DayOne Family Healthcare Clinic, in Battle Creek, MI*

∽

I love reading, and I try to read some before I go to bed each night. It's nice to have a quiet activity for myself. There aren't many other times in my life that are quiet.

Also, prayer is a wonderful time to be quiet and focus on what's really important. Prayer helps remind me that my little problems are nothing in the scheme of life and eternity. I also feel like I'm getting support from God—support outside of the people around me. I feel that God, who has so much more wisdom than I do, is helping me to be a better mom.

—*Melody Derrick, MD, a mom of a two-year-old daughter who's expecting another baby and a family physician in private practice with Cadence Physician Group, in Winfield, IL*

∽

We moms have very high standards for everything we use, demanding products that are easy and safe to use, as well as super effective. So it's not any different when it comes to choosing something to recharge my batteries!

Especially as a single, working mother, "recharging my batteries" becomes critical to my survival. I knew the things that used to work for me (shopping, getting my nails done, meeting up with friends) didn't anymore, and the things that normally work for people (watching a movie, going to the gym) just make me feel more agitated, so I started looking for a specific method to refill my reservoir.

I tried different hobbies and activities, including knitting, playing the piano and the ukulele, taking art classes, going to large outdoor markets, undertaking arts and crafts projects, yoga, going to lectures, meditating, and writing, but I just couldn't quite figure out which one activity worked best for me.

Finally, I realized that that was *exactly* what I needed: to always look for new and different things to do, so my mind is constantly challenged and feeling refreshed. That way, when I get home to my son, I can come up with interesting things to keep him and myself entertained, as well as have the activity reservoir and energy to patiently deal with him.

> —*Cheryl Wu, MD, a mom of a four-year-old son, a pediatrician at LaGuardia Place Pediatrics in New York City, and a pediatric emergency physician at the Joseph M. Sanzari Children's Hospital of Hackensack University Medical Center, in New Jersey*

❧

It amazes me that as a pediatrician, I take care of so many critically ill children, but now I'm challenged to care for my own two healthy children. As a doctor, you go off shift, but as a mom, your shift never ends.

The level of emotional fatigue surprises me. You always have to be emotionally available to your children, and I find that more draining than I had expected.

I learned early on that I needed to pay attention to my own emotional needs. I set aside a little time each day for myself. I try to get in 5 to 10 minutes of exercise each day. When my kids are older, I'll have more time, but for now I do the best I can. Also each night before I go to sleep, I read about 10 minutes of a Dilbert comic book or some Mommy Lit.

I've also learned it's important to adjust my expectations. Now that I have kids, my life isn't going to be the way it was before! I don't spend too much time pining for my pre-kids life. (My husband does, though!)

> —*Kate Tulenko, MD, MPH, a mom of four- and one-year-old girls, the author of* Insourced: How Importing Jobs Impacts the Healthcare Crisis Here and Abroad, *and a pediatrician and global health specialist with IntraHealth, in Washington, DC*

I think Mom's needs so often shift to the back burner, and when my kids were toddlers, I was no exception. I was working full-time all along as I was having babies, nursing babies, and taking care of babies. I just didn't have much time to take care of myself.

I tried to keep up with my hobbies, mainly needlework. That's relaxing for me. I've made many lovely things, many of which I hung in my kids' rooms.

I also love to read. I didn't have much time to read for myself, but I also enjoyed reading to my kids. That was relaxing for me, and my kids loved being read to. That's how I kept my sanity.

—*Susan Besser, MD, a mom of six grown children, ages 27, 25, 23, 21, 20, and 18, a grandmom of two, a family physician, and the medical director of Doctors Express-Memphis, in Tennessee*

One of the big challenges of being a mom is that I'm always feeling guilty about something. If I'm working, I worry my kids are suffering. If I'm with my kids, I worry that my work is.

To make matters worse, for the past 2½ years, I don't feel that I've done anything for myself. My career has been on autopilot. I didn't have the time to write papers or attend conferences. I felt like I needed to get back on the right track with my job, but at what cost? Even though I was only away for a few days for conferences, one of my daughters said, "Mom, you're always gone."

I try to manage my time—and my guilt—as effectively as I can. I focus on whatever is the priority of the moment. For example, this past week I had to stay late at work for a meeting with my accountant. But then the next evening I made sure to be home at 5:00 pm so we could have dinner together and decorate the Christmas tree.

I also do yoga, and I run during my "golden hour" of 5:45 to 6:45, when no one else is up. I had to train myself to be a morning person. By nature, I'm a night owl.

—*Brooke A. Jackson, MD, a mom of 4½-year-old twin girls and a 2½-year-old son, a dermatologist, and the founder and medical director of the Skin Wellness Center of Chicago, in Illinois*

It's so critical to take care of yourself. One of the many reasons for this is that you should never underestimate how in tune your children are with you. Even when children are little, they are very insightful and emotionally connected with how their parents (particularly Mommy) are feeling.

I take care of myself, so I can take care of my daughter. To do this, I have to make sure that I exercise. This helps me in so many ways, both physically and emotionally. I love cardio! It really helps me feel better by helping me to sleep better and improving my mood. I try to incorporate at least 30 minutes of cardio a day, five days a week. I try to keep it simple. Most days I hop on my elliptical machine. When the weather is nice, I enjoy walks outside.

I also try to minimize the number of tasks I place on my to-do list in a given week. I use an electronic calendar on my phone that merges both work and personal commitments. I usually will not schedule more than one or two business appointments in a given day. I also block out my time with my husband (we call this "Tad Time") as well as our family time on my calendar. I try not to be too structured, but I do try to consciously tell myself that "x" or "y" will be the main task I will focus on today.

Additionally, I try to ensure that I incorporate a little me time throughout my week. I have tea time two or three times per week and drink a cup of chamomile or lavender tea. I enjoy writing in my journal, listening to music, singing karaoke, and reading daily devotionals.

—*Tanya Douglas Holland, MD, a mom of a two-year-old daughter, a women's health advocate, and a consultant in medical affairs to a pharmaceutical company, in Atlanta, GA*

⌐∽⌐

I quickly realized that my children absorb all my emotions. If I am stressed, they get stressed.

I could not stay up all night for several days in a row with sick children and function well. The resulting lack of sleep and muscle aches would make me irritable. I had to dip into my savings and hire help. With the twins, it was even more important that I got help and plenty of sleep. I would say I greatly underestimated how much help I would need.

The smartest thing I did was to hire a happy, energetic sitter with a loving pair of arms to hold my children and play with them so I could get some much needed rest. Having twins at age 44 was tough, and it took me much longer to recover physically than it did with my first child. I was lucky I had the resources. I would tell anyone who is pregnant or planning to have children to make sure that they have several wonderful people as support for the first three years. My sitters were my angels!

The other thing I learned to do was to cut back on my responsibilities outside of the home. For a physician, that was tough. I thought I could just keep on working the same schedule I always had! But having children is just like having to be on-call 24 hours a day, seven days a week. I did have to let some things go, but then I was able to pick them back up later when my children went to grade school.

—Laura M. Rosch, DO, a mom of a 12-year-old daughter and 7-year-old boy-girl twins, a board-certified internist who works at Central DuPage Hospital Convenient Care Centers in Winfield, IL, and an instructor in the department of family medicine at the Midwestern University/Chicago College of Osteopathic Medicine, in Downers Grove, IL

RALLIE'S TIP

Moms who are too pooped to pop crave the very foods that will make them feel worse in the long run! We're often drawn to foods that are loaded with sugar, salt, unhealthy fats, and empty calories. Carbohydrate cravings are common in women, and for a good reason. Carbohydrate-laden foods are known to help increase levels of serotonin, which is a mood-enhancing neurotransmitter in the brain, so when you crave carbs, you're innately trying to self-medicate.

Although chips, chocolate bars, giant bowls of pasta, and deluxe, double-crust pizzas might be your first and favorite choices of high-carbohydrate foods, eating too many can make you feel tired, not to mention more likely to gain weight.

When my youngest boys were toddlers, it was especially challenging to get them out of the house during the winter months when it was freezing cold outside. I found myself snacking almost nonstop to deal with the stress of being cooped up so much. I've always been susceptible to the winter blues, and the short days and lack of sunshine made me feel even gloomier—and hungrier. I knew that if I didn't do something to lift my spirits and suppress my appetite, I was going to end up gaining a ton of weight, and of course that would make me feel even worse!

Because I had to spend so much time indoors, I decided to work on brightening up my living space. If you think of the words you use to describe low moods and feelings (bleak, black, gray, blue, dim, dark, lifeless, silent), you realize the importance of surrounding yourself with cheerful sounds, living things, bright light, invigorating scents, and warm, vibrant colors. I kept the curtains and blinds open during the winter days to let in as much sunlight as possible, and I kept the overhead lights and lamps turned on in the rooms I was using. I bought a few bright green houseplants and put them out of reach of my boys so they couldn't eat them or mangle them. Even though it felt like a minor hassle, I made a point of putting my favorite CDs in the stereo, so I could listen to music that I knew would energize me and lift my spirits.

I found that when my surroundings were brighter and more cheerful, I didn't feel the need to snack on junk food as much to try to lift my spirits. My youngest sons are teenagers now, but I still use these tricks to stave off the doldrums—and the munchies—during the winter months.

༄

My life when my twins were toddlers wasn't as balanced as it should have been. I tried to get back into jogging and going to the gym, but it was very hard. I was also working full-time, so it was hard to squeeze in time for my family, let alone for me.

If I had to do it over again, I would have taken more time for myself. I should have gone on walks and met friends for lunch. I should have felt a little less guilt when I was away from my twins and realized it's healthy to be away from your children and that it revitalizes you to do things for yourself occasionally. This is the hardest job there is, and sometimes it's necessary to have a little break. It's so important to make time for yourself.

—*Ann Contrucci, MD, a mom of 13-year-old boy-girl twins who works as a pediatric emergency physician, in Atlanta, GA*

Nurturing Your Relationship with Your Spouse

Fewer and fewer families are made up of two parents, two kids, and a minivan. More than 44 percent of Millennials (twenty-somethings!) say that the institution of marriage is becoming obsolete. That's compared with 37 percent of people age 30 or older.

If you have a spouse, that relationship is critical, both for setting the tone of your home and also for setting an example. It's a scary, oft-quoted stat that the divorce rate in the United States for first marriages is 41 percent. It's even higher for second marriages: 60 percent; and highest still for third marriages: 73 percent. Take some time to improve the state of your union!

∽

Just as it's important to be generous to your kids, it's important to be generous to your spouse with affection, love, support, and listening. Hug your husband and say "good morning" to him each day!

> —*Elizabeth Chabner Thompson, MD, MPH, a mom of 13- and 8-year-old daughters and 12- and 10-year-old sons, a radiation oncologist with 21 C. Radiation Oncology, and the inventor of the Mommy Bag, filled with supplies for moms-to-be having C-sections, in Scarsdale, NY*

∽

My parents never argued in front of my siblings and me, especially not about how to discipline us. It is very important to me that my husband and I are on the same page for disciplining our children. If parents have disagreements about this, it's amazing how quickly kids pick up on it—and can manipulate the situation.

If you and your partner have different ideas, you should talk about it alone, without the kids hearing. Then present a united front to your children!

> —*Sadaf T. Bhutta, MD, a mom of a six-year-old daughter and four-year-old triplets and an assistant professor and the fellowship director of pediatric radiology at the University of Arkansas for Medical Sciences and Arkansas Children's Hospital, both in Little Rock*

My husband is from another culture, and he is more old-fashioned than I am. Especially when our sons were toddlers, my husband had a difficult time being patient with them.

I respect my husband, but I sometimes had different opinions than him about things. During the toddler years, I made efforts for us to go on "dates," which were important for our relationship. Now working with parents of young children, I encourage them to make time for their spouses. For families who continue to do the family bed approach, I like to see one of the parents (usually Mom) in the middle of the bed. The parental relationship is sacred, and it requires work to keep it that way.

—*Lauren Feder, MD*

It's hard to make the time to go out on "dates," so my husband and I buy season tickets to the theater each year. This way, six times a year, we get tickets in the mail. This gives us the motivation to get dressed up and go out! Some years, those were the only six times we got to go out.

Having season tickets makes going out with your spouse a planned, scheduled event. It's not like a vague "we should go for dinner sometime" or a more isolated "our favorite band is coming to town." We buy these tickets each fall, and it puts our date nights on autopilot.

—*Kate Tulenko, MD, MPH*

Recently, my husband and I took our first trip without our daughter. We jumped in with both feet. We didn't just go to the next town; we went to Mexico!

It was hard to go, and we were gone for four days, but when we got home, I thought to myself, *Thank goodness we did it*. I really needed some time with my husband to recharge. It's very important to remind ourselves of the relationship that started our little family in the first place.

—*Jennifer Bacani McKenney, MD, a mom of a one-year-old daughter and a family physician, in Fredonia, KS*

When kids are toddlers, it's so important to take time for yourself and for your husband. We forget these things a lot, but it makes you a better parent.

Not every couple is able to pull this off, but if you have a parent or friend whom you trust to watch your kids overnight, it's great to go away for an overnight stay. I'm lucky enough to have parents who are willing and able and excited to watch my kids when we want

Plan a Date Night

A nice dinner that you don't have to cook is always a welcome idea for date night. But when you're in the mood to do something different, here are some date night ideas that are sure to ignite a romantic spark.

- Go to a karaoke bar and sing a duet.
- Search your local paper for free outdoor concerts or Shakespeare in the park. Make it even more special by bringing a blanket and a picnic with a bottle of wine.
- Hold hands while you watch a movie at the drive-in. Find drive-in theaters near you at DriveInMovie.com.
- Take dance lessons together. Try ballroom, salsa, swing, tango, Latin, or country.
- Work up a sweat while you conquer a rock-climbing wall. High-five each other when you reach the top.
- Re-create your very first date.
- Head to an amusement park and ride all of the roller coasters together.
- Rent a two-person kayak and take a trip down a river, to the middle of a lake, or along the coast of the ocean.
- Get some laughs at a comedy club.
- For a very special occasion, take a ride in a hot-air balloon. Many companies offer couple's packages and include a champagne toast while you're in the air.

to go away. My husband and I try to get away once a year at least for an overnight, and we've been lucky enough to take full-week vacations without the kids several times. It's good for everyone.

We did check in frequently, especially when our children were little. We have gone away for varying distances, from one hour away to overseas!

—*Heather Orman-Lubell, MD, a mom of 11- and 7-year-old sons and a pediatrician in private practice at Yardley Pediatrics of St. Christopher's Hospital for Children, in Pennsylvania*

I think some parents are so focused on their children that they lose their relationship with each other. My husband and I are very much in love, very mushy. We met in the emergency department and got married later in life. We have a lot in common; we love to spend time together fishing, hiking, skiing, and talking.

As often as we can, my husband and I take part of the day just to spend time together doing something we enjoy. Rather than date nights, which are difficult to schedule, we have date days. It's hard to leave our daughter with the nanny to do it, but it would be harder *not* to. We were pretty pathetic, though, when she was little. Neither of us wanted to be away from her for too long. We'd schedule the babysitter for five hours and be home in two!

—*Lisa Campanella-Coppo, MD, a mom of a three-year-old daughter, an emergency physician, and the emergency department director of academic affairs at Monmouth Medical Center, in New Jersey*

I believe the tradition my husband and I started when our daughter was an infant of having a date night is just as important during these toddler years. As a full-time doctor, I feel that when I come home, I need to give my daughter all my attention. And she and I do spend quality time together.

I also find it so helpful to spend time *away* from home with my husband. We both feel that we can recharge and connect as husband

and wife and parents again. Sometimes it means doing something like going to a movie where we can sit and relax and be entertained for a few hours. Sometimes we go for a quick cup of coffee where we can just have one hour of *uninterrupted* talking time! And other times we run errands together. Either way, it's always helpful to have some adult time away from the house.

—*Melody Derrick, MD*

Once when I was in a mall, I saw a weeping toddler and his mother, who had stopped to help her son pull himself together. Five paces ahead marched the father, who turned to bellow over his shoulder with deep sincerity and anguish, "Don't *baby* him!"

Raising toddlers can be rough on the parents' relationship with one another. Dads are often more in tune with the demands of the "real" world, and naturally they want to carry this metaphor over to the "management" of their toddler offspring. Moms, in contrast, tend to have more empathy with the toddler's tendency to take forever to do things, and the toddler's need for emotional support when he falls apart. This conflict between the parents can't be resolved in the midst of a crisis. Being in tune with the toddler's needs might need some explaining. Talking it out can help couples gain more understanding both of their toddler and of each other.

It's important that parents of toddlers find a way to be a couple, alone, without children from time to time. Many parents like to hire a sitter on a regular basis, or build in some sort of grown-up scheduled activity, which allows the parental relationship to equilibrate.

A certain gender-based distress occurs frequently in couples raising toddlers. Mothers, who typically spend many more hours doing the labor-intensive and exhausting work of responding to children at this age, might feel neglected by their husbands if they are not given breaks from these responsibilities and routines. Dads, on the other hand, might feel neglected by their wives—who once were entirely and alluringly focused on their wonderful husbands at 5 pm, and who are now utterly frazzled by cranky tots and covered with splattered oatmeal at that time of day. This is hard! Before everyone feels hopelessly neglected, a night out is in order.

—*Elizabeth Berger, MD, a mom of a 29-year-old son and a 27-year-old daughter, a child psychiatrist, and the author of* Raising Kids with Character, *in New York City*

RALLIE'S TIP

To prevent feeling depleted, I think prioritizing is the key to nurturing all of the relationships that are important to you. I often ask women to list 5 to 10 areas of their lives that are most important to them. I refer to this list as their "gardens" in life, because like gardens, these areas have to be regularly tended to thrive and flourish. Most women list things like this: children, relationship with their partners, health, spirituality, fun, career, community service, friends, and parents.

Once the list is created, I ask women to list the activities they do on a regular basis to nurture these gardens. If they're not doing something very regularly to nurture their gardens, those gardens will never bear fruit, and even worse, they'll shrivel up and die. If you list "community service" as one of your gardens, for instance, but you never make time to get involved with your community, you risk feeling sad and unfulfilled because you don't feel as if you're making a contribution to something that's very important to you. If your relationship with your partner is important to you, but you never make time for fun and intimacy, you won't succeed in having a good relationship.

Understanding and listing your priorities makes it easier for moms to avoid giving too much of themselves to activities that don't support their health and happiness, and it helps them make the right decision when they're forced to choose between activities. If, for example, your son's teacher invites you to her sister's baby shower, you might find it easier to say no when you realize that this activity doesn't support any of your priorities in life. You can say, "No, I'm sorry I can't come, but thanks for inviting me!" and go have a night out with your husband instead, which is an activity that supports one of your life priorities: your relationship with your partner.

When my youngest sons were toddlers and my oldest son was a teenager, I realized that my husband and I weren't going to get to spend time alone with each other unless I planned for it. We were so busy working and taking care of our children that we never seemed to have time for each other. Our solution was to plan a date night twice a month. We'd hire a babysitter and slip away for a few hours to eat dinner and watch a movie. Those date nights kept our romance alive and our relationship strong through the crazy toddler years.

Nurturing Your Relationships with Your Children

A child's first relationships provide the foundation for her social-emotional development. This in turn helps her to form healthy relationships with others and to understand social rules and standards.

Loving, nurturing relationships enhance emotional development and mental health. When infants and toddlers are treated with kindness and encouragement, they develop a sense of safety and emotional security. A nurturing, caring relationship provides a "secure base" from which children can begin exploring the world, frequently checking back for reassurance. The more they explore and try new things, the more success they experience.

Kind, nurturing relationships also teach children how to treat others. Children watch adults and copy them. Good relationships help children feel valued. Children who feel loved and cherished grow up to be adults who care about others.

∽

When my second daughter was born, we were concerned that our two-year-old would feel neglected. We knew that we would be getting many visitors who would arrive with presents for our newborn, so we bought and wrapped a few little gifts for our older daughter prior to my delivery. That way, she would have a gift to open while we were opening our new child's gifts. This worked well, and we told her that these little gifts were from her little sister. She loved that the presents were from her new sister!

We also planned a few trips to the movies and park for some

"alone time" when my second daughter first came home. These were mostly daddy time, and she loved every second.

—*Jeannette Gonzalez Simon, MD, a mom of three- and one-year-old daughters and a pediatric gastroenterologist in private practice, in Staten Island, NY*

I think the most important message about parenting is to be generous to your children—with love, hugs, attention, and food. My father, a medical oncologist, told me that the fastest way to make rounds in the hospital is to sit down at the patient's bedside. This relaxes the patient and you. An impatient doctor or parent leads to needy patients and children.

I think it's important to hug your children as much as possible. Every morning, say "good morning" and give your kids hugs.

—*Elizabeth Chabner Thompson, MD, MPH*

My daughter and I are very close. I'm a very busy person. I started my practice after my daughter was born, so ironically I work even longer hours now than before she was born. I really capitalize on the time that I do get to spend with my daughter. Every chance I get, I tell her that I love her. I want her to take that love for granted and really feel it in her heart.

—*Dina Strachan, MD, a mom of a six-year-old daughter, a dermatologist and director of Aglow Dermatology, and an assistant clinical professor in the department of dermatology at New York University, in New York City*

When my daughter was a toddler, I stayed at home in the mornings. My daughter and I either went to Pike Place Market, a children's museum, the zoo, or an aquarium, or we spent several hours coloring or doing art projects together. One of our favorites was to pick garbage up off the street for a garbage collage.

When my daughter was 2½, she often woke up and asked what the schedule was for the day. We lived only a few blocks from Lake Union, and feeding the ducks every evening was a reward for good behavior. This was also a relaxing time for both of us.

—*Stuart Jeanne Bramhall, MD*

Even though I'm very busy and I wear a lot of different hats, I protect my family time on the weekends. I consider that to be special time with my daughter. At the crack of dawn on Saturday mornings, my daughter gets up and asks, "What are we going to do today?" My daughter and I love to go to the park, watch a movie, or just spend time together. It's very important to me that my daughter knows that she is my priority.

I leave my phone on, but my work colleagues all know that my weekends are sacred. They know not to call unless it's an emergency.

—*Christy Valentine, MD, a mom of a six-year-old daughter, a specialist in pediatrics and internal medicine, and the founder of the Valentine Medical Center, in Gretna, LA*

Because my kids are 22 months apart, I had two toddlers at the same time. It's funny looking back: So many people had told me it would be easier to have my kids close together. Really? Who were they kidding? I learned that was not true. It was very difficult to have two kids who were so dependent upon me and my husband.

I tried to make the extra effort to spend individual time with each of my toddlers. Yes, it would have been easier and more convenient to spend time with them together! There's a tendency to want to group siblings together in the same activities, going to the park together, and planning playdates together. Sometimes, that's fine. But I also tried to make time with my kids individually, especially for my daughter to reassure her that she hadn't been displaced by my son. We had a lot of issues with that when my son was born, but by the time my daughter was around 31 months old, she was verbal enough that she could tell me how she was feeling.

I really enjoyed these special times with my kids. On days that my husband was able to watch our son, my daughter and I would play dress-up. Then on other days, my husband would watch our daughter, and I'd take our son outside to play. It didn't cost any money to do these things—only time.

—*Ann V. Arthur, MD, a mom of a 10-year-old daughter and an 8-year-old son, a pediatric ophthalmologist in private practice at Park Slope Eye Care Associates, and a blogger at WaterWineTravel.com, in New York City*

～∾～

When my children were infants, I used a sling to hold them, comfort them, and keep them close—especially if I had to run errands, cook, or work. I remember teaching an exercise class for pre- and postnatal moms while wearing a sling to hold my three-week-old daughter.

When my kids got older, but were still light enough to carry, I found I could still put them in the sling and walk around to comfort them. For some reason, even as they got a bit older, they would still run to the closet for the sling if they wanted me to hold them. The toddler years were no exception.

My seven-year-old daughter will deny this, but last week she had a rough day at school and went to the closet in the front hall.

"Mom, where is the sling?" I heard her ask from the kitchen.

It brought a tear to my eye!

—*Laura M. Rosch, DO*

～∾～

The larger goals of parenting should always be a priority. During the toddler years, the child's sense of security in the world, and the child's self-esteem, are being developed.

Toddlers, by definition, are just becoming mobile and testing whether independence is safe. Margaret Mahler, a pioneer in child psychology, called this the rapprochement phase of development. Kids toddle away, explore, toddle back to get mom's reassurance, toddle away, and so on. If a good sense of security is established during this time, all else will be easier in life, for the child and for the parents too. The child will be more secure and independent. The child will have less anger and less need to act out. So parenting will also be easier, with fewer battles.

For example, if a child toddles away, and returns to find a grumpy mom who wishes the child would stay away, the child will carry that impression of the world for a long time. It will impact the child's sense of security.

When my daughter was a toddler, I tried to never give her the sense that she was interrupting or bothering me. It's very important to be emotionally present for a child. I tried to work when she was asleep, so that I could focus on her when she was awake.

If a child has a secure attachment to a parent, the child will likely be less anxious in the future, less prone to emotional problems, and even less prone to disease. When a child is anxious, stress hormones are released. This can interfere with immunity. The body's proneness to release stress hormones is established early in life. A secure attachment to a parent can decrease the risk of disease for the rest of a child's life.

—Dora Calott Wang, MD, a mom of a nine-year-old daughter, a psychiatrist and historian at the University of New Mexico School of Medicine, and the author of The Kitchen Shrink: A Psychiatrist's Reflection on Healing in a Changing World, in Albuquerque, NM

RALLIE'S TIP

My oldest son was nearly 13 years old when his baby brother was born, and then he got another baby brother just a year later. He went from being an only child who was a little set in his ways to being the big brother of two wild and crazy toddlers. It was a huge change for him, but he took it all in stride.

Naturally, babies and toddlers demand a lot of attention, but I didn't want my oldest son to feel that he had been forgotten or neglected by his parents. Once a month or so, my husband and I did something really special with him, and we left his two little brothers with a sitter. We'd take him skiing, to a pro basketball game, or to a concert. I think that because he got our undivided attention every once in a while, he was perfectly happy to share his parents with his little brothers. Sometimes, older kids really like it when their parents aren't completely focused on them!

We'd also encourage my son to have his friends over to our house fairly often, so he wouldn't always feel that he was living in a day care. My husband would take him and his friends camping and fishing, or we'd just let my son and his friends hang out and play video games.

I made sure that my oldest son realized how much his little brothers loved him and looked up to him, and encouraged him to be a good role *model. He took his big brother responsibilities very seriously, and I think that helped him gain a lot of maturity as a teenager.*

Although having a teenager and two toddlers certainly wasn't sunshine and roses all the time, I tried to make sure that having two little brothers wasn't a negative experience for my oldest son. I tried not to ask him to make huge sacrifices, like giving up his room or any of his favorite activities. I let the toddlers know that their big brother always had seniority, and he was second in command to Mom and Dad. I didn't ask my teenager to do a lot of babysitting, and I tried not to use having two toddlers as an excuse to stay at home or to avoid certain activities. Sometimes it was a bit of a hassle to bundle up two toddlers and take them out to watch my oldest son's football games, but I did it anyway. I always wanted him to know that he was just as special and as important as ever to me and to the rest of our family.

Thinking about Having Another Baby

If you're thinking about having another baby, you might have less company today than in past generations. The number of American women having only one child has doubled over the past two decades.

How long is the optimum time between children? That depends on your particular family situation! There are benefits to having children close in age, and there are benefits to having more time in between.

An interesting study, conducted by researchers at Notre Dame University, found that when age gaps between siblings were greater, the older child performed better on math and reading achievement tests. Interestingly, the spacing between children doesn't seem to affect the achievement of the younger sibling.

If you are thinking about having another baby, one thing to consider, whether or not you considered it with your first baby, is banking your baby's cord blood. Deciding whether or not to bank your baby's umbilical cord blood is a very personal decision. Because you have only one opportunity to bank your baby's blood, on the day she's born, it can also be a very difficult decision to make. The blood in the umbilical cord contains stem cells, which have the potential to treat leukemia and some inherited disorders now and have the possibility of treating more diseases in the future.

When the baby is born, the doctor or midwife collects the cord blood from the part of the umbilical cord that is attached to the placenta. Normally, this blood would be disposed of as medical waste. The blood is placed into collection bags and carried by courier to a cord blood bank. There the sample is given an identifying number and frozen in liquid nitrogen. Researchers have examined 20-year-old samples and found no loss of viability. They also went a step further and transplanted stem cells from the units into laboratory animals and found no change in the rate of engraftment, showing that stem cells stored under proper conditions have no expiration date.

Cord blood banking comes with a cost, around $2,000 for the initial collection and processing and an annual storage fee of around $125. You can donate your baby's cord blood to a public bank for

Mommy MD Guides-Recommended Product
Cord Blood Registry

Cord Blood Registry (CBR) is the world's largest and most experienced cord blood bank in the United States, entrusted with storing more than 400,000 cord blood units for individuals and their families.

CBR's laboratory in Tucson, Arizona, was the first family cord blood stem cell bank in the world. Inside, the lab is an amazingly high-tech facility, with the most advanced technologies to save the maximum number of stem cells. But outside, the building is nondescript and secure from natural disasters such as tornadoes and hurricanes.

In its 20-year history, CBR also helped more clients use their cord blood stem cells for lifesaving transplants and experimental regenerative medicine therapies than any other family bank.

Visit **CORDBLOOD.COM** to learn more about cord blood banking.

free, but it is not reserved for your family's use. If you're considering donating it, a new program at Duke University, the M.D. Anderson Cancer Center, and the Texas Cord Blood Bank is providing a special free mail-in kit for parents anywhere who want to work with their doctors to donate their baby's cord blood. For more information, call 919-668-2071 at least six weeks before your baby is due.

My son is one year old, and my husband and I are thinking about having another baby. While I love that idea, I also understand how much work it is to have a baby, and now a toddler. My husband doesn't want our son to be an only child. My sister and I are five years apart, and my husband and his siblings are two years apart. We are thinking about meeting in the middle, and having our children be around three years apart.

—*Michelle Davis-Dash, MD, a mom of a one-year-old son and a pediatrician, in Baltimore, MD*

When thinking about having another baby, it's so important to plan to bank each of your children's cord blood. The newest uses for cord blood, called regenerative medicine, can only be done with your child's own cord blood. Regenerative medicine involves using cord blood to help regenerate damaged organs, such as the brain, heart, and pancreas. I would tell my patients, "You wouldn't just buy one car seat if you had two children who needed them, so why bank only one child's cord blood?"

—*Marra S. Francis, MD, a mom of eight-, seven-, and five-year-old daughters and a gynecologist, in San Antonio, TX*

My older son was a fertility drug child. Although we wanted to have a second child, my husband and I were not sure if we could handle the stress of a toddler and the emotionality of fertility drugs. They made me very difficult to be married to for about a week each cycle. I would be so emotional that there was nothing my husband could do that was "right" in my mind. My younger son was a complete surprise. We did not use any sort of contraception after child one because we didn't think we could have another child.

My husband and I were overjoyed, but not overwhelmed, by the thought of another child, and our older son was almost as excited as we were about having a baby. We didn't tell him until I was almost 20 weeks pregnant because we didn't want to have him get excited until we were sure the pregnancy would work out. Several of the other kids in my son's day care had younger siblings, and he was happy to be part of the crowd.

Regarding cord blood banking, many companies offer cord blood banking that you pay for and get your own child's cord blood back if you need it later down the road. This would be a good answer if you have two children who could benefit if one needed cord blood from the other. North Carolina had a public program where you could bank cord blood for research or to be given to another person in need. We went that route as it was free and would help others if they needed cord blood.

After my younger son was born on Friday, my older son was happy to go back to class the following Monday with cupcakes to celebrate his baby brother's birthday.

—*Carrie Brown, MD, a mom of eight- and six-year-old sons and a general pediatrician who treats medically complex children and specializes in palliative care at Arkansas Children's Hospital, in Little Rock*

Nurturing Your Relationships with Your Friends

The philosopher Aristotle said, "In poverty and other misfortunes of life, true friends are a sure refuge. They keep the young out of mischief, they comfort and aid the old in their weakness, and they incite those in the prime of life to noble deeds."

With all due respect to Aristotle, we would like to add, "They prevent moms from losing their marbles, murdering their husbands, and eating an entire super-size bag of potato chips in a sitting."

A lot of my friends started families at the same time I did, so we have children the same ages. This makes it very easy to keep in touch and get together. Often when we want to get out of town, we'll leave early in the morning when my daughter is still sleeping and drive over to visit some of our friends with children. We all spend the day together, catching up while we have our kids in the middle so we can all help keep an eye on each other's children.

—*Jennifer Bacani McKenney, MD*

❧

When my kids were toddlers, I shared lots of common time with other parents, exchanging experiences and approaches. This was healing and helpful for my personal growth. We'd plan playdates. We'd meet in a kid-friendly environment and offer lots of safe items for the kids to stay busy with while we would discuss issues and share ideas. Sometimes, one mom would watch all the kids, and the other moms prepared snacks while we shared experiences. We often would invite moms with older kids, who had more experience. We respected these older moms, and we could learn from them.

—*Hana R. Solomon, MD, a mom who raised four children, a grandmom of three, a board-certified pediatrician, the president of BeWell Health, LLC, and the author of* Clearing the Air One Nose at a Time: Caring for Your Personal Filter, *in Columbia, MO*

❧

It's easy to become so consumed by working, running the household, and caring for children that you lose your friendships. You have to constantly work at maintaining your friendships, like any other relationships. I try to connect with my friends once a week, or at least once a month. With the best friends, even if months have gone by, it doesn't feel like that much time has passed. You pick up the threads right where you left them off.

My husband and I have a good social circle here in town. We often go to dinners with friends on weekends. But I also feel it's important to keep in touch with my friends in other cities and other countries!

—*Sadaf T. Bhutta, MD*

❧

I think it's important to maintain my relationships with my friends, who are outside of my family. Those are people I went to high school or college with, who knew me before I was a mother. I try to check in with them frequently, even if just by Facebook, to see what's going on in their lives.

I started to Facebook to market my practice, but it has really helped me to reconnect with old friends. Even though we might not get together often, Facebook helps me to feel connected with them.

Also, as often as I can, I make time to meet friends for lunch or for a quick visit one night after work.

—*Christy Valentine, MD*

MomMy TIME Plan a Girls' Night Out

Some quality girl time is just as important as quality time with the family. Here are some excuses to get out of the house with the girls.

- Start a book club with a small group of friends and meet at a coffee shop to discuss your recent read.
- Attend a "martinis and manicures" event at a local mall or restaurant.
- Put on your cowboy boots and go line dancing together. (Find free instructional videos on how to do it at HelenAnd NitaLineDancing.com.)
- Make it girls' night at a pottery painting store. Choose a slow weeknight when it will be quiet, bring a bottle of wine, and create a masterpiece while catching up with friends.
- Bring a friend to a yoga studio and pay a drop-in rate for a yoga or meditation class.
- Sign up for an art or cooking class together.
- Take an afternoon to visit some local vineyards and go wine tasting.
- Pretend you have a fancy party to go to and try on expensive gowns and dresses at an upscale department store. Model them for each other and then leave without spending a dime.
- Go roller-skating or ice-skating with the girls.
- Take a class together that's a little outside of your comfort zone, such as belly dancing.

Nurturing Your Relationships with Your Parents and In-Laws

The mother-daughter relationship is fragile, fascinating, and at times frustrating. Having children might have strengthened your relationship with your mom and dad and siblings, or it might have damaged it. It's humbling to think that just as you would step in front of a Mack truck to save your child, your mom and dad would likely do the same for you. That's unconditional love.

⌒⌒

I found it difficult sometimes to let my children's relationship with my parents grow, without hovering. I tried to take a step back and let them spend quality time together, without me. I would ask my parents to babysit. Then I'd go for a walk or run errands.

—*Eva Mayer, MD*

⌒⌒

When my girls were toddlers, they had a very special relationship with my parents and my in-laws, who watched them while I was at work. My daughters used to go to Bloomingdale's with my mother-in-law for salad and popovers. It was very nice and really helped them bond.

—*Siobhan Dolan, MD, MPH, a mom of 16- and 13-year-old*
daughters and an 11-year-old son, a consultant to the March of
Dimes, and an associate professor of obstetrics and gynecology and
women's health at Albert Einstein College of Medicine/Montefiore
Medical Center, in Bronx, NY

⌒⌒

When my kids were toddlers, we moved and were only three hours away from my mother. She was happy that we lived closer and didn't hesitate to drive three hours to spend weekends with us. This was terrific because she got to spend big chunks of time with my kids, and my husband and I got to have evenings out! The kids love hanging out with her because she does different things than "Mommy" does. They do practice workbooks and play lots of games.

—*Antoinette Cheney, DO, a mom of a seven-year-old son and*
a six-year-old daughter and a family physician with Rocky Vista
University College of Osteopathic Medicine, in Parker, CO

I'm very close with my parents and in-laws. My dad and I work together in our family practice, and my mom goes to my house to visit my daughter during the day. My husband's parents live only a few hours away. It's funny, my dad is a doctor, but when he's with my daughter, the doctor part goes out the window, and he's Grandpa. He loves to try to give my daughter treats like cookies and ice cream. It's a joy for me to see their grandparent-grandchild bond grow.

It's important to me that my daughter has a close relationship with my parents and in-laws. I do everything I can to make my parents and in-laws feel welcome in our home and a part of our lives. For example, I remind them that they don't need an invitation to come over, just come over. Also, if my husband has to be gone for a few days for work, we invite his parents to come and stay to help out with our daughter.

For the first time recently, my husband and I went away and left our daughter with my parents. It was a very special time for them to spend several days together. My parents absolutely loved dressing her up and taking her for walks. They had so many fun stories to tell us when we got home!

I had left my parents a whole list of instructions for what to do if our daughter had any trouble while we were gone, but I'm pretty sure they just laughed it off. They like to remind me that they raised all of us and know what they're doing!

I always thought it was just a cute saying that "it takes a village to raise a child." But now I understand. I am very grateful for my family's love and support.

—*Jennifer Bacani McKenney, MD*

Encouraging Sibling Peace

Around 80 percent of Americans have at least one sibling. No one knows what percentage of them actually *like* those siblings, however.

A recent Gallup poll asked Americans what they thought was the ideal family size: 56 percent think it's best to have a small family of one, two, or no children; 34 percent think it's ideal to have a larger family; 9 percent have no opinion. Were they awake?

The average response was 2.5 children, which hasn't changed much since the 1970s. Prior to that, Americans were more likely to have larger families.

No matter how many children you have, keeping the peace can be difficult. That might explain some of our fascination with reality shows like *Quints by Surprise*. *If Ethan and Casey Jones can keep it together with six kids, surely I can keep the peace in my house,* you might think.

❧

Sibling squabbles can be very frustrating to parents. My husband and I have learned that leading by example is the best teaching guide. We treat each other and our children with respect, and they have learned to do the same.

— *Aline T. Tanios, MD, a mom of nine- and three-year-old daughters and a seven-year-old son and a pediatric hospitalist at Arkansas Children's Hospital, in Little Rock*

❧

My younger daughter and son are only 20 months apart. To this day, we call them the "little ones." Having two very small children was hard when they were babies and toddlers. But now they're inseparable. They can't live together, but they can't live apart either. One minute, they'll kick and trip each other; the next minute, they'll hug and play together. It's very cute.

— *Siobhan Dolan, MD, MPH*

❧

One of the biggest challenges during my kids' toddler years was sibling rivalry. The constant fighting was so annoying. I found a book called *How to Talk So Kids Will Listen and Listen So Kids Will Talk* and its sequel, *Children without Rivalry*.

When I told my brother about that first book, he joked, "What is that, a novel?" But the books really helped me. I often found books held the solutions to my difficult parenting challenges.

— *Dana S. Simpler, MD, a mom of 25- and 20-year-old girls and a 23-year-old son and a specialist in internal medicine in private practice, in Baltimore, MD*

We had a challenging dynamic in my family. My oldest three children are very close in age, and my second child could be very ornery and irritable. Looking back, I think it was because he often didn't feel well. He was often sick with recurrent sinus infections.

Fortunately, my daughters, one of whom was older than my son and one of whom was younger, were very accommodating to and forgiving of him. It was almost as if they understood that he wasn't feeling well and that was why he acted that way. I rewarded my daughters by giving them lots of praise.

"Thank you for being so kind to your brother," I'd say.

—*Ann Kulze, MD, a mom of 23- and 17-year-old daughters and 22- and 20-year-old sons; a nationally recognized nutrition expert, motivational speaker, and physician; and the author of the best-selling book* Dr. Ann's Eat Right for Life, *in Charleston, SC*

My sons generally get along very well. When one son is up before the other, he can't wait until his brother wakes up too.

When kids argue, it can be tempting to take pity on the younger child and presume that the squabble was the older child's fault. I'm careful not to do that. My younger son can be bossy. He can be the instigator just as often as his big brother. I try to figure out exactly what happened to make sure that I'm disciplining the right son.

—*Sharon Boyce, MD*

My son is six years older than my daughter. Yet they are very close. One way that I fostered their relationship was to involve my son in his younger sister's care. For example, when she was a baby and toddler, I asked my son to read to her. This was great for both of them. Also, when I was attending to my daughter, such as changing her diaper, I'd enlist my son's help to go get me the new diaper.

Today, my kids are very close. My son plays basketball, and my daughter is a cheerleader for his team.

—*Teresa Hubka, DO*

My sons get along very well on the whole. My older son gets frustrated sometimes when his little brother messes up his toys. But they care deeply for each other. The other day, my older son was tired, and he was lying on the couch. My younger son got a blanket and gently placed it over his brother.

Over the holidays, my older son was home from school for their 2½-week break. My younger son was so used to having him around that after the first day back to school, he spent most of the morning looking around the house for his brother!

We are a very affectionate family, so I think this is just mostly learned behavior. My older son loves to sit with me on the couch in the evening, so his little brother just learned to do it. My younger son wasn't very affectionate until he got old enough to really pay attention to what his older brother does.

—*Rebecca Reamy, MD, a mom of seven- and two-year-old sons and a pediatrician in emergency medicine at Children's Healthcare of Atlanta, in Georgia*

With four active boys in the house, there's often a lot of wrestling around. Our kids have taken martial arts for years, and we have a rule that any boy can tap out at any time. That means you tap the other person on the shoulder twice, or if you can't do that, you tap the floor. When someone taps out, all wrestling stops right away. We chose not to make it a verbal cue, like saying "stop," because you can't always speak.

We also have a rule that if the boys decide to wrestle, that's like giving informed consent that you could get hurt. We don't want them to come tattling to us if they get a bump, though a kiss and a cold pack are always available.

—*Deborah Gilboa, MD, a mom of nine-, seven-, five-, and three-year-old sons, a parenting speaker whose advice is found at AskDoctorG.com, and a family physician with Squirrel Hill Health Center, in Pittsburgh, PA*

With two toddlers at the same time, there was always plenty for them to argue about: Who gets to pick the show to watch on TV, gets into the car first, gets to take the first bath, and on and on. I modified a system that our preschool had used with great success to my home: the Star of the Day.

I bought a double-sided photo frame, and I put a photo of my daughter on one side and a photo of my son on the other side. I rotated kids, so one day my daughter was the Star of the Day, the next day my son was. The photos helped me to keep track of whose day it was!

As long as the Star of the Day had good behavior, he or she would get to go first, or choose first, on things all day long. For example, I'd ask the Star, "Do you want to take your bath first, or second?" This strategy prevented tons of disagreements.

—*Eva Mayer, MD*

∽

Three is the new terrible two. Three-year-olds have more independence and a greater demand for attention. When my twins turned three, I really began to see their independence growing in two different directions. That was also the beginning of competition, and my girls would say things like, "She has more grapes than I do," "I want to wear the shoes that she has on," and "My favorite color is blue, not hers."

To make things even more interesting, when my girls were toddlers, we brought home their new baby brother. My solution was toddler dates. I spent some quality one-on-one time with each one. My husband and I try to do this once every two to three months. My husband and I each take one of the twins for a toddler date of about 45 minutes, and then afterward we meet up for lunch or dinner and they can share their date. This helps to shore up the relationship with the parent who is currently not the "Velcro" parent.

—*Brooke A. Jackson, MD*

∽

My kids are just over a year apart. A big challenge for me was having two toddlers at the same time. Both of my kids are very strong-willed. Especially as toddlers, they both wanted what they wanted, when they wanted it. That was very difficult at times.

People told me my kids would be playmates, and that really has been the case. My kids get along very well.

As toddlers, it helped that they both like to do different things, so they weren't arguing over toys. My son loved to read early on, and my daughter preferred to do artistic things.

It's fascinating to watch my kids' relationship change over time. My daughter used to be the more laid-back one, and my son took charge. Now my daughter rules the roost! When they do imaginative play, she's the teacher, the head chef, or the CEO! I'm very curious to see what happens next in their relationship as they grow.

—*Antoinette Cheney, DO*

My children were born a year apart, and they were generally very devoted to one another throughout their lives. However, intense discord was apparent at times. I often felt very helpless and anxious when war broke out. In retrospect, I think the best approach for parents is to try to walk the fine line between too much sibling intervention and too little. When the stronger, older, or more intimidating child seems to be truly victimizing the other, naturally the parent needs to step in and break it up. But often it's best to calmly tell the squabbling offspring to work it out themselves. Encouraging endless "tattling" and micromanagement of your brood are bound to backfire.

The aggressive sibling might be the one who actually "needs more," because the aggression directed toward the other sibling is really an expression of jealousy and anger at the parent, who is too big to take on as an enemy. The older child resents the need to "share" the parent; there doesn't seem to be enough parent to go around. Thus meeting the aggressive child's need for security in the parent's love might be much more effective than insisting all the more firmly that the aggressive child has to "share." Of course, this is somewhat counterintuitive, because the parent is likely to feel like doing just the opposite: comforting the victim and glaring at the aggressor, who is in the dog house. A more helpful approach is often for the parent to take the calming stand—"There's enough love to go around"—rather than reinforcing the idea that the embattled tots must "share."

—*Elizabeth Berger, MD*

Teaching Character, Values, and Manners

The folks at Parents.com asked parents, "What value do you most want to instill in your children?" Here's what they said.

- 54 percent: Kindness/compassion
- 22 percent: Responsibility
- 10 percent: Respect
- 8 percent: Honesty
- 4 percent: Other
- 2 percent: Tolerance

When your child is around 18 months old, she will start to understand that there are certain accepted social graces. She'll hear you say "please" and "thank you," and she'll be eager to please and to be like you, so she'll start to do the same. Because toddlers are great imitators, there's no better time than now to model your best manners. She's watching!

From a very early age, I taught my kids to say key words and phrases, such as "please" and "thank you." I believe if you start early enough, these habits become ingrained in them.

    —*Aline T. Tanios, MD*

The toddler years are the "no" age. My husband and I are strict about this: We don't allow our sons to tell us "no." They may say "no thank you" or "I'd rather do . . ." But they cannot look at us and proclaim "no." When our kids have tried to "no" us, we sent them immediately to time-out on our stairs.

    —*Deborah Gilboa, MD*

Each night as part of our bedtime routine, my husband and I ask our kids to name one thing that they are thankful for. It can be something as simple as, "I'm thankful that I got to go to the park." We began this tradition when our kids were toddlers, and we continue doing it today.

    —*Ann V. Arthur, MD*

I teach my children to make people feel safe and welcome when we're with them. My sons pick up on words and phrases at preschool that aren't nice. I tell my sons, "You might hear other kids say these things at school, but you shouldn't say them."

I really work with my sons to teach them to say, "Yes, Ma'am," "No, Ma'am," "please," and "thank you." These basics lay a foundation for good manners.

Also, each night at dinner, I ask everyone questions such as, "How was your day?" Even now at age three, my middle son asks, "Mommy, what was your favorite thing today?" I want to teach my sons to be kind and to take an interest in other people. It's working well for us.

—*Amy Thompson, MD, a mom of five- and three- and two-year-old sons and an ob-gyn at the University of Cincinnati College of Medicine, in Ohio*

Nothing is transmitted via diffusion; you have to teach things intentionally. I believe that as a parent, you should think about what you value, and then work on transmitting those values to your children.

For example, languages are important to me, so I focus on teaching my daughters foreign languages. There are other things I value less, such as music classes. My daughter took a music class once, wasn't ecstatic about it, and that was it. Not everything in life can be a priority; you have to make choices.

—*Kate Tulenko, MD, MPH*

When my daughter was a toddler, I didn't so much teach her about values and manners as I did set a good example. Sometimes I worried that it wasn't working, though.

At home, my daughter could be a terror. Yet in preschool, she would help the teachers, organize the other kids, and be the most polite child imaginable. One of her teachers told me, "I'm so glad I met your daughter. It makes me so glad I became a teacher."

If you don't always see the behavior you want at home, don't dismay. Kids can behave completely differently at school than they do at home. A friend of mine who's a psychiatrist once told me that it's good for kids to feel comfortable at home so that they can be themselves.

—*Debra Jaliman, MD, a mom of a 20-year-old daughter, a dermatologist in private practice, and an assistant professor of dermatology at Mt. Sinai School of Medicine, in New York City*

⁓

My daughter's very first sentence was spoken as a response to me, as I wailed to no one in particular, "Oh, I'm so cold in this house" one wintery day in Ohio. She beamed up at me and declared triumphantly, "I make you warm, Mommy!"

I believe that the empathy that children show for people whom they love forms the building blocks of children's eventual character. The child's empathy in turn is a response to the parent's overall devotion to the child, part of the give-and-take of their relationship. It isn't a curriculum, and parents don't need to worry about composing artificial lessons, speeches, and reminders that impart values.

Parents who are trustworthy, generous, and respectful will find that their children grow to inherit these qualities through the workshop of everyday interactions. Even "please" and "thank you" are taken in by children amidst a home atmosphere that is gracious and kind. Parents can have faith in the child's capacity to absorb, naturally, the tone that the grown-ups set for human relationships.

—*Elizabeth Berger, MD*

Building Your Toddler's Self-Esteem

Self-esteem is your armor against the unkindnesses of a not–always-so-nice world. If you feel good about yourself, you're better at handling conflicts and resisting negativity. Kids with greater self-esteem smile more, are generally optimistic, and enjoy life more.

Self-esteem is one of those concepts we've read about in 326 self-help books and articles, but it can be hard to wrap your brain around what it actually *is*. Self-esteem is the collection of beliefs and feelings that you have about yourself. It's your self-perceptions, how you define yourself. Your self-esteem influences your motivations, attitudes, and behaviors.

A child's patterns of self-esteem begin very early in life. When your toddler took her first steps, and she heard your praise, saw your smile, and felt your arms embrace her in a hug, that bolstered her self-esteem. Every day, dozens of times a day, your child measures her accomplishments against an internal yardstick. As she tries, maybe fails, tries again, maybe fails again, tries again, and then succeeds, she's developing a sense of her capabilities. She looks to the people around her to gauge their responses. Healthy self-esteem is generated when a child who's happy with an achievement feels loved and supported.

Here's a simple trick to model self-esteem for your toddler: Sit up straight. A new study showed that people who sat up straight, with their backs straight and chests pushed out, reported higher confidence than people who slouched. Polish up your own self-esteem armor a bit today!

⁓

One thing I felt strongly about was that my children's caregivers not say that a child is a "bad" child. Instead, I asked them to say things like, "I don't like what you did."

—*Cathie Lippman, MD, a mom of 31- and 29-year-old sons and a physician who specializes in environmental and preventive medicine at the Lippman Center for Optimal Health, in Beverly Hills, CA*

⁓

I'm a huge believer in the importance of labels. You are what you think you are. So I always tell my girls, "You're such a smart girl," "You're such a pretty girl," You're such a thoughtful girl."

By doing this, you're teaching your children to think of themselves as the people you want them to be.

—*Eva Ritvo, MD, a mom of 21- and 16-year-old daughters, a psychiatrist, and a coauthor of* The Beauty Prescription, *in Miami Beach, FL*

⁓

I don't focus on trying to raise "happy" kids. I hope for their happiness, but I focus on raising kids with these four Rs: respectfulness, responsibility, resilience, and responsiveness. With that foundation, my kids can accomplish anything.

—*Deborah Gilboa, MD*

There's a lot of good evidence that rather than praising a child for being smart, it's better to praise her instead for being persistent. Kids can think they're smart, but if they encounter something challenging, they'll stop doing it. The fact that they're not able to accomplish something goes against their self-image. But if they believe they're persistent, and they encounter a challenge, they'll keep trying because that's consistent with their self-image.

—*Kate Tulenko, MD, MPH*

I try to limit phone conversations and texting when I have my children with me. It's rude to talk on the phone or text in front of someone else. So I don't do it in front of my children or husband—or my friends.

—*Elizabeth Chabner Thompson, MD, MPH*

A toddler's self-esteem is based on his pride in his own mastery and on his love relationships. The first of these is naturally somewhat shaky,

MomMyTIME Take a Martial Arts Class

Exercise is well known for boosting self-esteem, and what better way to feel strong and confident than to take up martial arts? Martial arts help improve your cardiovascular conditioning, strength, and flexibility, and they have the added benefit of teaching you self-defense. You could try literally dozens of different types of martial arts, including karate, tae kwon do, krav maga, and kung fu. If none of those appeal to you, simply try a kickboxing class. Many martial arts studios even offer classes for kids three and up *and* moms, which means you can get your workout and confidence boost while your three-year-old learns kung fu.

because toddlers are very liable to run into frustrating situations that they cannot master. In fact, the toddler's day often must seem like an unending series of ambitions foiled by an uncooperative reality: things they can't reach and things that don't obey the toddler's will.

Parents can build their child's self-esteem by trying to arrange matters so their child doesn't experience too much frustration and disappointment, to the degree that this is possible. The parent who helps the child attain the ambition of the moment, so that the toddler has the illusion of mastery and success, is building the child's self-esteem. There are a thousand ways to help a child do things "all by myself," such as getting into a difficult sweater, that illustrate this principle.

The ordinary devotion and love that parents extend to their children is also the bedrock of a child's self-esteem. There is nothing wrong with directly praising a child's actual achievement in words, but the real message of devotion is conveyed through actions, gestures, and looks, which are more eloquent than words. The parent's heart says, "You're the best little girl in the world," or "That's the most beautiful crayon picture that I ever saw." These are not administrative assessments, which might or might not be accurate, but statements of devotion.

It helped me so much to recognize that being rigid as a mother often undermines the sense of pride toddlers take in doing things "all by myself." I could insist on bundling my toddler into a jacket before we walked out the door—when it made no sense to the child, who already felt warm enough indoors. A power struggle about jackets was certainly one option. Another was to suggest a jacket to the toddler but let her go outdoors into the snow without a jacket if the suggestion about the jacket met with resistance. After a minute outdoors, the child was happy to put on the jacket (with a little help) "all by myself!" Then the memory of the day is "I had fun in the snow with Mommy" not "I had a fight with Mommy about a jacket." Very soon, the toddler can anticipate the cold weather and begins to see the wisdom of putting on jackets beforehand. The toddler then owns the experience, rather than being the humiliated loser in a power struggle.

—*Elizabeth Berger, MD*

Chapter 15
Helping Your Toddler Become Self-Disciplined

YOUR TODDLER'S DEVELOPMENT

At two, a child has a very limited understanding of "good" and "bad." He doesn't yet understand rules and warnings. So when you tell him, "It's bad if you grab the cat's tail because she might bite you," your toddler hears something akin to the teacher in *Peanuts* cartoons, "Wah, wah, wah, wah, wah, wah, wah." Instead of simply telling your toddler not to grab the cat's tail, it's necessary to *show* your toddler how to gently pet the cat. If your toddler still insists on manhandling your pet, your best bet is to remove your child—or the cat—from the situation. At this age, your toddler needs gentle guidance and constant supervision.

Your two- and then three-year-old might often melt into temper tantrums. Toddlers, with limited ability to communicate verbally, sometimes resort to pushing and shoving to get their own way. Toddlers are very physical beings! It's very difficult, some might say impossible, to reason with a young toddler. They view things in simple terms.

The most important things to do are to guide your toddler with kindness, focus on his safety, and model the behavior that you want from him. This is what will help your child to develop the self-discipline he needs as he grows.

TAKING CARE OF YOU

A popular discipline strategy for toddlers is time-out. Bet you could use a time-out yourself! Make yourself a special, Mom's time-out place. Choose a favorite spot in your home, preferably by a sunny window, where you can place a comfy chair, a small table for a cup of tea, and a basket for books, notepaper, and pens. Now go have a time-out!

JUSTIFICATION FOR A CELEBRATION
Anytime your child really pushes your buttons, but you keep your cool and speak softly and kindly, give yourself a huge pat on the back.

Considering Your Options
Google "discipline" and "toddlers" and you'll find more than 7 million results, ranging from ignoring bad behavior to spanking, and everything in between. Whatever strategy you try, experts suggest giving it about three weeks before you expect to see an effect. Some strategies to consider include the following.

Positive reinforcement: Praise and encourage the behavior that you like.

Extinguishing: Ignore the behavior that you don't like.

Time-outs: Give the child one minute of time-out for each year of age.

Logical consequences: Connect the behavior with an outcome, such as having your toddler pick up the blocks he just dumped onto the floor.

Never resort to punishments that emotionally or physically hurt your child. Harsh spanking, slapping, screaming, and swearing will damage your relationship with your child. Break the cycle of abuse if you have to: As recently as 1998, the American Academy of Pediatrics reported that 90 percent of U.S. parents spanked their kids at some time. According to a more recent *Pediatrics* study, 80 percent of preschool kids have been spanked. In another study, kids who had been physically disciplined were almost 50 percent more likely to be physically aggressive. Don't be a statistic.

When my children were toddlers, I found that taking away a privilege was an effective method of discipline. Kids are very smart and are talented in manipulating their parents' attention, which makes it harder to discipline them. When you take away from them—even for just a few minutes—anything they enjoy playing with, they will start realizing that there is a consequence for bad behavior. This will allow you to avoid other methods of discipline that can be more harmful and less rewarding.

Far more effective than discipline, though, was giving my toddlers praise when they did something good.

—*Aline T. Tanios, MD, a mom of nine- and three-year-old daughters and a seven-year-old son and a pediatric hospitalist at Arkansas Children's Hospital, in Little Rock*

When my kids were toddlers, we used time-outs. I gave them one minute of time-out for each year of age. A challenge was that my son wouldn't sit in the time-out chair! He'd sneak away from the chair to play with his toys. So I would sit and hold him on my lap for the time-out. My son didn't like it, but he made it through the time-outs that way.

—*Eva Mayer, MD, a mom of an eight-year-old daughter and a six-year-old son and a pediatrician with St. Luke's Pediatrics Associates, in Bethlehem, PA*

Our middle child is very strong-willed. Generally, we use time-outs. But we do spank for severe things, such as safety issues.

—*Amy Thompson, MD, a mom of five- and three- and two-year-old sons and an ob-gyn at the University of Cincinnati College of Medicine, in Ohio*

My husband and I started to use time-outs when our kids were very young, around 18 months old. Our time-out place is on our stairs or on our shoe bench. These are singularly boring places without toys but without danger as well.

The parents have to be in charge. If you give a toddler half the chance, he will try to be in charge, even though he isn't most comfortable that way. I let my kids know that "Dad and I are in charge; you don't have to be."

—*Deborah Gilboa, MD, a mom of nine-, seven-, five-, and three-year-old sons, a parenting speaker whose advice is found at AskDoctorG.com, and a family physician with Squirrel Hill Health Center, in Pittsburgh, PA*

No matter what discipline techniques work for your family and each individual child, consistency is the key to disciplining your toddler. The minute you back down or don't follow through, you have destroyed any progress you made. All discipline needs some appropriate consequence, and that's obviously age and behavior appropriate. You need to tell the child what is going to be their consequence if they don't stop a particular behavior, and then you actually need to execute that consequence without letting the child bargain his way out of it.

My children knew what the word *consequence* meant at a very early age. It has helped now that they are older. I am carrying that through with the concepts of "consequences of their choices and living with them."

—*Marra S. Francis, MD, a mom of eight-, seven-, and five-year-old daughters and a gynecologist, in San Antonio, TX*

Instead of using time-out or grounding my children, I assign chores. I started as young as age two with chores such as putting away a toy and picking up trash. As my children grew, the chores advanced in complexity. Different behaviors get different numbers of chores.

This strategy helps to get my house clean, and also I believe it teaches an amazing lesson. We all make mistakes. We can make amends quickly and move on to the fun parts of life, or we can dwell on our consequences and make them seemingly last forever.

—*Jennifer Hanes, DO, a mom of a six-year-old daughter and a three-year-old son, an emergency physician, a certified forensic physician, and the founder of Empowered Medicine, PLLC, in Austin, TX*

When toddlers are misbehaving, it's often easy to distract them with a surprise. Everyone loves a surprise! It's a great motivator.

When my girls were two and three years old and I needed them to pay attention to me, I'd say, "Mommy has a surprise for you." Then the pressure would be on because I would have to come up with something novel to show them. Changing what you are doing can also help eliminate misbehaving. "It's time to go do something different," I would say. Toddlers have very short attention spans, and you can use that to your advantage.

—*Eva Ritvo, MD, a mom of 21- and 16-year-old daughters, a psychiatrist, and a coauthor of* The Beauty Prescription, *in Miami Beach, FL*

My daughter didn't go through a biting or hitting phase, thank goodness. But we did have the usual tantrums. When my daughter misbehaved, my strategy was to count to three.

"What happens when you get to three?" people have often asked me.

"We've never gotten to three!" I explain.

I think my daughter knew from a very early age that if we got to three, there would be a consequence, such as a time-out. But I never had to articulate that to her. She just knew.

—*Christy Valentine, MD, a mom of a six-year-old daughter, a specialist in pediatrics and internal medicine, and the founder of the Valentine Medical Center, in Gretna, LA*

I used to hold my son's hand at the curb and say, "Now, let's look both ways." Later on, I would hear him say to himself under his breath, "Now, let's look both ways." Of course, I wouldn't let him run into the street. The grown-ups need to keep toddlers safe until they are old enough to keep themselves safe reliably. But my son's statement revealed the way that the child who feels loved and protected by the parent gradually takes on the parent's role in his own self-management.

A toddler's growing capacity to manage himself is based in part on the parent's controlling the overall situation so that actual danger simply doesn't arise. But once the parent has controlled the situation and made it safe, the toddler develops self-control through admiring the parent and wanting to be like her. Toddlers are eager to put on your glasses, to wear your shoes, and to copy your tone of voice. The drive within toddlers to imitate people whom they love is immense. This drive forms the core of the child's ambition to manage himself one day, the way the parent used to do.

—*Elizabeth Berger, MD, a mom of a 29-year-old son and a 27-year-old daughter, a child psychiatrist, and the author of* Raising Kids with Character, *in New York City*

Parenting each of my four children offered unique challenges. Finding effective ways to discipline each of them was one of the hardest. Each child was like a new chapter in a book. For example, time-out worked well for two children, but not at all for the others. The trick was finding out which technique worked for each child.

One technique that was *not* helpful was sending my daughter to her room. A child's room should be a sanctuary, not a place of punishment. But my husband and I were desperate, and we couldn't think of anywhere else to put her. To this day, she's challenging to discipline!

When a toddler is acting out, it's not so much misbehaving as it is challenging you. If what the child was doing was dangerous and it was a safety issue, I stopped whatever I was doing, held the child close to my face, and said "No" in a very harsh tone. That way, the child knew this "no" was different from the hundreds of other "nos" he heard.

—*Victoria McEvoy, MD, a mom who raised four children; a grandmom of six-, four-, and two-year-old grandsons; an assistant professor of pediatrics at Harvard Medical School; the medical director and chief of pediatrics at Mass General West Medical Group; and the author of* 24/7 Baby Doctor, *in Boston, MA*

We're not spankers or yellers; we're a big time-out family. My husband and I started to give time-outs when our sons were around a year old. When our sons misbehave, we send them to have a time-out away from everyone else, usually in their rooms. My kids don't have a lot of toys in their rooms; they pretty much just sleep in there.

Our older son was very rambunctious, and he had lots of time-outs. On the other hand, our younger son has probably only been in time-out a half dozen times in his entire life. The length of the time-out varies. The key is, they have to be quiet in time-out, not shrieking. Sometimes, if my older son was quiet for 30 seconds, I was happy and let him out. But of course if he turned around and did the same thing again, then I'd keep him in time-out a little longer.

My husband and I also give our sons' toys time-outs, when appropriate. For example, if one of our sons threw a toy, that toy would go into time-out on top of the fridge for a while. We still do this. The Wii was on time-out recently because it got a little too much love over the holidays.

—*Carrie Brown, MD, a mom of eight- and six-year-old sons and a general pediatrician who treats medically complex children and specializes in palliative care at Arkansas Children's Hospital, in Little Rock*

∽

When my sons were toddlers, spanking wasn't my approach. But over the years, I've started to realize that I'm not totally opposed to spanking anymore. I know spanking isn't politically correct, but in my experience, when a child is acting in a way that you cannot reason with him, and he could do harm to himself or others, spanking might be a viable option. I know some people consider all spanking to be abuse, but I think there are many fine lines in life in general, and in parenting in particular. Spanking is one of them.

One thing that I see more often these days is children abusing their parents. It's heart-wrenching for me to see a child calling all of the shots and seeing the parents acting spineless or weak. I wonder if those parents were too tightly controlled by their parents, and now they have gone the other way and are too permissive with their own children. Children need to have boundaries.

I believe that many behavioral issues can be treated with homeopathy: from violent behaviors to impulsiveness and hyperactivity. These deeply rooted conditions can be treated by a holistic practitioner, who might recommend holistic medical treatments and also dietary changes. In homeopathy, there are dozens of different medicinal choices for these types of behaviors. The correct medicine is chosen following an in-depth consultation for each individual.

—Lauren Feder, MD, a mom of 18- and 14-year-old sons, a nationally recognized physician who specializes in homeopathic medicine, and the author of Natural Baby and Childcare *and* The Parents' Concise Guide to Childhood Vaccinations, *in Los Angeles, CA*

Coping with Criticism

Parenting isn't for wimps. And that's on a good day. Certain parenting topics—such as circumcision, bed-sharing, and spanking—are minefields because they touch upon passionate, deeply held beliefs and feelings. Plus, they're polarizing, leaving little room for middle ground. It's difficult if you disagree with your partner, your parents, or even your physician about deeply held convictions regarding discipline.

If a friend told me she didn't approve of how I was disciplining my children, I would probably walk away and think, *You cannot tell me what to do.*

—Sadaf T. Bhutta, MD, a mom of a six-year-old daughter and four-year-old triplets and an assistant professor and the fellowship director of pediatric radiology at the University of Arkansas for Medical Sciences and Arkansas Children's Hospital, both in Little Rock

When my younger daughter was a toddler, I got a lot of criticism from family for carrying her around too much.

"Why are you carrying her? She's old enough to walk," they'd say.

I simply ignored those comments. When kids are two and three years old, they still need a lot of physical contact, hugging, and kissing. Love triggers the secretion of good chemicals such as serotonin and oxytocin that make people feel happy, safe, and connected. I spent as much time as I could close by my daughters, such as sitting close to them and reading. Now my younger daughter rows crew, and I barely see her. I am glad for the extra time we spent together when she was young. Carrying her as a toddler certainly didn't hurt her motor skills or independence!

—*Eva Ritvo, MD*

My mother has never approved of the way that we discipline our children. When my sons were toddlers, my mother repeatedly told me that they were "out of control."

My husband and I received no complaints from the day care, and our sons seemed to behave about as well as the other children we spent time with. I chose to ignore my mother, which wasn't too difficult because we saw her only once or twice a year.

When my mother visited most recently, she commented about how well my now eight- and six-year-old sons behaved. She said that maybe she had been wrong to judge them—and my parenting—when she saw them only a few days a year.

It can be hard for children to be on their best behavior when they are very young and excited to see a new person or to be in a new environment. My best advice is to have confidence in your parenting style and to not let the feelings of others change how you do things if your children do well in their usual environments. Consistency is the most important thing for kids.

—*Carrie Brown, MD*

When it comes to child-rearing practices, China and the United States differ in many ways. In China, for example, parents are much more likely to pick up their babies when they cry. When my daughter was a baby and toddler, some of my husband's Midwestern relatives told me, "She needs to cry it out, become more independent, and take care of herself."

I disagreed with them. Allowing my daughter to cry, to not soothe her, would have meant bathing her brain and body in stress hormones at crucial stages of their development. How can that be good?

I always thought of my child first. I did what I knew was best for her, no matter what others said.

As a psychiatrist, I know that a child learns to cope emotionally by having that image of a loving parent to carry around for the rest of life. Babies and toddlers need to know that their needs will be met. I always did my best to soothe my toddler, no matter what.

These same relatives have commented on how "easy" my child is now, and how she's not obstinate. It's no coincidence. She learned early in life that she's important and worthy. She doesn't have to keep testing us, to reassure herself. People have also commented on how alert my child is, and how well she concentrates. I believe it's because during her earliest years, I made sure that her brain was not scattered by anxiety.

> —*Dora Calott Wang, MD, a mom of a nine-year-old daughter, a psychiatrist and historian at the University of New Mexico School of Medicine, and the author of* The Kitchen Shrink: A Psychiatrist's Reflection on Healing in a Changing World, *in Albuquerque, NM*

RALLIE'S TIP

My husband and I didn't see eye to eye when it came to disciplining our children. He believed that spanking was necessary from time to time, especially when one of our toddlers was defiant or blatantly disobedient. I wasn't a big fan of spanking; I thought it was kind of a parenting shortcut. We had a few heated debates about this, but we finally agreed that we would each discipline our toddlers as we saw fit, as long as the discipline was age appropriate and administered with love and compassion. We also agreed that we wouldn't argue about methods of discipline in front of our children. My goal was to teach our sons right from wrong ahead of time, rather than punish them for doing something that they didn't know was wrong in the first place. My husband had the added goal of teaching them to respect authority from an early age.

By the time my two youngest sons were toddlers, I'd already been through the toddler years with my oldest son. I learned from experience that as a parent, I could usually prevent my toddler from disobeying me if I redirected his attention early enough. If he wanted to climb the stairs but I wanted him to stay in the living room with me, I could usually entice him to step away from the stairs if I asked him to come and play a game or sit down and read a book with me. This took a lot more effort than just saying, "No, don't go up the stairs," but it also was much more effective in getting my son's cooperation and helped us sidestep a battle of wills.

The trouble with this approach is that at some point, for toddlers' own safety, they need to know that no means no. Parents don't always have time to redirect a child's attention, such as when the child is running toward a busy street or reaching to pet a snarling dog. Giving toddlers an unpleasant consequence, such as a spanking, for being disobedient might protect them from far worse consequences down the road. That was my husband's philosophy, and although I saw the wisdom of it, I still wasn't willing to spank my toddlers. And as it turned out, my husband is very kind and gentle and has tons of patience, so he rarely spanked any of our boys. I think that just knowing that Dad was perfectly capable of administering a spanking made our toddlers mind him a little more quickly than they minded me.

Resolving Your Toddler's Negative Behaviors

What's your child's most annoying behavior? In a poll, 33 percent of parents said whining, 22 percent said tantrums, 20 percent said refusing to listen, 15 percent said talking back, and 10 percent said other. For those vastly different frustrations, it's probably best to have a range of discipline options from which to choose.

❧

I don't so much believe in tough love, but I do believe it takes a certain amount of maturity to say, "This is the way we do things." I think it's important to set clear limits for children. There are no magical answers, and I don't pretend to be the best at it.

I received a wonderful gift a few years ago when my older son thanked me for being so strict. He told me that he didn't like it at the time, but looking back, he appreciates it.

—Cathie Lippman, MD, a mom of 31- and 29-year-old sons and a physician who specializes in environmental and preventive medicine at the Lippman Center for Optimal Health, in Beverly Hills, CA

⁓

When my daughter misbehaved, I always gave her the benefit of the doubt. First, I thought about her physical needs. Was she hungry? Tired? Sometimes misbehavior is simply an indication that a child's physical needs aren't being met.

Next, I wondered if my daughter's emotional needs were being met. I tried to address her emotional needs—did she feel slighted, ignored, or wronged somehow? I would redirect and educate her about her misbehavior. Along with redirecting, I'd also often hug her and give her reassurances that I knew she was trying hard.

—Dora Calott Wang, MD

⁓

Sometimes when my younger son gets very angry, he bangs his head on the floor. This concerned me. I worried that he might hurt himself.

But my son doesn't bang his head too many times before he realizes it hurts. I imagine he probably thinks, *Ouch! That was dumb!*

—Rebecca Reamy, MD, a mom of seven- and two-year-old sons and a pediatrician in emergency medicine at Children's Healthcare of Atlanta, in Georgia

⁓

When my son was born, my daughter was almost 2½ years old. When I breastfed my son, my daughter acted out to gain my attention.

To remedy this, I bought a hat at the craft store. My daughter and I decorated the hat with gems, feathers, and stickers. We called it her "attention hat." When my daughter was feeling left out, she would put on her hat to let me know. Usually all I had to do to ward off a tantrum was acknowledge my daughter's feelings.

—Jennifer Hanes, DO

⁓

One of the biggest challenges with my toddlers, and now my "grand-toddlers," began when they learned the word *no*. Even after they understand what "no" means, they will give you that look that says, "Yeah, I know you said 'no,' but I'm going to do it anyway." Even more interesting is when they "no" you right back.

Of course you have to be firm, but I found that it helped me to reserve the word *no* for when I really needed it, such as "No, don't put your hand on the hot stove. It's dangerous." Otherwise, I'd try to reroute them rather than saying "no" all of the time.

—*Susan Besser, MD, a mom of six grown children, ages 27, 25, 23, 21, 20, and 18, a grandmom of two, a family physician, and the medical director of Doctors Express-Memphis, in Tennessee*

My older son was a head banger. From about the age of 13 months, when he got frustrated or angry, he would throw himself to the floor forward and hit his head. I have always told parents that if you ignore the behavior and the bruises, the head banging will stop. His did not.

When my son was about 14 months old, I asked the day care teacher if he was doing anything like that at day care because he never came home with new bruises, although he often arrived at day care with new ones. Turned out, she was catching him when he threw himself down and then giving him something different to play with, because she didn't want him to get injured at day care. I asked her to please let him fall because that would help stop the behavior, but she stated that she could not unless I had a note from his doctor saying that it was the correct thing to do in that situation. My son's pediatrician wrote the note. He came home from day care with new bruises twice the following week and never threw himself to the floor again.

—*Carrie Brown, MD*

Tackling Tantrums

Tantrums are often described as "emotional storms," implying that they're chaotic and uncontrollable. New research published in the journal *Emotions* might have proved that wrong. Scientists listened to high-fidelity audio recordings of more than 100 tantrums. (No amount of money could have adequately compensated them for that.) The scientists discovered that the tantrums weren't chaotic at all. Instead, they followed distinct patterns and rhythms.

Also, the scientists disproved the age-old theory that tantrums begin in anger and end in sadness. Instead, the scientists found that tantrums are anger and sadness *intertwined*.

The researchers suggest that the trick to ending a tantrum is to diffuse the child's anger by not reacting to the tantrum. This way, the child is left with sadness, and sad children instinctively reach out for comfort.

◇

My daughters never had tantrums. They hardly ever even cried. People have this notion of the terrible twos, but they don't have to be that way.

? When to Call Your Doctor

The toddler years are a time when kids start becoming independent, and that means you'll be hearing the word *no* more often and temper tantrums might make an appearance every day. What's most important might be to remember that children tend to continue doing something they're rewarded for and stop doing things when they're being ignored.

According to the American Academy of Family Physicians, you can approach negative behavior three ways. You might decide that it's not a problem because it's typical behavior for a toddler; you might try to stop it by ignoring it (which will work over a period of time) or punishing it with a time-out; or you could redirect your child to do something more appropriate (such as throw the ball outside instead of inside the house). When your child does show good behavior, reward him with praise, a hug, an extra bedtime story, extra time before bed, a favorite snack, a star sticker or stamp on his hand, or another treat that will make him happy.

If you're not able to find discipline strategies that work, try asking your doctor for advice or to recommend a parenting class at a hospital, community center, or school.

I don't think it's normal for kids to have tantrums. Perhaps they're hungry or upset about something, alone too much, or not getting enough sleep. Try to get to the root of the issue.

If your child's twos are terrible, think of the basics: HALT. Is your toddler hungry? Angry? Lonely? Tired?

—*Eva Ritvo, MD*

My daughter didn't have a lot of tantrums, fortunately. One of my child-rearing goals is for my child to feel like we're on the same side—that she doesn't need to fight me.

I try to see tantrums as opportunities. A tantrum is an opportunity to better understand a child. It's also an opportunity to teach a child about better methods of expression.

—*Dora Calott Wang, MD*

Temper tantrums in public were a big challenge during my daughter's toddler years. This problem was solved by pure luck. My daughter was lying in the middle of the sidewalk kicking and screaming when her favorite male babysitter walked by and asked what she was doing lying on the sidewalk. Totally humiliated, my daughter got right up. That was the last public tantrum.

It was around this age that my daughter began to understand that she could earn a reward for "acting good" in stores and other public places. We would have a little talk, and I would remind her about this before getting out of the car.

—*Stuart Jeanne Bramhall, MD, a mom of a 31-year-old daughter and a child and adolescent psychiatrist in New Plymouth, New Zealand*

If a toddler is just starting to misbehave, he can often be distracted or redirected. ("Hey, what's that over there?")

But if a toddler is having a full-out tantrum, I found walking out of the room was often effective. One time, my husband and I decided to give our children some culture. So we took them to a very sophisticated art museum in Boston. One of our sons, who was two years old at the time, decided to have a full-on meltdown. He was on the floor screaming. My husband and I were so mortified that we left the room! That worked. Our son stopped screaming. He was probably wondering, *Where'd my audience go?*

—*Victoria McEvoy, MD*

∽

In general, I'm a big fan of positive feedback and encouraging positive behaviors and discouraging or ignoring negative ones.

For tantrums, for example, I'd make sure my sons were safe, and then I'd walk away. Then after they were done having a tantrum, I'd give them hugs and kisses. If you do a lot of yelling when they're yelling, you're giving them attention. If they don't get attention, the behavior will extinguish.

Toddlers don't have a lot of control in their lives. They have control over their pooping, eating, and falling asleep. That's where you're going to have the battles.

—*Heather Orman-Lubell, MD, a mom of 11- and 7-year-old sons and a pediatrician in private practice at Yardley Pediatrics of St. Christopher's Hospital for Children, in Pennsylvania*

∽

As adults, my husband and I do not have tantrums. You'll hear no yelling and screaming from the adults in our family. We ask that there be no yelling and screaming from the children either. When my toddlers had tantrums in public or at home, I'd always convey the same message: Your tantrum will not change my behavior, and it's undignified. So stop it.

Children always seek positive attention, but second best is negative attention. I try not to make "no" a reflex answer to the kids. Most children will push back against a "no," but there are clever ways around every situation that you want to "no."

—*Elizabeth Chabner Thompson, MD, MPH, a mom of 13- and 8-year-old daughters and 12- and 10-year-old sons, a radiation oncologist with 21 C. Radiation Oncology, and the inventor of the Mommy Bag, filled with supplies for moms-to-be having C-sections, in Scarsdale, NY*

Most adults "lose it" and go to pieces from time to time, and small children—who are much less expert at managing themselves and at managing the world—are particularly vulnerable to feeling overwhelmed by hopeless frustration at times, a kind of falling apart that is sometimes captured by the word *tantrum* or *meltdown*.

I remember very well feeling very sad, anxious, and bewildered when my own toddlers collapsed in this manner. What helped me was the conviction that providing a soothing comfort to the child was the shortest path to children pulling themselves back together. Whatever other agenda had occupied me the moment before had to give way. Providing a lap, a voice that said, "There, there," and a relief from whatever pressure had precipitated the breakdown had to come first.

A parent who frames these moments as a power struggle with the child is in for a very hard time. The struggle is within the child. The parent's job is to help the child settle the raging war inside, so that the child can pull himself together and move on, supported by the parent's empathy.

—Elizabeth Berger, MD

❧

My daughter is very strong-willed. Even as a toddler, she had an opinion about everything. Some days, when her regular babysitter was on vacation, the temp would bring her to my office at the end of the day, and then I'd take her home with me.

One day, my daughter decided she didn't want to take our usual subway train home. She wanted to take a different train, never mind it was going in the wrong direction. My daughter became very upset when I explained that wasn't the right train. Her tantrum was so extreme that I grabbed her and held her close because she was becoming so explosive. People were staring at us! I had to hold her tight all the way home on the train.

We got through that phase, and today my daughter is the happiest person I know.

—Dina Strachan, MD, a mom of a six-year-old daughter, a
dermatologist and director of Aglow Dermatology, and an assistant

clinical professor in the department of dermatology at New York University, in New York City

⌒

One of the hardest times with my daughter was the terrible twos. She was very high strung, determined, strong-willed, and opinionated. When we were out in public, sometimes my daughter would throw a tantrum. I'd want to crawl under a rock. Once my daughter threw a tantrum at a dinner party, and a friend who's a clinical psychiatrist said my daughter was the most strong-willed child she'd ever seen!

I weathered my daughter's emotional storms as best I could. I think that kids are the way they are, and we can't do much to change their personalities. Even when my daughter was a toddler and it was challenging, I tried to look at her personality traits in a positive light. Teachers would tell me what a natural leader she was.

Now that my daughter is grown up, her determination isn't a bad thing. Really, it's a good trait. My daughter excelled in school, and she was accepted into her first-choice college. Sometimes the qualities in a toddler that drive you nuts become tremendous assets as kids grow up.

—Debra Jaliman, MD, a mom of a 20-year-old daughter, a dermatologist in private practice, and an assistant professor of dermatology at Mt. Sinai School of Medicine, in New York City

RALLIE'S TIP

Sometimes, children feel completely overwhelmed emotionally, and they just don't have any good ways to express how they're feeling or to relieve the tension. A temper tantrum is often the result. It seems that kids often have tantrums when parents are least prepared to deal with them—when we're in a hurry, trying to accomplish something, or stressed out. That's probably not a coincidence. Our emotions undoubtedly contribute to our children's state of overwhelm.

As toddlers, all of my boys had temper tantrums from time to time, but fortunately they were few and far between. My middle son had an especially memorable tantrum in the parking lot of the Riverbanks Zoo in Columbia, South Carolina. We had been traveling for a few hours beforehand, and the weather was hot and humid. While my husband and I were strapping our boys into their stroller, my two-year-old had a complete meltdown right beside the car.

My husband and I stood close beside him to make sure he was safe and didn't hurt himself, but we didn't try to reason with him. We just let him scream and cry and roll around until he got all of his frustrations out. We got a few questioning looks from other adults, but we tried to ignore them. After a few minutes, our son's fury and frustration were spent, and my husband picked him up, and we hugged him and comforted him. By then, my son was ready to go and see the animals in the zoo.

I think that it's far better to focus on preventing tantrums rather than punishing children for having them. It's our job as parents to make sure that our children don't become so tired, hungry, or emotionally overwhelmed that they end up having a tantrum. It might take your child having a tantrum or two for you to figure out what his triggers are. Once you do, you'll have a much easier time preventing them.

Curbing Whining

"But Mommeeeeeee…" Some toddlers aren't whiners. If your child is part of the other 99 percent, hopefully you can come up with a strategy to wind down the whine.

∽◌

Whining is my pet peeve. What I want to do is yell, "Stop whining, now!"

What I *actually* do is explain to my children that if they stop whining and ask for what they want in a "regular" voice, they are more likely to have the desired outcome.

—*Sadaf T. Bhutta, MD*

∽◌

My toddler hasn't really learned to whine, but his seven-year-old brother whines a lot! So I know it's coming.

I think sometimes it helps if you ignore the whining. By that, I mean the whining shouldn't get a positive reaction, or you reinforce it.

—*Rebecca Reamy, MD*

Every now and then, my daughter's speech turns into a bit of a whine, especially if she wants something that I don't want her to have. When this happens, I'm pretty good about distracting her and focusing her attention on something else, like a toy or game, so she forgets what she was whining about. My sister and I like to call this her "Goldfish memory": She's easily distracted and forgets if we make her focus on something else!

—*Jennifer Bacani McKenney, MD, a mom of a one-year-old daughter and a family physician, in Fredonia, KS*

My son became incredibly whiny and clingy as a toddler. He would cry and whimper for hours on end sometimes. I initially made an effort to cater to his whims, but that was giving reinforcement to this behavior. Ignoring my son did not particularly help. He eventually outgrew this stage, so I would say patience was what helped.

—*Bola Oyeyipo-Ajumobi, MD, a mom of four- and one-year-old sons, a family physician in private practice, and the owner of SlimyBookWorm.com, in Highland, CA*

My daughter started to whine when she was around three, after she began pre-K. When she talked to me in that whiny tone of voice, I simply would say, "What? I can't understand you when you speak like that. When you were a baby, I was your Mommy, and I could understand your baby talk. But now that you are a big girl, I need you to speak 'big girl.'"

My daughter pretty quickly realized that whining wasn't having the desired result, and so she stopped. Every now and again, she'll whine, but if I consistently remind her that I can't understand her whining, she'll stop.

—*Christy Valentine, MD*

Stopping Biting and Hitting

Children bite and hit for several different reasons. These reasons change as children grow through different ages and stages. One-year-olds, for instance, might bite or hit as they learn about cause and effect. *What happens if I hit the wall? The cat? My brother?*

Children between 18 months old to two years old might bite or hit for attention. *Mom's on the phone. Hey, pay attention to me!*

Older toddlers might bite or hit because they're angry or frustrated. *That's MY toy! Give it back!* Communicating can be difficult for toddlers, and that can be frustrating. It can be especially challenging for a child to express how he feels. A child might resort to biting and hitting when words fail him.

Fortunately, most children outgrow biting and hitting by age three. By then, they have better control over their feelings—and more words to express them.

∽

My boys did not bite out of anger but rather because they were teething. I tried to remember that they were just looking for anything to chew on. A common phrase in our home is "No biting."

—*Sharon Boyce, MD, a mom of three- and one-year-old sons and a family physician at DayOne Family Healthcare Clinic, in Battle Creek, MI*

∽

My daughter sometimes bites my fingers when I brush her teeth. I think she does it to be more playful than hurtful. But it does hurt! At this point, I think that she's just learning about having free will, and she loves it. We tell her "No," but she'll smile and do it anyway. I know she'll eventually learn to stop, so we just try to be consistent and tell her "No" each time.

—*Jennifer Bacani McKenney, MD*

∽

When my younger son gets frustrated, he bites. Not people, but whatever it is he's mad at, like a toy or the couch. To discourage that behavior, I say to him, "Now that didn't really help, did it?"

—*Rebecca Reamy, MD*

∽

I had the very challenging situation of other people's children biting and hitting my kids. When my Mommy instinct takes over, it can be hard to keep calm and react appropriately. I lifted the offending children up and said, "No, we do not bite/hit" in a very loud voice, being sure that the parent who was responsible for the children would hear me and hopefully intervene.

—*Carrie Brown, MD*

Keeping Your Cool

Thomas Jefferson said, "When angry, count to 10 before you speak. If very angry, count to 100." Whether or not Jefferson's six children inspired him to say this, we can only imagine.

〜

When my son misbehaves, such as by doing something he's not supposed to be doing, I try very hard not to get upset. Instead, I sit down on the floor and look him directly in the face. Then he knows that I'm serious, and he really listens. I change my tone of voice and say "no," and I encourage him to go do something else instead.

—*Michelle Davis-Dash, MD, a mom of a one-year-old son and a pediatrician, in Baltimore, MD*

〜

A very helpful book for me was *1-2-3 Magic*. It was a godsend. The book advocates that when a toddler or child misbehaves, you slowly, calmly count, "1, 2, 3," explaining that the toddler has that time to change his behavior, or else he will receive a consequence, such as a time-out.

What I really liked is that counting "1, 2, 3" also helped me to remain calm as well! Sometimes, I counted very, very slowly!

—*Eva Mayer, MD*

〜

I have learned that kids don't want to be bad. So often, they want to play. This understanding has really helped me to be more patient. For example, if I'm trying to get my son dressed, but he won't listen to me, it's not that he wants to misbehave, but rather that he doesn't want to stop playing.

When this happens, I try to take a deep breath and a step back to figure out what my son needs. Then I try to meet that need before I try to get him to do what I want him to do.

—*Sharon Boyce, MD*

It can be challenging to keep your cool when children misbehave, such as when they have a tantrum. I think the key to dealing with a tantrum, especially when it is in the middle of a public place, is to realize that nearly every adult has had to deal with this with their children or they will be dealing with it once they have kids. Once you overcome the initial embarrassment that you might feel, you can't give in to your child. You don't want to reinforce this behavior with your toddler because then he will attempt it every time he wants something when you are out in public.

Most important, you should keep calm, remove your child from the situation if you feel it's necessary, and let him cry it out. Don't try to reason with a three-year-old having a tantrum.

After your child is done crying, kicking, and screaming, then you can tell him that he should not do that and discuss what happened.

—*Jeannette Gonzalez Simon, MD, a mom of three- and one-year-old daughters and a pediatric gastroenterologist in private practice, in Staten Island, NY*

∽◌

Keeping my cool when my kids are misbehaving is hard for me. Just the other day, I was driving my kids home from school. Two of my kids were talking and playing in the backseat, which quickly escalated to arguing and singing very loudly. I asked them to stop. They didn't. I asked them to stop again. They still didn't.

"If you don't be quiet, I will stop this car and let you out, and you can walk the rest of the way home," I yelled rather loudly. Then I pulled the car over. That got their attention.

—*Sadaf T. Bhutta, MD*

∽◌

I think each stage of childhood has its own challenges. In the toddler years, the challenge was stimulating and motivating our child to listen and behave without having a meltdown every hour! My daughter was developing normally, and she had her own ideas about life and wanted to be independent and assert her own authority.

I knew all this was normal, but it was a challenge to be constantly giving my daughter attention, interacting and playing directly with her, and trying to figure out what discipline was best at the time. Basically, it was mentally draining!

To keep my cool, sometimes I would have to take a deep breath and walk away for a few seconds. Sometimes my daughter would do something that was naughty but so funny I couldn't help but laugh. I didn't want to encourage the behavior, but sometimes it's hard to not laugh at some of the things these toddlers come up with!

Also, it always helped to be around other moms or other families and realize that this challenging behavior is just part of normal development. It helped me to see that other toddlers were acting the same way and moms and dads were experiencing the same frustrations. It's normal!

I think working was also one way I kept my sanity. I felt that being able to go to work and have "adult time" made me a better parent when I came home to my toddler. It was less quantity of time with her, but much higher quality of time.

—*Melody Derrick, MD, a mom of a two-year-old daughter who's expecting another baby and a family physician in private practice with Cadence Physician Group, in Winfield, IL*

Disciplining Other People's Children

Disciplining one's children is hard enough. If you ever find yourself in the difficult situation of having to discipline someone *else's* child, that's really tricky. An online poll of more than 2,000 parents asked moms and dads if they thought that it's okay to discipline someone else's child. More than half of the parents said, "Uh, I dunno," 28 percent said "yes," and only 16 percent said "no."

❧

If other people's children were in my house, they were expected to follow our "house rules." I'd be nice about it and say things like, "That isn't how we treat each other in this house, and if you want to play here, then we need to play nicely." If a child refused to follow the house rules, then she didn't come back to play.

—*Marra S. Francis, MD*

Every summer, we vacation with family, including my kids' cousins. Sometimes, one of my nieces or nephews would break a rule that I saw but their parents didn't. I feel when it is a safety issue and someone gets hurt or has the potential to get hurt, it's important to speak up and discipline the child if need be. It never hurts to give a gentle reminder to the child.

I always made sure to follow up with the parents to let them know what happened.

"I had to tell my little niece to stop doing this," I'd say. "I hope that's okay with you."

—*Eva Mayer, MD*

❧

Having to discipline another person's child is a tough one. Many times, my family is at a park or playground, and we see a child cutting the line for the swings or slide, with no parent around. If I don't know the child, I'll let the first infraction slide—while trying to figure out which parent is his. If the behavior happens again, I calmly tell the child to wait his turn and that he should not cut in line. I also make sure that my daughter knows it is not appropriate behavior.

—*Jeannette Gonzalez Simon, MD*

❧

I recall a few times when I had to react to other children who were putting themselves in danger, such as climbing the outside of a play structure at the playground. I would say, "No, that is not safe" in a very loud voice, so that the adult who was responsible for the children would hear me. A few times, the other mothers took their children and left the park or play area, but I can live with that more than I can live with broken limbs and head injuries.

—*Carrie Brown, MD*

❧

Disciplining other people's children was very easy—until I had children of my own. My friends' kids, my brother's kids—I used to discipline them all the time. But ever since I had kids of my own, I have greater tolerance and patience.

It bothers me when I'm at a friend's house, and I see children misbehaving. I love to see children having fun, but if they cross that line into bad behavior, someone has to say something. My parents freely reprimanded my siblings and me for bad behavior in front of other people anytime, anywhere. And we never developed any complexes. Kids are more resilient than we give them credit for. Many parents these days are more concerned about their kids' psyches and the negative effects their disciplining is going to have. We are raising a whole generation of ill-mannered kids who will grow up to be rude and ill-mannered adults.

—*Sadaf T. Bhutta, MD*

⋐⋑

When my kids were toddlers, I often took them to nearby parks and playgrounds. Sometimes I'd observe another child doing something potentially dangerous, to himself or to others. For example, I'd see children intentionally bumping into other children or jumping out from behind equipment to try to scare other kids.

If I could tell that the parent hadn't noticed and so wasn't likely to intervene, I would speak up.

"Let's try a fun way to do what you are doing," I'd say gently.

I didn't scold the child or draw too much attention to the behavior. But I wanted to prevent anyone from getting hurt.

—*Teresa Hubka, DO, a mom of a 14-year-old son and an 8-year-old daughter, an ob-gyn and the medical director of Comprehensive Wellness Care in Chicago, and an associate professor of obstetrics and gynecology and the chairman and residency program director of the department of obstetrics and gynecology at the Midwestern University/Chicago College of Osteopathic Medicine, in Downers Grove, Illinois*

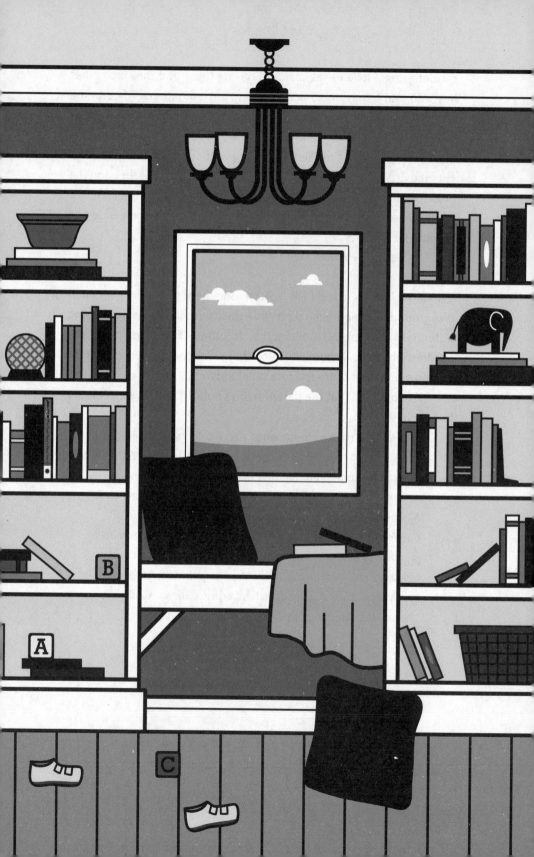

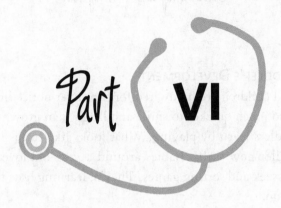

Part VI

LEARNING AND FUN

Chapter 16
Celebrating and Having Fun

YOUR TODDLER'S DEVELOPMENT

Babies and children are hardwired for fun. Ever notice how children are so much quicker to smile and laugh than grown-ups?

Toddlers learn by playing. What looks like fun is teaching your toddler new skills. Babies around a year old love to play hide-and-seek and sorting games. They're learning how to kick a ball and run.

Around 18 months, babies begin to playact, and the magic of make-believe play begins. Your toddler might pretend a banana is a phone or make believe she's eating a book. She's probably able to ride a tricycle now and climb on the play equipment at the park.

By age three, your child's play becomes more complex. You might see her act out her day in play, such as waking her doll up, dressing her, and feeding her "breakfast."

All through these ages and stages, your child's favorite thing to play with is *you*!

TAKING CARE OF *YOU*

Take some time to plan a playdate for yourself. Schedule lunch, shopping, or a movie with a friend.

JUSTIFICATION FOR A CELEBRATION

Someone, somewhere has proclaimed practically every day of the year a holiday for some reason. Why not celebrate some of these unique holidays—or make up one of your own?

- January 3: Festival of Sleep Day (Sleep in!)
- February 7: Send a Card to a Friend Day
- April 2: Children's Book Day (Mark the birthday of Hans Christian Andersen.)
- May 6: No Diet Day (Celebrate with a sundae!)
- June 8: Best Friends Day
- September 21: World Gratitude Day
- October 19: Evaluate Your Life Day
- December 26: Boxing Day (Fill a box to donate to the needy.)

Celebrating Birthdays

Birthdays take on a whole new meaning after you have children. Your children's birthdays are milestones for you too. When your child turns two, that means you've been a mom for two whole years. Happy MomDay!

When my sons were toddlers, we had family parties to celebrate birthdays. When kids are two and three years old, I don't think they need to have elaborate parties with ponies.

—*Heather Orman-Lubell, MD, a mom of 11- and 7-year-old sons and a pediatrician in private practice at Yardley Pediatrics of St. Christopher's Hospital for Children, in Pennsylvania*

The best birthday party we've had so far was when my younger son turned one. Our neighbors had just bought a new chest freezer that came in an enormous box. They gave us the box. I cut out holes for windows and a door, and I even put a battery-operated touch light inside.

At my son's party, I let all of the kids decorate the box as a playhouse. The kids spent more than an hour decorating and playing in that box! And it cost nothing!

—*Carrie Brown, MD, a mom of eight- and six-year-old sons and a general pediatrician who treats medically complex children and specializes in palliative care at Arkansas Children's Hospital, in Little Rock*

Celebrate MomDay

What? You haven't heard of MomDay? We think that it should be a national holiday! MomDay is your child's birthday, but the celebration is for *you*. MomDay serves as a reminder to take some special time on your child's birthday to sit back and reflect upon its significance for you. You've been a mom for two or three years now. *That's* truly something to celebrate!

For my older son's first two birthdays, we've had low-key celebrations at home with our family. My son loves to blow out the birthday candles and eat cake! He's just happy to be surrounded by our family. At this point, he doesn't really pay much attention to his birthday gifts. He just loves the togetherness.

—*Deborah Kulick, MD, a mom of two-year-old and eight-month-old sons, a child and adolescent psychiatrist at the Everett Teen Health Center, and an instructor in psychiatry at Harvard Medical School and the Cambridge Health Alliance, in Boston, MA*

I'm from a large family, and birthday celebrations are big. Our family and extended family get together for a big party. The birthday girl picks out her own cake, and we all sing and have a great time together as a family.

We don't exchange birthday gifts. I've explained to my daughter that some families exchange birthday gifts, but in our family it's about the family, not presents.

—*Christy Valentine, MD, a mom of a six-year-old daughter, a specialist in pediatrics and internal medicine, and the founder of the Valentine Medical Center, in Gretna, LA*

When my kids were very small, we started a special birthday tradition. The night before each child's birthday, we ask the birthday boy or girl what he or she wants to do the next day. Then the whole birthday is about the birthday child, who gets to choose what we eat, where we go, and what we do. My son usually chooses outdoor activities like going to a park. My daughter usually picks things like going to a local arboretum.

—Teresa Hubka, DO, a mom of a 14-year-old son and an 8-year-old daughter, an ob-gyn and the medical director of Comprehensive Wellness Care in Chicago, and an associate professor of obstetrics and gynecology and the chairman and residency program director of the department of obstetrics and gynecology at the Midwestern University/Chicago College of Osteopathic Medicine, in Downers Grove, Illinois

∽

A fun part of the toddler years is when your children get invited to other kids' birthday parties. Our schedule is so crazy that it's really hard to keep everything straight. About a month ago, I went to the wrong birthday party. We got to the party at the jumpy place, and I was looking around for the birthday girl.

"Where's Nadia?" I asked. "I don't know," replied the birthday girl's mom! Uh-oh.

By this time, my kids were already quite invested in the party and having a great time. I wasn't sure how I was going to calmly extract my kids from the party! I went to the right location, but Nadia's birthday party was the day before. I was a day late.

The mom was so gracious, and she invited us to stay.

"We can stay, but we're leaving before they hand out the goodie bags!" I whispered to my kids.

I asked the mom for her e-mail address so we could invite her daughter to our twins' party, which was a few weeks later. After the party, I sent her a huge box of chocolates! As life gets crazier and crazier, I just try to maintain a sense of humor.

—Brooke A. Jackson, MD, a mom of 4½-year-old twin girls and a 2½-year-old son, a dermatologist, and the founder and medical director of the Skin Wellness Center of Chicago, in Illinois

Celebrating Holidays

Holidays are some of the best parts of life, and they're even more special when you get to enjoy them—and see the wonder and excitement—through your child's eyes. Happy day!

We celebrate major holidays with family, and that means taking a trip. With kids, I have just come to expect that I am going to forget to bring something. I just bring what I can, and I figure that unless we're going somewhere really remote, I can buy whatever it is I forgot.

—*Heather Orman-Lubell, MD*

⌒⌒

One of the most fun holidays I remember celebrating when my daughter was a toddler was Easter. When my daughter was two years old, a friend of mine had an Easter egg hunt, using plastic eggs in her backyard. My daughter had so much fun looking for those eggs, and I had such a great time watching her!

—*Christy Valentine, MD*

⌒⌒

This year for Halloween, my older son wanted to be an astronaut. It was very cold here on Trick or Treat night, so we decided not to go out, although I had been looking forward to meeting more of our neighbors.

Rather than walking around outside in the cold, my son was happier staying home and handing out candy to the kids who came to our door. He was so excited to see them all dressed up in their costumes.

—*Deborah Kulick, MD*

⌒⌒

Ever since my kids were babies, I've had this lovely Christmas tradition. I put each of their baby hats on the Christmas tree. I have two tiny pink hats and one tiny blue hat hanging on my tree.

—*Siobhan Dolan, MD, MPH, a mom of 16- and 13-year-old daughters and an 11-year-old son, a consultant to the March of Dimes, and an associate professor of obstetrics and gynecology and women's health at Albert Einstein College of Medicine/Montefiore Medical Center, in Bronx, NY*

⌒⌒

When my oldest child outgrew her toys, I cleaned them and stashed them away in our basement. Then when our youngest child was ready for those toys, I wrapped them up and gave them to her for Christmas! She was only two years old and had never seen those toys, so they were all brand-new and exciting to her, and I was glad to recycle the older toys.

—*Dana S. Simpler, MD, a mom of 25- and 20-year-old girls and a 23-year-old son and a specialist in internal medicine in private practice, in Baltimore, MD*

From the time my daughter was a toddler, I wanted to encourage the spirit of giving over receiving. So my daughter and I would make crafts for her to give as gifts, such as to my mom. My daughter really enjoyed choosing what to make, shopping for the supplies, making the craft, and then, of course, giving her gift to her grandma.

—*Christy Valentine, MD*

My mom has always written a poem and enclosed it with her holiday cards. I adapted that tradition a bit. Throughout the year, I write down the funny things my kids say in books that I call my "Isms Books." Each year at Christmas, I enclose a list of the "Top 10 Isms of the Year." They're filled with witty, wise Wilder women quotes!

—*Susan Wilder, MD, a mom of a 17-year-old daughter and twin 13-year-old girls, a primary care physician, and the founder and CEO of Lifescape Medical Associates, in Scottsdale, AZ*

At Christmastime, we bought a beautiful fresh tree and set it up in our living room. With a toddler in the house, my husband decorated only the top half of the tree.

This is silly, I thought, and so I started to put decorations on the bottom too. As quickly as I put them on, my younger son took them off!

One day, I was at work and my husband was in another room of our house. He heard a loud crash in the living room. When he went to investigate, he found that the Christmas tree had tipped over! We'll never know if our younger son knocked it over, or the cats, or a combination of the two. The good news is that no one was hurt.

—*Rebecca Reamy, MD, a mom of seven- and two-year-old sons and a pediatrician in emergency medicine at Children's Healthcare of Atlanta, in Georgia*

Toddlers love to be a part of things, rather than just watching them happen. My son loves to cook, so a way to help him to be a part of our Hanukkah preparations was allowing him to help me to make cookies. I bought premade dough, and my son stamped the cookies with cookie stamps. He loved to help make the cookies, and, of course, he loved to help eat them too!

Before Hanukkah, I got out all of our books about the holiday and read them to my sons. We also started to play with the dreidel and sing the traditional songs. This is the first year that my older son was starting to understand a bit of what was going on.

I decided to try to separate the gift aspect of the celebration from the spiritual part. So each night, we'd light the candles and sing, but I gave my son gifts sporadically and not at those times. I didn't say, "Here's your Hanukkah present!"

—*Deborah Kulick, MD*

? When to Call Your Doctor

A big, white-bearded man in red, a funny-looking Easter bunny, or Halloween costumes that are scary enough to make adults shiver with fear can certainly take a toll on a toddler who doesn't understand the difference between reality and make-believe. It's normal for a child to be fearful in these situations (the plethora of pictures of terror-stricken kids sitting on Santa's lap can tell you that), but a child will usually settle down after being comforted by a parent.

Kids with anxiety disorders, however, will be so fearful, nervous, and shy that they may want to avoid some places and activities altogether, such as a Halloween party at school or a visit from Santa.

One in eight children has an anxiety disorder, according to the Anxiety Disorders Association of America. Those children who don't get treated might end up struggling later in school, have trouble in social situations, or abuse drugs when they're older. If you think your child is unusually anxious, call your doctor to get help earlier rather than later.

I'm Hindu, and we celebrate Diwali, which is an Indian holiday. It's the festival of lights and is celebrated the two or three days before the Hindu New Year. It's a time of great celebration. We have our family over and enjoy elaborate Indian dinners. My children love it because they get to wear Indian clothes.

As a first-generation American, I enjoy having my family celebrate all of the Christian holidays as well. My son especially enjoys celebrating Christmas. For example, this year my son really loved setting cookies and milk out for Santa.

—*Shilpa Amin-Shah, MD, a mom of a two-year-old son and a one-year-old daughter and an emergency physician at Emergency Medical Associates, in Livingston, NJ*

When my kids were growing up, my husband and I didn't want to get a babysitter so that we could go out. Instead, we did things together as a family and often with other families. I remember one night in particular that was so fun: We had three families with kids over to celebrate New Year's Eve. We gave the kids streamers, and they threw the streamers off of our balcony at midnight. It was a big mess and a wonderful memory that I'll never forget.

—*Dana S. Simpler, MD*

Finding Fun in Quiet Times and Keeping Kids Busy

You might already have noticed how fast the weeks, months, and years with a child fly by. Paradoxically, some days, especially blustery winter days, go by at the speed of molasses in January. It can really be a challenge to keep kids busy, and out of mischief, on quiet days at home.

My daughter loves music. We sing and dance a lot together, and we also enjoy our home karaoke machine. Using it actually encourages her reading, or at least word recognition, as well.

—*Tanya Douglas Holland, MD, a mom of a two-year-old daughter, a women's health advocate, and a consultant in medical affairs to a pharmaceutical company, in Atlanta, GA*

On quiet days when my girls were younger, we'd go out and explore our neighborhood. They loved to collect things, like acorns. I still have a stash of them in my freezer!

I sometimes made up scavenger hunts, such as finding three different-colored leaves. These activities are fun—and free!

—*Cathy Marshall, MD, a mom of 28-, 14-, and 11-year-old daughters and a pediatrician in private practice, in Encino, CA*

When I needed to prepare a meal, make a phone call, or do something else in the kitchen fairly uninterrupted, I came up with an easy way to keep my kids busy. I'd place a large piece of brown craft paper on my kitchen table. I'd tape the edges down with painters' tape so it wouldn't affect the finish. Then I'd let my kids draw all over it while I was right there in the kitchen.

—*Jennifer Hanes, DO, a mom of a six-year-old daughter and a three-year-old son, an emergency physician, a certified forensic physician, and the founder of Empowered Medicine, PLLC, in Austin, TX*

Where we lived in Germany, the winters were long, cold, and dreary. We were lucky that there are a lot of indoor aquatic complexes. They were so inviting and warm. I spent many cold winter days with my kids in those complexes. They were a godsend for me. I think even here in the United States, you might be surprised to find local indoor pools that are open to the public in the winter.

—*Ann Kulze, MD, a mom of 23- and 17-year-old daughters and 22- and 20-year-old sons; a nationally recognized nutrition expert, motivational speaker, and physician; and the author of the best-selling book* Dr. Ann's Eat Right for Life, *in Charleston, SC*

In the middle of winter, when it's too cold or snowy to go outside to play, it can be hard to keep toddlers busy. One winter, I brought our water activity table inside. Instead of filling it with messy water or sand, I filled it with dried beans. (Of course, you don't want to do this if your child still puts small objects into her mouth.)

My kids loved it! It was such an unusual toy to have inside that they played with it for hours.

—*Eva Mayer, MD, a mom of an eight-year-old daughter and a six-year-old son and a pediatrician with St. Luke's Pediatrics Associates, in Bethlehem, PA*

Believe it or not, the iPad is a must-have product. It's great for movies, games, and educational apps, and it is a perfect, compact helper for Mommy! My sons use educational (and fun) apps on the iPad when I need to get something done at home.

We never use our iPad in the car, or at the kitchen table, and I never let my sons use it for more than 30 minutes at a time.

—*Mona Gohara, MD, a mom of five- and three-year-old sons, a dermatologist in private practice, an assistant clinical professor in the department of dermatology at Yale University, and a cofounder of K&J Sunprotective Clothing, in Danbury, CT*

The biggest challenge I faced was keeping my kids active in the winter. They could spend only so much time playing with the same toys in the same room each day. All three of my children were very active, and they needed to have physical playtime as much as possible.

I purchased a play tent and made a makeshift napping and imagination area. I set up a small desk with supplies, including a broken cell phone for my oldest daughter that she would play with next to me when I had to do paperwork.

—*Laura M. Rosch, DO, a mom of a 12-year-old daughter and 7-year-old boy-girl twins, a board-certified internist who works at Central DuPage Hospital Convenient Care Centers in Winfield, IL, and an instructor in the department of family medicine at the Midwestern University/Chicago College of Osteopathic Medicine, in Downers Grove, IL*

One of my favorite quotes is from Thoreau: "I wanted to live deep and suck out all the marrow of life." Not every part of raising children is positive, but I try very hard to make as much of it as positive and fun as possible and to learn from the difficult parts. It's certainly made me a better, more empathetic person.

We have so much fun at home. Sometimes we put our iPod on speakers and dance. I believe that an important part of parenting is active brainwashing. You want to get your children to enjoy doing what you enjoy so that you can all share the fun together. My older daughter was barely one week old when we took her to her first art show. That's something my husband and I enjoy doing, so we want our girls to like it too. Our younger daughter was only a few months old when we put her into a Baby-Björn and took her hiking for the first time.

My husband and I want to expose our daughters to our favorite activities when they're babies and toddlers, so they'll never remember *not* doing them. I think many parents introduce both potentially enjoyable activities such as sports as well as responsibilities such as household chores too late and are surprised when their children resist. Children develop their preferences and habits very early, and you have to introduce your values early.

—*Kate Tulenko, MD, MPH, a mom of four- and one-year-old girls, the author of* Insourced: How Importing Jobs Impacts the Healthcare Crisis Here and Abroad, *and a pediatrician and global health specialist with IntraHealth, in Washington, DC*

Making Family Traditions

Perhaps you come from a family that celebrated wonderful, rich traditions. Or perhaps you come from a family that didn't. Either way, it can be a joy to celebrate traditions with your own family—either continuing your parents' traditions, making up new ones, or both.

❧

Each week, we try to have a family game night. We started this when my kids were toddlers. We'd play simple games like Candy Land.

We also try to do fun things more spontaneously throughout the year. For example, sometimes we have an Opposite Day where we eat breakfast meals for supper.

—*Eva Mayer, MD*

⤜⤏

In our house, Sunday was family day. We'd cook a big breakfast, and then we'd all do something fun together. It didn't have to be a big expedition or even cost any money. Our kids were happy to just go ride bikes at the park.

> —*Lisa Dado, MD, a mom of 23- and 20-year-old daughters and an 18-year-old son, a pediatric anesthesiologist with Valley Anesthesiology Consultants, and the cofounder and CEO of the nonprofit organization the Center for Humane Living, which teaches life skills with an innovative approach to traditional martial arts training in six centers in and around Phoenix, AZ*

⤜⤏

When my older son was younger, my husband, our son, and I went out to eat every Sunday morning. We went to the same restaurant every week, so the people there knew us, and they helped to expedite our meal because we had our son with us. But really my son did fine. He was used to eating out at the restaurant, and he was very comfortable there.

It was such a wonderful tradition. I work Sunday mornings now, and I miss those breakfasts.

> —*Sharon Boyce, MD, a mom of three- and one-year-old sons and a family physician at DayOne Family Healthcare Clinic, in Battle Creek, MI*

⤜⤏

Family traditions and rituals are so valuable for toddlers, who are seeking security and a sense of belonging. They also crave that understanding of what's coming next.

I love to establish new traditions and rituals. For example, each night when my husband and I tucked our toddlers into bed, my husband would touch the Winnie the Pooh figures that my daughter kept on her dresser. My husband would touch Pooh and say, "Good night, Pooh," then "Good night, Tigger," and "Good night, Piglet."

Have Breakfast in Bed

You've been making sure your kids enjoy family traditions all year long, but once or twice a year, make sure you throw in a tradition that pampers you. Start a tradition that you get to sleep in on Mother's Day or your birthday (or both) while Dad and the kids take their time and make you breakfast in bed. It's the perfect start to a day that honors you.

My daughter is now 11 years old, and she still has those figures on her dresser, even though she's long ago given up many other toddler toys. I think it's because those figures evoke such a positive memory for her.

—*Cathy Marshall, MD*

My parents had so many wonderful traditions that I've continued, so I haven't felt the need to come up with any new traditions of my own. My family now celebrates our Muslim holidays. For example, my daughter and I put henna on our hands the night before Eid, one of our major religious holidays. For the holiday, we wear traditional Pakistani clothes and bangles. We visit friends to exchange gifts, and we eat traditional foods, such as vermicelli soaked in milk or lamb roast.

I enjoy sharing these traditions with my children, and I hope they'll pass them on to my grandchildren and great-grandchildren.

—*Sadaf T. Bhutta, MD, a mom of a six-year-old daughter and four-year-old triplets and an assistant professor and the fellowship director of pediatric radiology at the University of Arkansas for Medical Sciences and Arkansas Children's Hospital, both in Little Rock*

Going to Parks, Playgrounds, and Play Places

In the United States, there are 397 National Parks. Add to that state parks, city parks, and playgrounds, and that's a lot of places to play. New York City, for example, boasts 19 percent of the total city area as parkland, San Diego has 23 percent, and New Orleans has 25 percent.

When we play outside, it's a hard sell to put sunscreen on my son. Yet I know it's critical to protect his skin from the sun's damaging rays.

My son loves animals, and I found a way to use that to my advantage. When I want to put sunscreen on my son, I tell him that the sunscreen is cream for whatever animal is his favorite at the time. For example, I call it "elephant cream" or "octopus slime." That really helps.

—*Lennox McNeary, MD, a mom of a three-year-old son, a specialist in physical medicine and rehabilitation at Carilion Clinic, and a cofounder of the Mommy Doctors Bakery (makers of Milkin' Cookies), in Roanoke, VA*

When my boys were toddlers, they loved to go to the park and playground. Unfortunately, many of the parks near our home have little or no shade. While I was happy that my boys were playing outside, I worried about their sun exposure.

To make matters worse, it was harder to put sunscreen on my boys as toddlers than it was when they were babies! I had bought some sun-protective clothing, but I didn't like the fact that most of them contained chemicals to block out the sun.

My sons were my inspiration for creating my own line of sun-protective clothing, K&J Sunprotective Clothing. My boys were my models and first "customers."

Our T-shirts, which are made for everyday play, are 100 percent cotton, chemical free, and made with UPF 50 fabric. Standard cotton shirts do not protect adequately from cancer-causing UV rays. So parents can rest assured that their kids are protected when they play while wearing these hip graphic tees that block out 99 percent of the sun's harmful rays. They're available in sizes up to 6T. (You can purchase them at KJSunProtectiveClothing.com.)

—*Mona Gohara, MD*

When I take my four sons to the playground, I'm outnumbered. So I try to go to playgrounds that have only one exit. If that's not possible, I at least choose playgrounds that are on level ground, with no hills, so I can see very clearly what all of my kids are doing.

—*Deborah Gilboa, MD, a mom of nine-, seven-, five-, and three-year-old sons, a parenting speaker whose advice is found at AskDoctorG.com, and a family physician with Squirrel Hill Health Center, in Pittsburgh, PA*

When my son was a toddler, we lived very close to a beautiful park. When I took him there to play, I kept him very close to me every second. I never let him wander off by himself. We tried to always play in wide-open spaces, so there was never a tree or hill that might impede my view of my son.

—*Sigrid Payne DaVeiga, MD, a mom of a six-year-old son and a two-year-old daughter and a pediatric allergist with the Children's Hospital of Philadelphia, in Pennsylvania*

My sons have a five-year age difference, and something that always works well for both of them is going to a playground. They can each be playing on different pieces of equipment, but close to each other, and have a great time.

An elementary school very close to our house has a great, fenced-in playground. Anyone is allowed to play there after school hours. We love to take our sons there because my younger son can run around, and he can't easily escape.

Fortunately, he doesn't really try to run away. He loves to climb, so he's happy as a clam on the playground, where there are so many pieces of equipment to climb on.

—*Rebecca Reamy, MD*

～✑～

We're very fortunate to live close to several parks and playgrounds. When we go, we always see lots of kids of various ages. The challenge, though, is that sometimes the kids get overexcited, bump into each other, and get hurt.

I am always the "attentive parent" at the park. I stand quite close to the playground equipment so that I can keep a close eye on everything and everyone. It's surprising how many parents aren't paying attention to their kids at the playground. Instead, they're talking on the phone, reading, or socializing with other parents.

When my kids were toddlers, I talked with them a lot about holding onto the equipment tightly, being strong, and being careful. I taught them how to use the equipment correctly, to minimize their chances of getting hurt.

—*Teresa Hubka, DO*

～✑～

When I took my toddlers to indoor play places, I always made sure to abide by the rule of keeping their socks on! After my kids were done playing, I wiped down their hands with alcohol wipes, and I also wiped the soles of their feet. Even though my kids had socks on, often those play places have water in them, and then their socks get soaked. I felt it was important to wipe down their feet before I put their shoes back on.

Wet surfaces are a great place for kids to pick up the virus that causes plantar warts. Cleaning their feet with alcohol wipes helps prevent this.

—*Jennifer Hanes, DO*

Planning Playdates

Young toddlers are just learning how to play with other children. It's wonderful to encourage your child to play with other kids by planning playdates. Even if the kids don't play together, don't get discouraged. Two hours seems to be the "golden" length of playdates. It's long enough to have fun, time to play and have a snack, but not so long that the toddlers get bored and cranky.

∽

When my daughter was a toddler, we made lots of playdates. My daughter was always much less demanding and better behaved when she had a playmate.

—*Stuart Jeanne Bramhall, MD, a mom of a 31-year-old daughter and a child and adolescent psychiatrist in New Plymouth, New Zealand*

∽

Since my older daughter was born, we've been a part of a playgroup. It's great! A bunch of us get together, and the parents get the chance to talk, and the kids run around and play. Sometimes when it's just our family, the kids are constantly looking to my husband and me for attention and help. But when we're with the playgroup, they're busy with other kids, which allows the adults to relax.

—*Kate Tulenko, MD, MPH*

∽

My younger daughter was shy as a toddler, but she always had some best buddies she played well with. I think for toddlers, less social activity is more. Rather than planning frequent, formal playdates, we had a very house-centered life when she was a toddler.

There was a big grassy circle in our neighborhood where moms and nannies took their kids. We spent a lot of our days outside, interacting with other children. My daughter had very wholesome early years before she started school.

—*Eva Ritvo, MD, a mom of 21- and 16-year-old daughters, a psychiatrist, and a coauthor of* The Beauty Prescription, *in Miami Beach, FL*

My sister, who is a special education teacher, told me one of the most important things children can learn during the toddler years is socialization. I made sure all of my children had ample opportunity to socialize and to learn to cooperate with other children during the first several years of life.

My toddlers had tons of playdates with planned activities, such as Play-Doh, finger-painting, dress-up, and playing house.

—*Laura M. Rosch, DO*

I love playdates. Many lifelong friendships developed through our children's playdates, both for the children and for me. But I did not do playdates with sick children. Many mothers I knew were so desperate for companionship that they would let their children play with sick children. As a physician, I could not bear it.

This brings me to the topic of sleepovers. As my children have gotten older, I've never been a big fan of sleepovers. I call them "no-sleep-overs." Kids always seem to come home tired, sick, and irritable after sleepovers.

I think some parents use sleepovers as a way to dump their kids at other people's houses so they can go out or have an hour to themselves. Not our style. We managed to have a great social and personal life, and we also took care of our children or hired a babysitter or asked my mother to come and stay with the kids.

—*Elizabeth Chabner Thompson, MD, MPH, a mom of*
13- and 8-year-old daughters and 12- and 10-year-old sons,
a radiation oncologist with 21 C. Radiation Oncology, and the
inventor of the Mommy Bag, filled with supplies for moms-to-be
having C-sections, in Scarsdale, NY

Going Shopping

Going to the grocery store might not be your favorite thing to do, but errands, even mundane ones, are great for toddlers. Going to different places and seeing new things is beneficial for toddlers. It might be easier—and surely quicker—to run errands without your toddler, but if you take her along, it might be more fun, for you both.

I actually enjoy grocery shopping. I usually go at 10 pm when my husband is at home, our daughters are asleep, and the store is empty. I enjoy the time to myself, plus, it's guilt-free shopping.

—*Kate Tulenko, MD, MPH*

When my three oldest kids were toddlers, we lived in Germany. We had no friends or family to help us. The only time I went shopping was when my husband could go with me. It was impossible to keep an eye on three kids and shop at the same time. Grocery shopping became a family event!

—*Ann Kulze, MD*

It's very challenging when you're in a store and your toddler throws a tantrum. People often say that you should leave the store immediately to end the tantrum. But I never did that. I just finished up my business as quickly as possible and pretended I didn't realize the entire store was looking at me.

—*Victoria McEvoy, MD, a mom who raised four children; a grandmom of six-, four-, and two-year-old grandsons; an assistant professor of pediatrics at Harvard Medical School; the medical director and chief of pediatrics at Mass General West Medical Group; and the author of* 24/7 Baby Doctor, *in Boston, MA*

When my twins were toddlers, I carried a bag of Cheerios everywhere we went. It was a handy distraction and also, of course, a healthy snack. I started very early not getting in the habit of buying them a treat every time we went shopping. This really helped later when they were older; there wasn't an expectation that they would get something. This made for a lot fewer meltdowns in "aisle 2."

—*Ann Contrucci, MD, a mom of 13-year-old boy-girl twins who works as a pediatric emergency physician, in Atlanta, GA*

With two young children, running errands was really a challenge. I bought a Sit and Stand stroller. It was terrific because my son could ride in the stroller, and my daughter, who was older, could either sit or stand as she wished. I kept the stroller in my car throughout my kids' toddler years.

—*Eva Mayer, MD*

⌇∽

When my son was born, I bought a double stroller. I thought it would be so handy to put both kids in there to go shopping. That didn't turn out to be the case! I could barely push the stroller through doorways! After I discovered that, I took only one of my toddlers shopping at a time, and I left my other child at home with my husband.

—*Ann V. Arthur, MD, a mom of a 10-year-old daughter and an 8-year-old son, a pediatric ophthalmologist in private practice at Park Slope Eye Care Associates, and a blogger at WaterWineTravel.com, in New York City*

Mommy MD Guides–Recommended Product
Gerber Graduates Grabbers Squeezable Fruit

"When I take my daughter with me to run errands, I bring lots of snacks," says Rachel S. Rohde, MD, a mom of a one-year-old daughter, an assistant professor of orthopaedic surgery at the Oakland University William Beaumont School of Medicine, and an orthopaedic upper-extremity surgeon with Michigan Orthopaedic Institute, P.C., in Southfield, MI.

"Gerber Graduates Grabbers are the travel miracle. They are awesome. I put some into my purse, and I always have something healthy to give my daughter when we're on the go and need something to prevent a meltdown."

No spoon required—and no mess! Each pouch has two servings of fruit, and some even throw in a vegetable. Your child simply squeezes the fruit into her mouth straight from the pouch. Flavors include banana blueberry and apple. You can buy them at supermarkets for about $1.79 per 4.23-ounce pouch.

Grocery shopping with my overactive toddler son was a huge chore. I used to joke that he was like a ticking time bomb with a 20-minute limit, which would start counting down as soon as I got to the store. If I overstayed that 20 minutes, I was sure to deal with a thrashing, screaming child, or an embarrassing announcement of "Cleanup in aisle 4!" (My son loved knocking everything off the lower shelves.) When my son was a toddler, I brought toys along to keep him entertained. I also made lists with "most needed" items at the top so I could abandon the rest if I ran out of time.

In-store clothes shopping was definitely out of the question for me. I ordered a lot of stuff online in those first two years. I just made sure I ordered enough to get free shipping, and that the store had a full-refund, three-month minimum return policy. When I got those clothes in the mail, my bedroom turned into a changing room, and I could try on all the clothes with all my shoes and accessories. The return trip to the store was much shorter, so I was able to take my son with me.

Now that my son is older, I've started to include him in the grocery shopping process. He loves riding in those shopping carts with a little car attached at the front. (He'll buckle his seat belt and pretend to "drive" the shopping cart!) I'll give him a list of groceries he needs to get, which he will bag himself and put on the seat next to him. And no, I still don't take him clothes shopping!

—*Cheryl Wu, MD, a mom of a four-year-old son, a pediatrician at LaGuardia Place Pediatrics in New York City, and a pediatric emergency physician at the Joseph M. Sanzari Children's Hospital of Hackensack University Medical Center, in New Jersey*

Shopping with my daughter has been super easy. I have to give some credit to the stores! My daughter loves to ride in the shopping carts shaped like trucks or race cars. I encourage her to "hop in and help Mommy drive." My daughter also loves to get a free balloon at the grocery store when they offer them. (Popped balloons are choking hazards; never let a toddler play with a balloon unattended.)

I often pick my daughter up from preschool, and we go straight to the grocery store. At that time, my daughter can be hungry, and maybe even a little cranky. I make sure to give her a nutritious snack to eat in the car on the drive from school to the store, such as some on-the-go applesauce. That won't fill my daughter up, but it will take the edge off her hunger.

If anything, my daughter enjoys shopping so much that she can get a little animated.

"Use your inside voice, please," I remind her. That usually does the trick.

—*Tanya Douglas Holland, MD*

When my twins were toddlers, they were full of energy, full of fun. One day I was in a store bathroom with my twins, and they escaped, right underneath the bathroom door! I didn't take my twins many places by myself. I usually went shopping when my husband could go too.

My husband and I used to fantasize about a make-believe store where they'd have a Velcro wall where you could put your kids in Velcro suits, stick them to the wall, and shop in peace.

—*Susan Wilder, MD*

I found going to the store was a fun thing to do together, but usually with only one or two children in tow.

Honestly, I would have to move through the store fast some days. My kids loved to be helpers, so I had to get very creative. I would play "I spy" and pretend we were looking for something red (and then I would get the apples). Sometimes I would have the kids "hold" an item for Mommy. They would feel like they were doing an important job, and they took pride in being helpful. It was too cute to see my twins trying to hold their items and do a good job!

It also helps if you go to the stores with the child-friendly carts that look like animals or race cars. I would then make car or animal noises and tell them to stop driving the car so fast.

On "bad attention" days, I would resort to bribes. I would tell them they could pick out one package of cookies or treats for the pantry if we got all of the shopping done.

Thinking back now, there are a ton of educational opportunities in a store! I really tried to get my kids as involved with the process as I could. Because I have a graduate degree in nutrition, I also started to teach them early on how to read food labels. My son knew that I would not buy things with hydrogenated oils in them. As a toddler, he knew how to recognize that word when he looked at ingredient lists. And my children first began to learn about money and numbers at the checkout.

But as with anything regarding children, you can't bring them to a store if they are tired or hungry or sick. That would make it very difficult to get through the store.

—*Laura M. Rosch, DO*

I will move heaven and earth to avoid going grocery shopping with a toddler. Grocery shopping is boring for them, and to make matters worse, the grocery store aisles are filled with bright, shiny objects that kids inevitably beg for. I try to grocery shop alone, either after my husband is home from work or when I have a babysitter. Why set yourself up for failure?

When I absolutely cannot avoid going grocery shopping with a toddler, I make my expectations clear up front. Sometimes, I tell my son that if he makes it to the checkout without asking me to buy anything, he will find that I've picked up a special treat for him. Other times, I'll set a limit, such as he can choose something that costs $5 (if we're at Target) or $1 (if we're at the grocery store). The rule is that at any one time, he can have one item in the cart. So, for instance, if he sees something in the produce section he likes, he can put it in the cart. But then if he sees something in the toy aisle, he can put that in the cart but he has to put the first thing back. That way, we don't wind up at the checkout with 17 kids' things in the cart.

—*Deborah Gilboa, MD*

Especially when my daughters were toddlers, I tried to make things fun, and to keep them positive rather than negative as much as possible. For example, when we'd go shopping at Target, my younger daughter would often ask me to buy her things that she couldn't have. Rather than turning this into a power struggle, I'd make it into a game.

"Show me how much you want it," I'd tell my daughter, to get her to raise her arms up to the sky and giggle.

"Let's make a list of the top 10 things you want and come up with ways to save for them," I'd say next.

While my daughter puzzled out the answer to that, I'd make a beeline far away from the toy department!

—*Cathy Marshall, MD*

Doing Arts and Crafts

What looks like scribbles on a page is actually important development for your toddler. Arts and crafts help to encourage and develop creativity. They also help kids to improve their motor skills, as they use pencils, scissors, and glue, and to learn dexterity. Older kids benefit from doing arts and crafts because it requires them to concentrate on a task, and sometimes even helps them to develop patience. Moms benefit from arts and crafts because they keep kids busy—and contained!

I found doing things like arts and crafts to be great opportunities to emphasize my girls' strengths and build their self-esteem. For instance, when they created a pretty picture, I'd say, "You are such a good artist. You are such a creative girl. I can't wait to see what you come up with next! You are so smart and learning so fast. Let's go learn something new. That was so much fun!"

—*Eva Ritvo, MD*

My daughter loves art. She's always been my crafty one. I'm a bit of a neat freak, and arts and crafts are messy, so I probably didn't foster that as much as I could have.

When my kids and I do arts and crafts, we usually do them outside on a picnic table. That way the finger paints, Play-Doh, and glitter all stay outside.

—*Antoinette Cheney, DO, a mom of a seven-year-old son and a six-year-old daughter and a family physician with Rocky Vista University College of Osteopathic Medicine, in Parker, CO*

Take Some Library Time

Give yourself a small break every day by designating 15 to 30 minutes of "library time" at home. Explain to the kids that it's time to sit down and look at books quietly, just as they do when they're in the library and can't make a lot of noise. While they look through their own books, pull out whatever you want to read, whether it's the newspaper, a paperback, your Kindle, or a magazine.

When my kids were toddlers, the house we lived in had a kitchen with an easy-clean, tile-type floor. It was great. On rainy days, I'd get out the arts and crafts supplies and spread them all over the kitchen floor. My kids would play there for hours, and after they were done, it was easy for me to wipe up.

We also had a child-size table and chairs. That was terrific when my kids were toddlers because I could move it from room to room. My kids could color or play on that table while I read or cooked.

—Ann Kulze, MD

We did lots of creative crafts when my kids were toddlers. I am naturally artsy, so anytime that I was beading, sewing, or gardening, the toddlers "helped Mommy."

Now, my adult kids are all crafty. I'm certain it's because they were exposed to all sorts of home projects all the time. Arts are ideal for teaching language, math skills, and the sharing tools of socialization.

—Hana R. Solomon, MD, a mom who raised four children, a grandmom of three, a board-certified pediatrician, the president of BeWell Health, LLC, and the author of Clearing the Air One Nose at a Time: Caring for Your Personal Filter, *in Columbia, MO*

Choosing and Caring for Toys

The toys will take over your house if you let them! Wrestle back control today.

When my kids' plastic toddler toys started to look dirty, I'd fill a bathtub with warm water, add a cup or two of bleach, and swish the toys around in the bleach solution.

—*Jennifer Hanes, DO*

My best tools for organizing my kids' toys were huge Tupperware containers with lids and my label maker! I had a bin for this, a bin for that. This system helped me to keep everything much neater.

—*Eva Mayer, MD*

I've had several different toy organization systems over the years. None of them work. For example, I used to carefully separate toys into their own bins: one for Legos, another for Hot Wheels cars, etc. But the toys all end up jumbled together anyway, so I gave up.

My sons keep most of their toys in their rooms, and throughout the day, those toys slowly migrate downstairs. The funny thing is, it's a one-way street. The toys never migrate back upstairs!

The best we can do is to keep several large baskets on hand. A few times a day, my husband fills a basket with toys and takes the toys back upstairs.

—*Rebecca Reamy, MD*

One great thing I did for myself was to build a good-size playroom in our home. This keeps my kids' toys out of our living room. The playroom has lots of shelves and cubbies to make it easier to organize toys. You can't ever have too many storage options with toys.

We keep almost all of our kids' toys in the playroom, rather than in their own rooms. This encourages our kids to play together in the playroom, rather than separately in their rooms.

A few times a year, I have my kids go through their toys and pick out any toys they've outgrown. We recycle those toys by donating them to charity.

—*Sadaf T. Bhutta, MD*

My husband and I try to raise our daughters in a gender-balanced way.

We buy them trains and construction equipment to play with. My husband does a lot of work around the house, and he encourages our daughters to put on their safety goggles, follow him around with a hammer, and help.

It upsets me that there's a wider variety of toys for boys. Girls' toys all seem to be animals and dolls, and they're all pink. When boys have dolls, they call them "action figures." Boys have so much more to choose from: maps, puzzles, trains, action figures, sports equipment, and more. My husband and I have tried to expose our daughters to all of these things too.

But even with all of our efforts to raise our daughters this way, my husband and I got a rude awakening when our older daughter came home from preschool and said, "Girls don't play with swords. Boys do." This was a shock especially to me, because I had participated in fencing when I was in school! We don't have a TV, so these negative gender sterotypes don't come from the TV. They come from contact with their peers in half-day preschool. It's amazing.

—*Kate Tulenko, MD, MPH*

Preserving Memories

Making memories with toddlers is so much fun. You think you'll remember them all, but memories are fragile. Preserve them and save them to savor later.

❧

When I was pregnant with each of my children, I bought a pregnancy book that also had space for me to journal. I wrote down my thoughts and feelings, and I also wrote down practical things such as questions I had asked the doctor and the doctor's responses.

When my kids were toddlers, they loved it when I read their baby books to them. This became a tradition that we did on their birthdays. In fact, even now, my kids enjoy it. They still ask to see their baby books on their birthdays.

—*Teresa Hubka, DO*

Since my daughter was born, I've kept a "Mommy journal." I keep a small notebook on my bedside table, and I love to write in it. It doesn't have to look pretty, so it's easy to jot something down before I forget.

Now that my daughter is older, she loves for me to read to her from the journal. It's amazing to read these things that I would have long forgotten had I not written them down!

—*Katja Rowell, MD, a mom of a six-year-old daughter, a family practice physician, and a childhood feeding specialist with TheFeedingDoctor.com, in St. Paul, MN*

I'm not a big photographer, and I haven't taken tons of photos of my kids. I might have 1,000 photos of my older daughter and 100 of my twins' entire lives!

When my kids were toddlers and starting to talk, I started a book for each of them. I call them my "Isms Books." I write the funny things my kids say in their books. I keep the books in my kitchen. When my kids say something funny, I write it down right away. You think you'll remember these things forever, but you won't. You'll forget them the next day.

Those books are the most fun thing to have. My kids love to get their books out and read them.

—*Susan Wilder, MD*

During my daughter's toddler years, I loved seeing what new skills she would learn. It seemed every day had a new excitement for her!

Our child's strength was talking and verbal skills. She would say new and funny things every day. I started keeping a journal, and it is still fun to look back and see what things she said. One of our favorites was when I was eight months pregnant. Out of the blue, my daughter turned to me and said, "Mommy, you look like a puffer fish!"

—*Melody Derrick, MD, a mom of a two-year-old daughter who's expecting another baby and a family physician in private practice with Cadence Physician Group, in Winfield, IL*

Chapter 17
Learning and Education

YOUR TODDLER'S DEVELOPMENT

The toddler years are a wonderful time. Toddlers learn by playing. What fun for your toddler—and for you!

The best way you can help your toddler learn is to play with him. Similar to how a varied diet of different foods offers different vitamins and minerals, varied play helps your toddler to learn many different skills. You can practically see the connections being made in a toddler's brain; certainly you can see the delight on his face when he learns something new!

Toddlers are tiny bundles of motivation. They always want to do more—to learn more. You'll likely notice your toddler focusing all of his concentration and energy on the task at hand and working at it until he gets it right. But playtime should be fun, not work. If your toddler gets frustrated because he isn't the playground Picasso he wants to be, it's a good idea to have a distraction at the ready. Hey, let's go blow some bubbles!

TAKING CARE OF YOU

As your toddler is soaking up knowledge like a little sponge, it's a great time to learn something new yourself. There's never been a better time than today, with thousands of online classes available.

JUSTIFICATION FOR A CELEBRATION

Anytime you hear your child say "I love to read," celebrate! Instilling a love of reading—of learning—is a great accomplishment.

376

Teaching about Computers

A generation ago, computers were barely in the workplace, let alone in the home. Today we have unlimited, near constant access to computers. This brings many benefits, such as making it easier to keep in touch with friends and family, but also tremendous responsibility, protecting our kids.

One study published in *Pediatrics* found that toddlers who used computers developed better learning skills than toddlers who didn't use computers. Experts caution, though, that too much screen time means less face time, playing with other kids.

∽

I let my daughter play with my iPad. I think of it as an interactive, educational TV.

—*Lisa Campanella-Coppo, MD, a mom of a three-year-old daughter, an emergency physician, and the emergency department director of academic affairs at Monmouth Medical Center, in New Jersey*

∽

My sons are very active, fit, and healthy, so I don't worry too much about policing their screen time. They're generally running around in the backyard, so if one of them wants to play a computer game for 15 minutes while my husband or I take a shower, that's great.

I think that computer games teach kids skills, such as math and reading, and they also improve hand-eye coordination and fine motor skills. Computer games keep kids busy to boot.

—*Rebecca Reamy, MD, a mom of seven- and two-year-old sons and a pediatrician in emergency medicine at Children's Healthcare of Atlanta, in Georgia*

∽

Computers have no place in the lives of two-year-olds. Yes, later they can be educational, and I don't know where I would be without my computer. But I didn't encourage my toddlers to use computers. Young kids need to play, be read to, and talk. They don't need to type.

—*Ayala Laufer-Cahana, MD, a mom of 16- and 14-year-old sons and a 12-year-old daughter, a pediatrician, and the founder of Herbal Water Inc., in Wynnewood, PA*

When my sons were toddlers, we didn't have any computer games. We didn't even have cell phones! They played the occasional game at the library requiring them to click and drag; it simulated cleaning up trash at a park. That was it. I still prefer and recommend that kids explore their world the old-fashioned way—playing with toys and physically manipulating their environment (blocks, etc.). The rest will come soon enough.

—Leena Shrivastava Dev, MD, a mom of 15- and 11-year-old sons, a general pediatrician, and an advocate for child safety, in Philadelphia, PA

Reading to Your Toddler

Reading to your child increases his vocabulary, memory, and attention span. Plus, it fosters creativity and a love of learning. Rhyming books can help with pattern recognition, peekaboo books can help teach cause and effect, and photo books can encourage object recognition. What wonderful gifts to give to your child! Plus, few things are sweeter in life than snuggling up with your child before bed to share a story.

Every night before bed, we read. It's amazing to see how much kids learn even in a day! I always choose books that have content that will interest my children; right now, it's Super Heroes! We always read after we do a dance party to their favorite songs, so reading is our cooldown.

—Mona Gohara, MD, a mom of five- and three-year-old sons, a dermatologist in private practice, an assistant clinical professor in the department of dermatology at Yale University, and a cofounder of K&J Sunprotective Clothing, in Danbury, CT

My daughter loves reading. We've purchased most of her books, and we keep them all over the house. She has books in her playroom downstairs, books in her bedroom, and books in the living room. We even keep books in the car, so she's really surrounded by books! She also has a Tag Jr. as well as a story reader. One habit that my husband and I consistently did when she was very little up until now is to have story time every night before she goes down to sleep. When she was younger, we chose the book, but now we let her choose which book we will read. I've also started to incorporate poems, such as those by Shel Silverstein. We also allow her the opportunity to "read" to us (in her own way, of course). This seems to encourage her to pick up a book.

> —*Tanya Douglas Holland, MD, a mom of a two-year-old daughter, a women's health advocate, and a consultant in medical affairs to a pharmaceutical company, in Atlanta, GA*

I own an online kids' bookstore, so we have an abundance of books in my home. I love books, and the apples don't fall far from the tree: My sons love books too. I think it helps to instill a love of reading in your children by being a reader yourself. Little kids still think their parents are cool, and your children will aspire to do the things that you do.

We buy our sons lots of books, and we allow them to select two books each night for bedtime reading. My kids look forward to bedtime for this reason.

> —*Bola Oyeyipo-Ajumobi, MD, a mom of four- and one-year-old sons, a family physician in private practice, and the owner of SlimyBookWorm.com, in Highland, CA*

Reading to my daughter each night before bedtime was a special time. My daughter really liked me to read chapter books from about age three on. Judy Blume's books about Fudge and his family were special favorites, as were *Winnie the Pooh* and two really old books from the 1930s my grandmother read to my mother: *Bertram and His Funny Animals* and *Bertram and His Fabulous Animals*.

Each night, my daughter and I would get in her bed together to read. She would get really sleepy after about 20 minutes, and we would turn the lights out.

> —*Stuart Jeanne Bramhall, MD, a mom of a 31-year-old daughter and a child and adolescent psychiatrist in New Plymouth, New Zealand*

The Froggy books were very helpful with tricky parenting situations. For example, my son never wanted to wear his coat. So we read the book *Froggy Gets Dressed*, which also talks about Froggy wearing a coat.

Jonathan London has written more than a dozen Froggy books, including *Froggy Goes to the Doctor*, *Froggy Goes to Camp*, and *Froggy Learns to Swim*.

—Teresa Hubka, DO, a mom of a 14-year-old son and an 8-year-old daughter, an ob-gyn and the medical director of Comprehensive Wellness Care in Chicago, and an associate professor of obstetrics and gynecology and the chairman and residency program director of the department of obstetrics and gynecology at the Midwestern University/Chicago College of Osteopathic Medicine, in Downers Grove, Illinois

My son is a book fiend. I think it's because we read to him so much as a toddler. We were living in Cleveland at the time. The winters were cold, and we stayed indoors a lot.

A few years ago, my son mentioned a book that he had enjoyed as a toddler, called *Goodnight Gorilla* by Peggy Rathman.

"I'm going to remember it for the rest of my life," he said.

That thought still brings a smile to my face!

—Sigrid Payne DaVeiga, MD, a mom of a six-year-old son and a two-year-old daughter and a pediatric allergist with the Children's Hospital of Philadelphia, in Pennsylvania

I'm a huge fan of the public library system. I've taken my kids to the library from a very young age. We go to story time, and we sign out books. We've signed out so many books over the years, it's sometimes a challenge to find books that we haven't read.

It's all free, and I think that going to the library is a wonderful experience for kids. It's a valuable lesson for them to learn they can borrow these books for free, take good care of them, return them, and then they can borrow more.

My son got his first library card this year. He was very excited about that!

—Antoinette Cheney, DO, a mom of a seven-year-old son and a six-year-old daughter and a family physician with Rocky Vista University College of Osteopathic Medicine, in Parker, CO

The Your Baby Can Read program was given to us for my first son. It really did help my son with sight reading. He's only three and if I turn off the volume or show him the words on a flash card, he can say them.

—*Sharon Boyce, MD, a mom of three- and one-year-old sons and a family physician at DayOne Family Healthcare Clinic, in Battle Creek, MI*

My toddlers loved being read to. We read whenever, whatever, wherever we could. We loved Dr. Seuss books—all of them. Also, *Goodnight Moon* was a favorite, as was *The Napping House*.

As my kids got older, books specifically for toddlers would bore the older ones, so we also read "big-kid" books at story time. Story time at my house was frequently for all the kids at once—sort of like library reading time.

—*Susan Besser, MD, a mom of six grown children, ages 27, 25, 23, 21, 20, and 18, a grandmom of two, a family physician, and the medical director of Doctors Express-Memphis, in Tennessee*

Reading to my kids was one of the dearest things to me. I think that reading should begin at age 0! And it should continue even after kids are able to read themselves.

I enjoyed reading some of my favorite books to my kids, and I also enjoyed discovering new favorites. The moment after my kids got out of the bath, when they were sleepy and snuggly, was such a great time to read to them.

We have books spread all over our home, not just in the playroom or family room. I think it's important that my kids see me enjoying books too. The books that you read—as well as the people whom you meet—are what make you wiser, at any age.

—*Ayala Laufer-Cahana, MD*

Organizing Books

If the toys haven't taken over your house yet, the books might. Organizing them helps to show your child that you value books— and that he should too.

We have a large bookshelf in the hallway outside our bedrooms. I encourage my kids to treat it like a library. Each night before bed, they choose the books they want to read and take them back to their bedrooms. The next morning, they re-shelve the books, or at least do so after some reminders.

—*Sadaf T. Bhutta, MD, a mom of a six-year-old daughter and four-year-old triplets and an assistant professor and the fellowship director of pediatric radiology at the University of Arkansas for Medical Sciences and Arkansas Children's Hospital, both in Little Rock*

We have two giant bookcases in our hallway that are filled with books. I put the picture books on the bottom shelves so even my daughter can take them off the shelves herself.

—*Sigrid Payne DaVeiga, MD*

We organized our books so that the books on some shelves were for everyone to read, and the books on other shelves were for Mom only to touch and read. It's hard to keep books looking nice after lots of use, but I would rather have scruffy, well-used books and kids who love to read than mint-condition gorgeous but untouched books.

—*Susan Besser, MD*

I really like my kids to interact freely with their books, and I am not at all bothered if they destroy their books in the process. We have books everywhere in our home: on bookshelves, in their rooms, on the floor, and even in the car. When kids are little, board books work well because paperback books are more easily damaged.

—*Bola Oyeyipo-Ajumobi, MD*

We have a lot of books. As with my kids' toys, I don't really have an elaborate strategy to organize the books either. The most important thing to me is that my boys have easy access to their books. I want to encourage their love of reading.

We have a bookcase in each room of our house, and they are all filled with books. I keep most of my kids' books in baskets, though.

This makes it easy for my boys to get a book out, and it's easy for them to put the book back too.

—*Rebecca Reamy, MD*

❧

Practically since my daughter was born, she has loved to look at books. She flips through the pages herself and looks at the pictures.

I don't have an elaborate organizing system for cataloging my daughter's books. I simply toss them into a big basket.

I'm a hand surgeon, and we tend to like everything "just so." A lot of that has gone out the window at home since my daughter was born. I have to leave that "just so" in the operating room!

—*Rachel S. Rohde, MD, a mom of a one-year-old daughter, an assistant professor of orthopaedic surgery at the Oakland University William Beaumont School of Medicine, and an orthopaedic upper-extremity surgeon with Michigan Orthopaedic Institute, P.C., in Southfield, MI*

Teaching ABCs and 123s

Our lives are so filled with letters and numbers we hardly even notice them, let alone can remember them all. (Quick: What's your ATM card PIN?) It's incredible to think back to a time before letters and numbers ruled our lives. Yet that's the world your toddler lives in. What an incredible opportunity you have now to teach him about letters and numbers—the building blocks of our lives.

❧

Life offers tons of opportunities to teach toddlers things like the ABCs and 123s. For example, when my girls were toddlers, each morning as we drove to preschool, they loved to count the school buses we passed along the way.

It's so fun how family traditions are borne out of these simple pastimes. One day, one of my daughters started to count the buses imitating the Count from *Sesame Street*: One! Two! Three! We still joke about that.

—*Cathy Marshall, MD, a mom of 28-, 14-, and 11-year-old daughters and a pediatrician in private practice, in Encino, CA*

A very excellent learning tool that parents might not think of is puzzles. My kids really enjoyed them. We had a puzzle of the United States, and each piece listed the state and its capital. We played with that puzzle

When to Call Your Doctor

A child with a learning disability is as intelligent as any other child, but his brain is structured differently or functions differently from the brains of other kids. That might affect the way he learns how to speak, read, write, memorize, reason, perform math problems, socialize, organize, or find learning strategies. He might also have problems with coordination.

If you suspect that your child has any type of developmental delay, it's best to act early because he'll perform better the sooner he receives early intervention services. One study by the National Institutes of Health found that 67 percent of kids who had trouble reading in school and received help in the early grades improved enough to become average or above average readers.

Call your doctor if you suspect that your child has any of the following warning signs of a learning disability among preschool children.

- Your child's speech is delayed compared to most children.
- Your child has trouble pronouncing words.
- Your child struggles to use the correct words or to expand his vocabulary.
- Your child has trouble rhyming words.
- Your child isn't learning numbers, the alphabet, the days of the week, colors, or shapes.
- Your child is distracted easily or seems very restless.
- Your child doesn't interact well with other kids his age.
- Your child doesn't follow directions well or stick to routines.
- Your child struggles with fine motor skills, such as reaching, moving things from one hand to the other, using the pincer grasp, or dropping and picking up toys.

while we were also reading a hilarious book called *The Scrambled States of America* by Laurie Keller. My son and I put that puzzle together so often that by age three, he knew all of the states' capitals.

—*Sigrid Payne DaVeiga, MD*

When my sons were toddlers, their grandparents bought them an easel with a chalkboard on one side and a dry erase board on the other. My sons loved to draw on that, and it was helpful for them to practice writing letters and numbers too. There's something special about writing on a chalkboard that made my kids more willing to do that than writing on paper. Plus, they had something to show off to their dad when he came home after work. As for me, I could get a few minutes of work done in the kitchen while they were busy writing and drawing.

—*Leena Shrivastava Dev, MD, a mom of 15- and 11-year-old sons, a general pediatrician, and an advocate for child safety, in Philadelphia, PA*

One of the best teaching tools my husband and I use is our iPad. I have found many wonderful educational games and programs. My three-year-old can count to 100, recognize two-digit numbers like 38, and identify all of the shapes and colors.

I believe that these games are especially helpful for boys because they engage several senses at once. My son is seeing the words and hearing them, and he's interacting by touching them on the screen. These games make use of how my boys think. They put all of their senses to work.

—*Sharon Boyce, MD*

My older daughter learned her ABCs and 123s just by going to preschool, without much teaching from me. Instead I focus on teaching my daughters the important things that aren't taught in the standard educational system, such as personal finance and economics.

My husband bought my daughter the Your Baby Can Read DVDs. I let him do what he wants. But if a child is going to learn something naturally or through the education system, I don't worry about it.

More than teaching my girls specific skills like ABCs and 123s, I focus on teaching them problem-solving. For example, if my daughter comes to me with a problem, such as her car is stuck underneath the couch, it would be easier for me to simply retrieve the car. But instead, I ask her, "What could we try to do to get the car?" I encourage her to brainstorm and come up with her own solution to the problem. I think a lot about what has made me successful in life and teach those lessons and skills directly to my daughters. They're never too young.

I also believe it's important to help kids set their life goals. Even as toddlers, I talk with my girls a lot about the future. We talk about them going to college as if it's a given, "You'll go to middle school, then high school, then college."

My sister struggled a bit in high school. Today she's a physician and a lawyer, but once she told our mom, "Thank you for talking about college as a given. Otherwise, I might not have chosen to go." That floored me and taught me an important lesson about making expectations explicit rather than implied.

—*Kate Tulenko, MD, MPH, a mom of four- and one-year-old girls, the author of* Insourced: How Importing Jobs Impacts the Healthcare Crisis Here and Abroad, *and a pediatrician and global health specialist with IntraHealth, in Washington, DC*

When my daughter was a toddler, people said parents shouldn't teach their kids to read. They believed that was the school's job. When my daughter was in preschool, there was a very disruptive child in class, and the other students never learned the alphabet. So my daughter missed out on those pre-reading skills in preschool. When my daughter started first grade, she didn't know how to read. I needed to get her tested and hire a reading tutor so that she could catch up. I should have checked to see that she was learning her ABCs in preschool so that she would have been better prepared for first grade.

—*Debra Jaliman, MD, a mom of a 20-year-old daughter, a dermatologist in private practice, and an assistant professor of dermatology at Mt. Sinai School of Medicine, in New York City*

Taking Classes

Taking a class with your toddler can be beneficial for many reasons. You'll expose him to something new, and maybe he'll make new friends. You'll meet new people too. And best of all, you'll enjoy time and making memories together.

When my kids were toddlers, we took quite a few classes, such as at Gymboree and at a wonderful, local music school. At these classes, my kids loved to play to the music, throw balls, and have fun with other kids. The classes were wonderful experiences for us all.

—*Teresa Hubka, DO*

Especially during the winter, it was challenging keeping my kids busy. I enrolled them in gymnastics, art classes, and music classes that had movement.

Taking classes is always best done when children are alert, fed, and well rested. It also helps if your children really love the activity that they are involved with, and for my children it helped if they had other children they liked in the class. I was lucky that my girls loved to go to music and dance classes.

I found that classes before lunchtime or naptime can be a disaster! I avoided the 11 am art class or the 3:30 pm gym class. These times didn't work for our schedule. I found it helped to be very organized for these classes. I still have a travel bag in the car with emergency items for my children. I always have water, juice, fruits, cereal, wipes, first-aid kits, books, toys, coloring books, markers, and a change of clothes. As my kids have gotten older, the contents have been modified, but we have the bag in our car to this day!

For every activity my child was involved with, I spent the extra money to have a separate bag packed with the necessary items for their class. My children are independent, and they're responsible for the items in that bag. I tried not to do everything for them, because I wanted them to learn how to prepare their things for the day so they could work independently on their executive function skills. Many two-year-olds are actually very good at planning and preparing simple activities independently. It is a life skill I wanted them to have because I have seen so many other children who can't organize themselves. Yes, there have been a few times when things were lost or forgotten, and we got frustrated. I can say that based on my experience, my children learned quickly how to be prepared. It has really been an asset to have this skill now that they are older.

I think the key goal for playdates and classes, in my situation, was to help my children develop socialization skills. I don't think there was any advantage to one over the other except that the classes can be expensive and somebody had to clean their house after the playdates! Chicago luckily has many family-friendly activities, and taking the kids out to see the world and experience new things was very exciting to me.

—*Laura M. Rosch, DO, a mom of a 12-year-old daughter and 7-year-old boy-girl twins, a board-certified internist who works at Central DuPage Hospital Convenient Care Centers in Winfield, IL, and an instructor in the department of family medicine at the Midwestern University/Chicago College of Osteopathic Medicine, in Downers Grove, IL*

I think a lot of parents feel pressured to sign their kids up for classes and then to be the one to go along to classes. I think that classes are wonderful for kids. I signed my older son up for plenty of them, but I hated going to them.

I realized later that going to classes wasn't a good use of my time. I signed my younger son up for classes too, but I had someone else take him! I enjoyed spending other time with him, doing things that I also enjoyed, such as playing with him on the playground.

—*Heather Orman-Lubell, MD, a mom of 11- and 7-year-old sons and a pediatrician in private practice at Yardley Pediatrics of St. Christopher's Hospital for Children, in Pennsylvania*

My husband did martial arts when he was a kid, and we started each of our boys in martial arts classes when they were three years old. We find it's excellent for developing discipline and self-confidence.

To keep the costs contained, we use economy of scale. Instead of sending each boy and my husband for individual classes, we pay for our own private group lessons. We do this with swimming also.

—*Deborah Gilboa, MD, a mom of nine-, seven-, five-, and three-year-old sons, a parenting speaker whose advice is found at AskDoctorG.com, and a family physician with Squirrel Hill Health Center, in Pittsburgh, PA*

I took my daughter to her first music class this morning. It was awesome! The kids were dancing, singing, and playing instruments. The class was held in this amazing, fun place. I had the fleeting thought, *I'm going to decorate my basement like this!*

I recently dialed back my work hours so that I can have more time at home to do things like this with my daughter. I've worked more-than-full-time hours my entire adult life. I finally decided that I am going to take Fridays off. I really enjoy this special time with my daughter. Toddlerhood goes by so fast. Once it's gone, you can't get it back.

—*Rachel S. Rohde, MD*

Monitoring TV Time

The American Academy of Pediatrics recommends that children younger than two watch no TV. Recent research supports the wisdom of this. A study found that watching TV can cause irregular sleep habits and schedules, and it can be linked with late talking.

My kids get a limited amount of screen time each day. But because you can watch TV while you exercise, if they're exercising, they can "buy" extra TV time.

—*Deborah Gilboa, MD*

I know that the American Academy of Pediatrics recommends no TV for kids under age two, but I think that's unrealistic. Certainly, I didn't let my sons watch four hours of TV a day! But I did let them watch

Enjoy Some ME-TV

Some years ago, researchers published a study in the journal *Science* about what makes people happy. Along with good times with friends and good sex with their partners, women said watching TV was one of those activities that helped them relax. In fact, they rated it as being more enjoyable than shopping and talking on the phone.

That's good reason to take some ME-TV time for yourself. When the kids are down for a nap or tucked into their beds for the night, say good-bye to *Sesame Street* and *Dora the Explorer* and take in a half-hour or hour of *Survivor*, *The Amazing Race*, *Grey's Anatomy*, or another prime-time show. Enjoy it uninterrupted and guilt free.

quality TV shows, such as *Sesame Street*, *Little Einsteins*, *Mickey Mouse Clubhouse*, and as annoying as they can be, Dora and Diego. I don't think TV is all evil. (Sponge Bob, maybe.) You just have to make good choices.

—Heather Orman-Lubell, MD

I let my daughter watch children's shows on TV, especially if I need a few minutes to do something without interruption. She likes to watch *Barney* and *Sid the Science Kid*.

I try to watch TV with my daughter, though, when she's watching. This is helpful when there's a lesson to point out, such as if a character is showing bad behavior. I also find that I feel more relaxed after watching an hour of *Sesame Street*!

—Lisa Campanella-Coppo, MD

My boys would far rather play than watch TV. But I have to admit, we do have the TV on as background noise much of the time. I don't worry about my kids' screen time, though, because very rarely do they sit and watch TV. For example, if *Sesame Street* is on, my younger son will play the entire time, oblivious to the TV, until Elmo's World comes on. He'll watch Elmo for a few minutes, and then he'll go right back to playing. At least for now, we don't have to restrict our kids' TV time. They restrict themselves plenty well enough.

—*Rebecca Reamy, MD*

❧

TV does have some value. I get ideas for craft projects and making smoothies from watching Sprout, for example.

When my daughter watches TV, I make sure to watch with her. That way, if she has a question about something, she'll ask it, and I can answer it right away.

I never have the news or prime-time television on when my daughter is in the room. That is not kid-friendly.

—*Christy Valentine, MD, a mom of a six-year-old daughter, a specialist in pediatrics and internal medicine, and the founder of the Valentine Medical Center, in Gretna, LA*

❧

Toddlers are so busy, so all over the place, that it's hard for parents to keep up. It can be tempting to plop toddlers down in front of the TV to get a break.

I tried not to do that. I kept TV a very, very small part of my kids' day. Instead I came up with ways to keep my kids busy. For example, I'd get out a big box of blocks for them to play with, we'd go outside and kick a ball, or we'd take a walk to pick up leaves. When kids are toddlers, parents need to lay down the framework for learning and encourage kids to explore their world.

Even now, my kids watch little to no TV. It's just never been a priority.

—*Ann Contrucci, MD, a mom of 13-year-old boy-girl twins who works as a pediatric emergency physician, in Atlanta, GA*

❧

If it's not Your Baby Can Read, my sons aren't watching it.

—*Sharon Boyce, MD*

I highly recommend playing a lot of music and dancing with your children instead of turning on the TV.

—*Elizabeth Chabner Thompson, MD, MPH, a mom of 13- and 8-year-old daughters and 12- and 10-year-old sons, a radiation oncologist with 21 C. Radiation Oncology, and the inventor of the Mommy Bag, filled with supplies for moms-to-be having C-sections, in Scarsdale, NY*

My husband and I got married in 1999. At the time, we were both living with other roommates, and neither of us owned a TV. We agreed not to buy one. Thirteen years later, we still don't have a TV!

I think we talk a lot more than other families do because we don't have a TV. We do have a DVD player, and we watch DVDs occasionally. But that's far less tempting because it involves more effort than simply pressing a button. I would very much like to never have a TV in our house.

—*Kate Tulenko, MD, MPH*

One of the challenges I found when my kids were toddlers was protecting them from advertisers and blocking the commercial messages that surround us. I felt that I needed to create a safe microenvironment for my kids, by blocking messages from the people who were trying to feed my kids rainbow-colored junk and get them nagging me for the advertisers' products.

Toddlers can't distinguish between ads and programming. And those advertisers are brilliant. Our power as parents is remote compared to theirs. We're really setting ourselves up for failure if we try to compete against them.

I support the American Academy of Pediatrics' guidelines for TV watching: No TV until age two years. Of course, let's be honest. All moms need a few minutes here and there, such as to take a shower. It's perfectly fine to put the toddler in front of a DVD so you can shower in peace. When my kids were toddlers, I occasionally let them watch carefully chosen Disney DVDs when I was alone with them and needed to take a shower.

I think it's important to lead by example. Before my husband and I had kids, we stopped watching TV. I discovered that I had much more time to read and to enjoy my husband's company. I didn't miss that TV one bit!

Over the years, the TV has crept back into our lives. It's in a remote room, but we do watch it on occasion, such as when my sons' favorite sports teams are playing. But we never watch TV during the school week.

—*Ayala Laufer-Cahana, MD*

Teaching Your Toddler to Help around the House

Many hands make light work, even if those hands are teeny tiny. The toddler years are a great time to get your child to pitch in around the house. Because your toddler wants to be like you, and to be with you, he'll be eager to help you sweep the floors, make dinner, and fold laundry.

Even a two-year-old can help pick up dirty clothes, match socks, and put away toys. Encourage his desire to be helpful now while it lasts.

∽

When my girls were helpful around the house, I would respond to them by saying, "Wow, you did such a good job. Mommy is so proud of you. Let's go get a reward."

—*Eva Ritvo, MD, a mom of 21- and 16-year-old daughters, a psychiatrist, and a coauthor of* The Beauty Prescription, *in Miami Beach, FL*

∽

When it was time to clean up around the house, I used to set the kitchen timer. We'd have races to see who could beat Mommy cleaning up the most toys. My kids loved these races, and of course they usually won. We started this when my kids were around two years old.

—*Eva Mayer, MD, a mom of an eight-year-old daughter and a six-year-old son and a pediatrician with St. Luke's Pediatrics Associates, in Bethlehem, PA*

I try to engage my daughter in the process of things as much as possible. During meals, lots of food falls to the floor. After we've finished eating, I get out dustpans and brooms, and my daughter helps me sweep up the crumbs.

—*Tanya Douglas Holland, MD*

Once my sons were old enough to carry something without dropping it, I gave them ways to help out around the house. For example, my sons carried their plastic plates to the sink after meals.

I find that it's helpful if you ask kids to do things that they find fun. For example, my kids loved to fling laundry from our second story to the first floor. To this day, it amazes me that even as toddlers they knew that it was okay to throw laundry down the stairs, but nothing else. A toy never sailed over the railing, but plenty of dirty clothes did.

—*Carrie Brown, MD, a mom of eight- and six-year-old sons and a general pediatrician who treats medically complex children and specializes in palliative care at Arkansas Children's Hospital, in Little Rock*

My husband and I used to get down on our hands and knees and pick up small toys like Legos in handfuls and throw them into a container. Then my husband came up with a genius idea: He sweeps them up in one fell swoop with a dustpan and broom! It's much quicker and easier, and my sons think it's fun to do too!

—*Rebecca Reamy, MD*

Early on, I established a simple rule: Any toys that were left on the floor at the end of the day, my kids must not value much. So I explained that I'd gather those toys and donate them to children who had no toys and would appreciate them.

I was a single mom for a long time, and I appreciate everything that I have. I want my kids to understand that you have to work for what you have. And you have to care for what you have.

—*Cathy Marshall, MD*

I found a simple way to get my toddlers to be more helpful around the house. Instead of giving them a long explanation about when, why, and how we needed to clean, I would break it down into a few words.

"Pick up blocks," I'd say while pointing to a stack of blocks.

Once that task was accomplished, we'd move on to the next one. Speaking in simple words, in a nonconfrontational way, was effective. Getting into a tug-of-war with a two-year-old is ridiculous.

—*Dana S. Simpler, MD, a mom of 25- and 20-year-old girls and a 23-year-old son and a specialist in internal medicine in private practice, in Baltimore, MD*

My husband and I started our kids with chores when they were around 18 months old, which is about when children can follow two-step directions. I believe that kids feel more connected to a group when they do something to help that group. So, for example, when we clean the house, our youngest son will sort and match up the big pile of shoes that gathers by the front door. Also, as soon as our kids are tall enough, they carry their plastic plates and silverware and put them into the dishwasher. Toddlers can reach the opened dishwasher long before they can reach the kitchen counter!

—*Deborah Gilboa, MD*

One way my older son helped me around the house was by helping me to empty the dishwasher. He loved to do this, and he liked to feel useful. He'd carefully pull the dishes out and hand them to me or put them on the counter.

When my son helped my husband or me to unload the dishwasher, it was also a great opportunity to teach him new words. As my son handed us things, we'd name them, "Fork, spoon, cup, plate," and he would repeat after us. This was also a fun bonding experience for us!

—*Leena Shrivastava Dev, MD*

Here's an easy way to get your toddler to help keep the house clean: Teach everyone to take their shoes off right inside the door.

Depending on your profession, this can be really critical. I'm absolutely adamant about not bringing work stuff home. While I'm relaxed about common germs in the everyday environment, the germs that I'm exposed to at work are typically serious germs, such as MRSA or C. difficile. I have a pair of clogs that I leave at work, my white coat stays on while I see patients and it stays at work, and my stethoscope stays at work. I have a separate backpack at work that goes in and out of the emergency department with me and stays in my locker. When I get home, I change my clothes immediately.

—*Lisa Campanella-Coppo, MD*

When children are toddlers, we are laying the foundation for all that is to come. For example, if you lay the proper foundation for their manners, work ethic, and safety, you're off to a great start.

In our home, we talked with our toddlers about how we all have jobs to do. As parents, our jobs are to work and to take care of our children. Their job is to learn and grow and to build relationships with their friends.

We also have chores that we do around the house. Even at two years old, my children were able to pick up toys and put them away. Now that my kids are older, they are able to unload the dishwasher, and everyone puts their folded laundry away. We work as a team: Five for one, and one for five!

I feel it's important to teach my children how to do these household tasks. Even if someone puts clothes into their drawer in a messy way, I'm grateful that the clothes were put away.

The points system has been working very well now that my children are older. Each of my three kids will have a new set of house chores (up to three) per week, such as picking up the trash, making their bed, unloading the dishwasher, brushing their teeth, picking up toys, saying "please" and "thank you," greeting people politely, not whining, etc. At the end of the week, my kids will add up the points they have earned daily for the chores they have fulfilled. The reward can be anything from having a friend over to going to the movies to receiving some pocket money.

> *—Aline T. Tanios, MD, a mom of nine- and three-year-old*
> *daughters and a seven-year-old son and a pediatric hospitalist at*
> *Arkansas Children's Hospital, in Little Rock*

∽◦

You wouldn't want a toddler using cleaning products, of course, but having children should cause you to reevaluate the cleaning products you use. I used a lot of Basic H Shaklee products. Today, there's an even greater variety of good products. A good rule of thumb is to check the ingredients list. If it reads like a chemical factory, put it back on the shelf.

> *—Cathie Lippman, MD, a mom of 31- and 29-year-old sons*
> *and a physician who specializes in environmental and preventive*
> *medicine at the Lippman Center for Optimal Health, in Beverly*
> *Hills, CA*

Taking Your Toddler to Church or Temple

According to the National Council of Churches, just under half of the American population attends church regularly. Who knows how many of the churchgoers with toddlers make it past the first hymn.

∽◦

We've only tried to take our son to church a few times, but so far he's done really well. We want him to start going to Sunday school early so that he can learn about religion on his level and also to be exposed to a school atmosphere.

> *—Michelle Davis-Dash, MD, a mom of a one-year-old son and a*
> *pediatrician, in Baltimore, MD*

∽◦

The earlier you expose a child to ideas and concepts, the more likely he'll be able to adapt to them. If your religious beliefs are important to you, you'll want to expose your children to them at a very early age. We aren't born with the concept of God, religion, and spirituality. We wanted to expose our children to these concepts early, so there will never be a time they don't remember knowing them. Both of my girls were in temple schools during their toddler years.

> *—Eva Ritvo, MD*

I live far from my family and friends, so we don't have a lot of play-dates. Instead, we take our sons to church. They are making new friends there, and they enjoy seeing other kids their own age at church.

Our church doesn't have a nursery. But the service is short, so my sons usually can make it through quietly.

—*Sharon Boyce, MD*

I want my kids to learn about my religion, and I try to take my son to temple each Sunday evening. Ever since my son was very little, I've played hymns for him in the car and at night before he goes to sleep. He's really starting to become very familiar with them. Last Sunday, my son started to sing the hymns all by himself! He was really enjoying himself and clapping along with the congregation.

Our service isn't long. It takes only about a half hour, so my son is able to sit through it.

—*Shilpa Amin-Shah, MD, a mom of a two-year-old son and a one-year-old daughter and an emergency physician at Emergency Medical Associates, in Livingston, NJ*

Fortunately, our daughter always loved going to church. She loved playing with the other kids in the nursery, and then she moved up to the toddler class and she enjoyed the crafts, activities, and Bible stories and songs that they offered.

We tried once to keep her in the adult church with us because we wanted her to see Mommy and Daddy participate in singing church songs and being a part of church also. My daughter was *not* interested in this! She just kept asking to go to her church class so she could play with her friends!

—*Melody Derrick, MD, a mom of a two-year-old daughter who's expecting another baby and a family physician in private practice with Cadence Physician Group, in Winfield, IL*

One place to keep a very close eye on is the church nursery. They don't have any regulations, and they might not even have policies on how many volunteers need to be present per child.

One time when my older son was 2½ years old, I dropped him off at the church nursery. At the time, there were only a handful of kids there. I went back to church. Soon after, my toddler wandered up a flight of stairs, through the building, and into the church sanctuary, all by himself, without the nursery volunteers even noticing he was gone! When I returned my son to the nursery, I found there were far too many kids per adult there.

If you get to the nursery and there are more than a few kids per adult, stay to help or don't leave your child there.

—*Carrie Brown, MD*

Planning for Your Toddler's Financial Future

Experts say it will cost more than $150,000 to raise a child born in 2010 to adulthood. You can find a really interesting, more detailed calculator at csgnetwork.com/childcostcalc.html. Time to ramp up your financial fitness. Consider checking out these websites, which all offer free financial advice and budgeting tools: LearnVest.com, DailyWorth.com, and WomenAndCo.com.

It's never too early to talk with your child about finances and to model good spending and saving habits. A study conducted at Washington University in St. Louis found that kids with a savings account in their names are about six times more likely to attend college than those without one.

My daughter has a couple of piggy banks. Even as a toddler, I talked with her about money. Any time she received money as a gift, I told her to put it into her piggy bank to save it for college. My daughter has done it so often now that she doesn't even think about it. The other day, she lost a tooth, and the Tooth Fairy brought her some money. Without hesitation, my daughter put it into her bank.

My daughter knows that the money in her piggy banks is for her education. She never asks to spend it on anything else, such as toys. She knows that she gets toys as gifts for special occasions, but that money is set aside for college.

—*Christy Valentine, MD*

When each of my girls turned one year old, we opened a kids' bank account at the local bank. They don't charge any fees for kids' accounts. My husband and I also gave them a piggy bank and a charity box, and we began talking with them about saving money and investing. We regularly take our girls' piggy banks to their bank so they can deposit their money. Every year around the holidays we help them make a donation to the charity of their choice. I also have some great children's books that explain the difference between needs versus wants and the value of saving for long-term goals.

My parents raised me to understand investing, and my grandmother was interested in the stock market as a hobby. When I met my husband, he knew so little about investing that he asked me, "What's a stock?" My mother took him under her wing and taught him about investing.

It was important to my husband and me that our girls knew about investing and were comfortable talking about it. I think that the lack of understanding about financial matters is a huge hole in most kids' education. It's very important to talk to them about finances and the economy. We talk so much about the importance of working hard. Why not teach them the importance of investing and saving the money they will have worked so hard for?

I often find everyday occasions where I can teach my girls about money. For example, at the grocery store, if my daughter asks for a fruit roll-up, I say, "You can buy a fruit roll-up or, for the same price, you could buy two apples." When she asks for something I don't want to buy her, I might say, "Next time we'll bring some money from your piggy bank to spend." That's a more useful answer than simply saying "no." This also helps her understand that everything we buy needs to be paid for with money.

—*Kate Tulenko, MD, MPH*

RALLIE'S TIP

When my children were toddlers, it was hard to imagine that one day they'd be ready for college. I could barely get them ready for day care! But I knew the day would come, and my husband and I wanted to be prepared for the expense of college for each of them. I knew how expen-

*sive it could be, since I graduated from medical school with around
$100,000 of student loan debt.*

*Whenever my husband and I had spare change, we'd give it to the
boys so they could drop it (supervised!) into a giant pickle jar that we
kept in our room. We'd tell them that the money was for college, even
though at that age, they had no idea what college was. My husband and
I wanted our boys to grow up with the knowledge that they would be
able to go to college if they chose to. We've never counted the money in
the pickle jar, but I'm sure there's at least several hundred dollars in it by
now. Maybe it will be enough to buy a textbook or two! Having my
toddlers put money into the pickle jar was more of a teaching exercise,
rather than an actual savings plan.*

*My husband and I have been really diligent about regularly putting
money into a savings account that's earmarked for our sons' college, even
when times were tough and it was really a bit of a struggle for us financially. My husband's parents had a great idea to help us save for the
boys' education early on. Since our kids were babies, my in-laws have
given them U.S. Savings Bonds as birthday gifts. These weren't exactly
popular items when my boys were toddlers, but now that they're older,
they're really starting to appreciate them.*

*The great thing about buying bonds as a way of saving for college
is that it takes a long time for the bonds to mature, so it's not very
tempting to cash them in right away. The easiest thing to do is just to
put them in a safe place and forget about them. By the time the kids are
ready for college, all of those U.S. Savings Bonds that they received as
gifts over the years will really come in handy. Combined with the money
in our college savings account and the pickle jar, we should be able to
finance the boys' educations without going completely broke!*

Encouraging Health and Fitness

Eating right, exercising more, sleeping well: As you do these
things, you're giving yourself the gift of great health, and you're
giving your child an example to follow. It's the ultimate two-for-
one deal!

I fit in some exercise time when my kids are at the playground by playing on the equipment with them. I also take a yoga class once a week.
I've lost more than 70 pounds since my son was born!

—*Jennifer Hanes, DO, a mom of a six-year-old daughter and
a three-year-old son, an emergency physician, a certified forensic
physician, and the founder of Empowered Medicine, PLLC, in
Austin, TX*

Right now, my goal is to fit in 5 to 10 minutes of exercise a day. I know
that's not a whole lot, but at least it's something! I work out on my
elliptical machine in the basement while my girls nap. Our basement
isn't finished, so it's not a place for toddlers to play. But I'm close
enough that I can hear them if they cry. Also, I do sit-ups in the living
room while I talk to them.

—*Kate Tulenko, MD, MPH*

I don't really have time to go to the gym, nor do I particularly enjoy
it. But I lead a very active lifestyle: I take my son out fruit or vegetable picking, to water parks, visiting friends, swimming, and more. I
also walk to my job (I work in a busy city), about an hour total each
day, so I'm going to count that as well. In fact, I recently went to a
gym on a guest pass with my childless, gym-bunny friend, and I
completely outpaced her in the back-to-back cardio classes we took!

I realized that my cardio was chasing after my son; aerobics was
going up and down the stairs because I was always forgetting something;
weight lifting was carrying my sleeping four-year-old son for three or four
blocks; agility and balance was putting away toys and doing laundry as
quickly as possible; and endurance was, simply, being a mom.

—*Cheryl Wu, MD, a mom of a four-year-old son, a pediatrician
at LaGuardia Place Pediatrics in New York City, and a pediatric
emergency physician at the Joseph M. Sanzari Children's Hospital
of Hackensack University Medical Center, in New Jersey*

I am very big on exercise. My daughter loves to be outdoors, so we
enjoy going for walks and getting her outdoors whenever possible.

She also loves to dance, so sometimes we will dance together to get the blood flowing. My daughter and I also like walking in the mall and playing at the Tot Lot in the mall.

—*Tanya Douglas Holland, MD*

Before I had kids, I was pretty fit. After my kids were born, I could not have lived without my double jogging stroller. I took it everywhere! When my kids were toddlers, my husband and I took them for walks in the stroller every night. It was a wonderful chance for us to talk, get some exercise, and also model for our kids the importance of exercise.

The double jogging stroller we had wasn't anything expensive or fancy. In fact, it had been a hand-me-down, but, boy, did we get our use out of it!

—*Antoinette Cheney, DO*

Finding time to exercise is so hard, but it's *so* important! I love to make it a family event. Then it feels like you're bonding as a family, not just exercising. We go on bike rides and walks together. I think it's also important for your kids to see you exercising. You have to model the good habits for them. Even when I'm doing something that my toddler can't do with me, such as running, I take her in the jogging stroller. It makes it more fun for me anyway!

—*Melody Derrick, MD*

When my kids were toddlers, I began taking Zumba. It's a wonderful stress reliever! Even now, every week Zumba is my me time. This helps to emphasize the importance of fitness to my kids.

—*Mona Gohara, MD*

We're a very active family. When I have the chance, I like to jog. My husband plays soccer three or four times a week. When our kids were toddlers, we played games such as kick-the-ball in the backyard. We were surprised at our son's coordination, so from an early age, we enrolled our kids in sports. Team sports have been invaluable in teaching my kids hand-eye coordination, agility, and also the importance of team spirit.

—*Teresa Hubka, DO*

As my children grew up, I considered it to be a fun challenge to come up with creative ways that I could exercise with them. This way, my exercising didn't take me away from my kids. When my kids were babies, I would hold them on my legs or in my arms and do "baby lifts." When my kids were toddlers, they loved to swing. We'd go to a playground, and I'd push them in the swing. As they were swinging, I'd run a circle around the swing set or run underneath the swing and yell, "Under Doggy!" If you do that for a half hour, you've gotten in some good exercise!

As my kids got older, we'd play kickball in the courtyard outside of our home. I'd be the pitcher, and when my kids kicked the ball, I'd sprint after it. The best part of this was it never felt like exercise. It felt like fun, and the kids had a great time too.

—*Dana S. Simpler, MD*

My family was blessed with an amazing dog who kept us enjoying the outdoors and active for many years. Being active with our dog became such a way of life for us that after he passed away, we found ourselves inviting a new four-legged friend, a Great Dane, into our home.

As my children get older and suggest they want to try any new activity or sport, I encourage it. I also make sure that they each have an opportunity to find out what they enjoy and will pursue in their own lives.

I'm a dancer, and I try to keep up with the art. I hope that modeling a love for something active will help my children stay active in their lives.

—*Sigrid Payne DaVeiga, MD*

When my kids were young, I took exercise any way that I could get it. Exercise is essential for my self-esteem and mental health.

When my oldest was a baby and then a toddler, I ran behind her pram in Central Park, and I walked everywhere with her in the Baby Björn. When we lived in the city, I only took a cab when it was absolutely essential. Otherwise, I walked everywhere.

When we moved to the suburbs, I figured out that exercise was just as important as eating and sleeping. I ran on a treadmill, and I walked as much as possible. My husband helped me to accomplish this. He would find time, even after work, to "liberate me" for an hour to exercise.

My daughter and I had a routine on the days that I didn't work: In the back of my mind, I figured that exercise made me feel good, so it would be good for our children as well. So it was my mission to wear them out physically, every day.

My husband and I were both early risers. He covered the Europe and emerging markets, so he was up and out around 5 am. I would feed my daughter and pack our pool bag, and we would go to Asphalt Green, where she loved swimming in the 90-degree rehab pool that was open to the public from 7 to 8 am. Then we would come home, she'd eat again, and by 10 am, she'd take a nap. I would work out on a Stairmaster in our living room and read.

By 12 or 1, my daughter was up again, and we would go outside and meet other mothers and run errands. By 3, she would be ready for another nap.

—*Elizabeth Chabner Thompson, MD, MPH*

When my girls were toddlers, I was very careful to impress upon them my core values. For example, when we'd see someone smoking, I'd say, "Smoking is bad. It harms your health. We need to move away from that person who's smoking."

When you introduce these concepts at such an early age, the child readily accepts your world view. This worked so well that when my daughter was six and we took her to a restaurant in Paris, so many people were smoking that we couldn't find anywhere to sit! When we found a table, the man at the next table was smoking. My daughter asked me if we could move, so we changed tables. The person at the next table there was smoking too.

"Mom, we have to move again," my daughter said. The message of smoking being bad was completely ingrained in her brain.

You can't tell a 14-year-old that smoking is bad. That can

actually backfire and make him want to smoke. You have to introduce concepts like this at a very young age. You can apply this to many concepts, such as not drinking and not using drugs, eating properly, being nice to others, embracing spirituality, and any of your core family values.

—*Eva Ritvo, MD*

RALLIE'S TIP

I can remember lying on the floor trying to do sit-ups with both my toddlers crawling on top of me for a horsey ride. Floor exercises definitely didn't work for me, so I ended up buying a double jogging stroller. I think I must have put several hundred miles on that stroller, and it gave me an incredible sense of freedom. With my babies in the stroller, I would jog around the bike path at a local park, and after I finished my workout, I'd let my boys run and play on the playground. It was great exercise for both of us. On rainy days, I'd put on some music, and my boys and I would dance together in the living room. Dancing is a great workout, and it's also a lot of fun for moms and kids.

If you're interested in working out with other moms and their children, you might be able to find (or start!) a Stroller Strides organization in your community. Stroller Strides offers several types of classes for moms who want to lose their baby weight or just stay in shape. Alternately, local gyms, fitness clubs, and community organizations sometimes offer Mommy and Me classes that help babies and toddlers—and their moms—stay active and fit.

Chapter 18
Travel and Trips

Your Toddler's Development

"To travel is to live."—Hans Christian Andersen

Although Hans Christian Andersen wrote more than 150 fairytales for children, he didn't have any children of his own, and he probably never traveled with any toddlers! Otherwise, he might have edited his quote to "To travel with toddlers is to wish that you had stayed home."

Traveling with toddlers is tricky, but it can be very rewarding. Studies have shown that vacations are good for your health.

Less tangible are the benefits to families from spending time making memories together, whether that's a day at the beach or a week in Paris. From the anticipation and planning of the vacation, to the actual trip, to reliving the memories by looking at photos and videos of the vacation for years after, vacation: It does a family good.

Taking Care of You

Whenever you plan a trip, whether it's a day trip to the zoo or a week at Walt Disney World, plan for a little post-trip downtime for yourself to regroup and relax.

Justification for a Celebration

When you're packing for a trip with your toddler, if you can get the suitcase to close, without jumping up and down on top of it, that's cause for a celebration!

Going on a Day Trip

Toddlers thrive on routine, so you might feel the need to stick to your routines like glue too. Day trips are pretty much the opposite of routine, but with some proper planning ahead of time, taking your toddler on a trip can be fun for both of you.

∽◦∾

Whenever we're going away with our kids, my husband and I make a packing list of everything we need to take. The night before, we pack everything up and load it into the car. That way, the next morning, we just have to get everyone up and dressed, and we can go.

My husband and I preplan a lot. We make a lot of lists. This helps life run much more smoothly!

—*Shilpa Amin-Shah, MD, a mom of a two-year-old son and a one-year-old daughter and an emergency physician at Emergency Medical Associates, in Livingston, NJ*

∽◦∾

Everywhere I go with my children, I bring a bag of supplies. It includes baby wipes, a change of clothes for everyone, and some antiseptic spray. That is very handy if someone falls and scrapes their knees. It stops the drama quickly.

—*Aline T. Tanios, MD, a mom of nine- and three-year-old daughters and a seven-year-old son and a pediatric hospitalist at Arkansas Children's Hospital, in Little Rock*

When I take my boys on a trip, such as to a museum, I don't necessarily dress them alike. But I do often dress them in the same bright color.

"Why do you keep dressing the boys in orange shirts?" my husband asked me once.

"Because I would like to bring all of the children home," I answered.

—*Deborah Gilboa, MD, a mom of nine-, seven-, five-, and three-year-old sons, a parenting speaker whose advice is found at AskDoctorG.com, and a family physician with Squirrel Hill Health Center, in Pittsburgh, PA*

My son loved animals, so we took him to the San Diego Zoo and the Aquarium of the Pacific. A lightweight collapsible stroller definitely made things easier for such trips.

My husband makes these types of purchases because he likes to research product features. I'm happy with a simple umbrella stroller!

—*Bola Oyeyipo-Ajumobi, MD, a mom of four- and one-year-old sons, a family physician in private practice, and the owner of SlimyBookWorm.com, in Highland, CA*

It's important to take toddlers places and to expose them to new experiences, but it's not easy. You need to bring a lot of food and toys. And you need to moderate your expectations. Your experience isn't going to be the same as it was before you had kids.

I find that it's helpful to go places with friends who also have kids. This gives us more adults to hold and distract the kids, and more hands to help. You can ask your friend, "How about if you hold the baby for 10 minutes while I watch the game, and then we'll switch?" Also, children entertain other children, and it helps to shift kids' attention to someone other than you!

—*Kate Tulenko, MD, MPH, a mom of four- and one-year-old girls, the author of* Insourced: How Importing Jobs Impacts the Healthcare Crisis Here and Abroad, *and a pediatrician and global health specialist with IntraHealth, in Washington, DC*

My husband is a big fan of road trips, so we go on a lot of day car trips. I'm a big fan of packing plenty of things to do. My kids don't play a lot of computer games, but in the car, their Leapsters were great. We saved them for occasions like long car rides.

Just be sure to bring plenty of extra batteries! I keep a spare package in my car's glove box. It would never fail, five minutes into a trip, I'd hear that familiar "beep, beep" that indicates the batteries are low. *Seriously?* I'd think. Then I'd have to stop at a gas station and pay a ridiculous price for new batteries.

—*Antoinette Cheney, DO, a mom of a seven-year-old son and a six-year-old daughter and a family physician with Rocky Vista University College of Osteopathic Medicine, in Parker, CO*

During the toddler years, I kept a schedule for the kids and myself. I planned outings almost daily Monday through Friday. We live in the Lincoln Park area of Chicago, so there are a million things we can do. We would go to the zoo (free admission!), park-district classes, planned playgroup, and swimming. Additionally, Chicago is filled with wonderful parks with things to climb on and play with. I would go online to find a park near our house and take the kids there for a picnic lunch.

On the days that I had to work, I asked my babysitter to follow the same schedule so that my children had something to do.

I wasn't a schedule freak, but I made loose plans in case of rain or illness. Toddlers can change moods like the weather in Chicago, and I needed to be flexible.

One of the fondest memories I have is taking the kids to the children's theaters and free book readings offered at the library.

My children love the arts to this day.

> —*Laura M. Rosch, DO, a mom of a 12-year-old daughter and 7-year-old boy-girl twins, a board-certified internist who works at Central DuPage Hospital Convenient Care Centers in Winfield, IL, and an instructor in the department of family medicine at the Midwestern University/Chicago College of Osteopathic Medicine, in Downers Grove, IL*

I always keep my eyes on my kids on day trips. When I was eight years old, I was abducted. I have a high sense of vigilance about my kids getting lost or abducted. In places like malls or parks, I held their hands or made sure they were strapped into their strollers.

> —*Susan Wilder, MD, a mom of a 17-year-old daughter and twin 13-year-old girls, a primary care physician, and the founder and CEO of Lifescape Medical Associates, in Scottsdale, AZ*

RALLIE'S TIP

When my middle son was a toddler, he used to get terribly car sick whenever we went on trips, so I would give him a bit of ginger candy. Ginger is one of the very best remedies I know for nausea caused by motion sickness. The results of several clinical trials have shown that ginger is safe and effective in alleviating nausea related to upset stomach, motion sickness, and morning sickness. Although moms today often use ginger ale to alleviate stomach upset and nausea, most varieties of modern-day ginger ale contain only ginger flavoring, rather than real ginger, so they aren't nearly as effective as beverages made with real ginger. If modern varieties of ginger ale are effective at all, it's likely because of the carbonation, rather than the ginger flavoring. (The fact that ginger is the key ingredient seems to have been lost in the translation when moms passed this remedy down through the generations!) To alleviate nausea, it's best to give kids a small piece of real ginger or ginger candy from a health food store, or to make them a nice cup of ginger tea.

Ginger's anti-inflammatory properties work wonders in the gastrointestinal tract. Long before commercially produced ginger ale became a popular remedy for stomach upset, ancient healers prescribed ginger tea to soothe a variety of digestive symptoms, especially nausea and vomiting.

In a study that included 80 inexperienced sailors, scientists tested the ability of ginger to reduce symptoms of motion sickness associated with travel at sea. The sailors who received powdered ginger experienced a significant reduction in nausea and vomiting compared to those who were given placebo powder. My husband and I didn't take our toddlers out to sea, but the ginger worked just fine for car sickness!

Going on Vacation

Whether you're going by plane, train, or automobile, taking a vacation with a toddler can really be a trip.

↪↩

After I had my second child, I loved my side-by-side double Maclaren stroller. It was light, maneuverable, narrow, and easy to travel with.

—*Marra S. Francis, MD, a mom of eight-, seven-, and five-year-old daughters and a gynecologist, in San Antonio, TX*

↪↩

We've traveled so much by plane that my kids each have their own frequent-flier numbers. When my kids were toddlers, I found it very helpful to give them a sippy cup to drink from during takeoff and landing to help their ears adjust to the changing air pressure. Now, because of the increased security measures at airports, you'd have to bring an empty cup, of course, and fill it with juice on the plane!

—*Antoinette Cheney, DO*

↪↩

I've taken my sons on quite a few plane trips. Even when they were young enough to sit on my lap, I bought them their own seats. It's more comfortable for both of us! I discovered that by calling the airlines directly, rather than booking online, I could sometimes negotiate a special reduced child rate.

Another thing I found to be very helpful is that I'd buy each of my boys a small, new toy at the airport, preferably something with lots of buttons. Sure, they were expensive. But my sanity is worth something!

*—Carrie Brown, MD, a mom of eight- and six-year-old sons and
a general pediatrician who treats medically complex children and
specializes in palliative care at Arkansas Children's Hospital, in
Little Rock*

Whenever I flew with my sons when they were toddlers, I always paid extra so they'd have their own seats on the plane. I also brought their car seats from home. They were used to sitting and sleeping in their car seats, so this worked out very well. I also tried to plan to fly at bedtime or at least naptime, so it was more likely they'd fall asleep.

I packed a lot of snacks, books, and toys. Later we started to bring a portable DVD player and DVDs too. I always brought a change of clothes for my sons. My kids never threw up on a plane, but I've seen plenty of other kids do it!

*—Heather Orman-Lubell, MD, a mom of 11- and 7-year-old
sons and a pediatrician in private practice at Yardley Pediatrics of
St. Christopher's Hospital for Children, in Pennsylvania*

When my kids were toddlers, we lived in Germany, where my husband was stationed with the Army. While we lived there, we did a fair amount of traveling. Germany is centrally located, and we were fortunate to be able to go to Paris or Belgium for a weekend.

We found that rather than flying, taking a train was a great way to travel with kids. On the train, our kids didn't have to be strapped into tiny seats. They could move around and play.

*—Ann Kulze, MD, a mom of 23- and 17-year-old daughters and
22- and 20-year-old sons; a nationally recognized nutrition expert,
motivational speaker, and physician; and the author of the best-
selling book* Dr. Ann's Eat Right for Life, *in Charleston, SC*

When we travel, I pack any over-the-counter medications that we've used in the past two years. Before we go, I check the labels to make sure that they haven't expired.

—Kate Tulenko, MD, MPH

RALLIE'S TIP

Traveling can be emotionally and physically stressful for kids and adults. It takes us away from our normal routines and gives us more to worry about. Travel normally requires a change in our diets, including timing and food choices, and it disrupts our normal sleep patterns. All this added stress can weaken the defenses of the immune system. The results of numerous studies have firmly established that any type of stress, whether emotional or physical, impairs immunity. Lack of sleep or a change in sleep pattern is known to weaken the immune system as well and dramatically increases the risk of succumbing to an illness, particularly colds and flu. To make matters worse, many families tend to eat more junk food when they're traveling. Eating fewer fruits and vegetables and more processed food means fewer vitamins and minerals, and more sugar, all of which compromise the immune system.

Some kids and adults tend to drink less water while they're traveling, and traveling by air can be especially drying. Even mild dehydration can weaken the immune system. The mucous membranes of the nose and throat are the body's first lines of defense, and if they aren't moist and sticky from proper hydration, they're not as capable of trapping and destroying germs before they travel deeper into the sinuses or lungs and set up infection.

Some children and adults don't feel comfortable using public bathrooms while traveling, or they might not have the opportunity to empty their bladders as often or as completely as they would if they were at home. This can increase the likelihood of acquiring a urinary tract infection.

While our immunity is compromised from the stress of travel, we're typically exposed to far greater numbers of disease-causing germs than we would be if we stayed at home in our normal environment. We often use public restrooms at airports or rest stops and gas stations. We are likely to be exposed to far greater numbers of disease-causing viruses and bacteria, and we're also exposed to different types. The strain of cold virus that's wreaking havoc in Kansas City, Missouri, where your in-laws live, might be completely different from the strain that just swept through your child's day care back home.

The following are a few steps you can take to keep your toddlers as healthy as possible while you're traveling.

- *Try to stick to a nutritious diet without a lot of sodas and sugary treats.*
- *Drink plenty of water.*
- *Take time for regular potty breaks.*
- *Avoid sharing straws and drinks.*
- *Encourage kids to wash their hands often and as soon as they can after playing in a public play space or traveling on any type of public transportation system. Lots of germs are lurking there, and kids typically wallow around in them. If the place was especially crowded or looked less than clean, it might be a good idea to take a bath when you arrive at your destination, or at least change clothes.*
- *Pack a travel bag with wipes, hand sanitizer, and a change of clothes. When you return home from your trip, it's time to clean out your travel bag and replenish supplies.*

With two toddlers, I learned quickly that you can't bring it all with you from home when you travel. Fortunately, many clever companies rent kids' equipment, such as strollers and Pack 'n Plays, when you arrive at your destination. This allowed me to avoid lugging tons of gear through airports. A good resource for renting baby items when traveling is BabyTravelPros.com.

—Ann V. Arthur, MD, a mom of a 10-year-old daughter and an 8-year-old son, a pediatric ophthalmologist in private practice at Park Slope Eye Care Associates, and a blogger at WaterWineTravel.com, in New York City

Each year since my kids were toddlers, we've gone on a summer beach vacation with their cousins. With so many other people around with different needs and wishes, our family's schedule pretty much goes out the window. For example, I didn't really expect my kids to nap at all.

We rented a pretty small house at the beach, considering all of the people we jammed into it. It could be very challenging to carve out our own space. Early on, I learned to say, "This is what we need to do for our family." Also, if we needed some space, my husband and I wouldn't hesitate to grab our kids and head out for a walk on the beach by ourselves.

? When to Call Your Doctor

Ever wonder why kids so often get sick on vacation? Part of the reason might be because their little bodies haven't adjusted to the food, water, and air in the new environment, something we're all exposed to when we're in a new place.

It can be particularly tricky deciding whether or not to call the doctor when you're away from home. A good rule of thumb is to call your insurance company before you leave home to find out if you'll have medical coverage in the place you're traveling to. If you don't, buy travel insurance, which will include medical coverage if you need it.

Also, be sure to have your pediatrician's phone number with you (enter it into your cell phone's address book) so you can call for advice about treating your child with over-the-counter medications, whether or not to see a doctor where you are, or if your doctor needs to call in a prescription to a pharmacy near you.

If you are traveling out of the country, find out the number for emergency services upon arrival.

A cold or cough, mild diarrhea, constipation, or sleep problems generally don't require a trip to the doctor's office. But you should have your child seen by a physician under the following circumstances.

- Vomiting and diarrhea last longer than a few hours.
- Repeated vomiting accompanies a fever.
- A rash occurs with a fever.
- A cough or cold gets worse or doesn't get better after several days.
- Your child has a deep cut that might need stitches.
- Your child is limping or can't move an arm or leg.

—*Eva Mayer, MD, a mom of an eight-year-old daughter and a six-year-old son and a pediatrician with St. Luke's Pediatrics Associates, in Bethlehem, PA*

Most of the trips we've taken have been to visit family. Generally, we stay with family instead of a hotel, which can be great but

- An earache accompanies a fever.
- There's drainage from the ear.
- Your child won't sleep.
- Your child has a severe sore throat or trouble swallowing.
- Your child has sharp stomach pains or stomach pains that don't go away.
- Your child has pain that gets worse or won't go away after several hours.
- There's blood in your child's urine or stool.
- Your child refuses to drink for more than 12 hours.

If your child has any of the following very serious symptoms, call 911 or the number for emergency services where you are traveling.

- Persistent bleeding that doesn't stop when you apply pressure
- Possibility of ingesting something poisonous
- Seizures
- Breathing difficulties
- Blue, purple, or gray skin or lips
- Neck stiffness with a fever
- A head injury followed by loss of consciousness, confusion, vomiting, or a change in skin color
- A sudden lack of energy or the inability to move
- Unconsciousness
- Changes in behavior, such as becoming withdrawn or less alert
- A large, deep cut or burn; a cut or burn on the head, chest, abdomen, hands, groin, or face; or a deep puncture wound

also challenging. One thing I found to be helpful is if you're going to a different time zone, remind your family of that up front. That way, they're not expecting your kids to sit quietly and eat dinner at 9 pm their time.

Also, when we stay with family, I always have a backup hotel plan. That way, if things don't work out, it's easier to move to a hotel for the rest of the visit.

—*Carrie Brown, MD*

∽

When traveling, we've had our best experience when staying in a hotel with either a family suite that had a small kitchenette or renting an apartment or a home. In addition to having private sleeping quarters, we often used the kitchen to prepare breakfasts and bag lunches, which also saved us money. For finding vacation homes and apartments to rent, I love to use Homeaway.com. Also, many of the big hotel chains have suites.

We also usually stay in a hotel with a heated pool. That way, even if the weather is terrible, there's a fun activity we can do as a family.

—*Ann V. Arthur, MD*

∽

I think that the worst time to take a vacation is when your child is a toddler. It's not really fair to your fellow travelers on the plane.

My family had a horrendous trip to Florida with all four of our children, who were very young at the time, and a babysitter. All of my kids caught a stomach bug. The babysitter, a pretty high school–age girl, attracted an "admirer," who tried to break into her room while she was sleeping. I thought that having a babysitter along would be helpful, but it was more trouble than it was help.

The trip was a nightmare. My husband and I vowed to stay home until all of our kids were past the toddler years.

—*Victoria McEvoy, MD, a mom who raised four children; a grandmom of six-, four-, and two-year-old grandsons; an assistant professor of pediatrics at Harvard Medical School; the medical director and chief of pediatrics at Mass General West Medical Group; and the author of* 24/7 Baby Doctor, *in Boston, MA*

Recently, I was invited to speak at a conference in Germany. I really wanted to go, but I didn't want to leave my family for that long. So I decided to take them all along.

The flight to Germany was the longest we had ever been on—eight hours! I booked a direct, overnight flight. I packed backpacks full of toys for each kid, and they also slept quite a bit.

I called the airline ahead of time to make sure that we could have kid-friendly meals. My kids aren't likely to eat beef stroganoff or other unusual things that the airlines might serve to adults. I also packed lots of snacks.

I asked the airline ahead of time if there would be age-appropriate movies playing on the flight. I knew that our portable DVD players' batteries would make it only for the first few hours of the flight.

I also paid our babysitter to go along. I didn't want my husband

Mommy MD Guides-Recommended Product
Kids Fly Safe CARES Airplane Safety Harness

"When I fly with my son, I buy him his own seat. But I also take a CARES Harness. It fastens to the seat belt behind my son, and it holds him securely with a four-point harness," says Lennox McNeary, MD, a mom of a three-year-old son, a specialist in physical medicine and rehabilitation at Carilion Clinic, and a cofounder of the Mommy Doctors Bakery (makers of Milkin' Cookies), in Roanoke, VA.

"I also bring toys and plastic toy clips, so that I can attach the toys, and even my son's sippy cup, to the harness," Dr. McNeary says. "This way, the toys don't fall onto the plane floor."

The CARES Harness is appropriate for toddlers who are one year old or older and who weigh 22 to 44 pounds. It's easy to install on an airplane seat, and it will keep your child secure during turbulence on routine flights and in emergency situations.

You can buy a CARES Harness at buybuy Baby or at KIDSFLYSAFE.COM/STORE for $74.95.

to have to entertain three kids in a hotel room in a foreign country by himself for the long hours I'd be at the conference. I had been banking American Express miles for years, and I was able to pay for five out of the six tickets with that.

—*Brooke A. Jackson, MD, a mom of 4½-year-old twin girls and a 2½-year-old son, a dermatologist, and the founder and medical director of the Skin Wellness Center of Chicago, in Illinois*

A product that has been invaluable at airports and on vacations is the Gogo Kidz Travelmate, which is a wheeled attachment you can use with children's and toddlers' car seats. My relatives live across the country, and we often travel to see them and for my work. The Travelmate has been worth its weight in gold. One time recently, we were flying out of a different city, so my routine was off, and I forgot our Travelmate. It was a miserable experience!

When we get to the airport, my son rides in the Travelmate. The last time we used it, my son sat there with his hands folded behind his head, just chilling. When my son is in the Travelmate, I know that he can't get lost, and I can zip through the airport much more quickly than if my son was walking. If my son falls asleep while he's riding, that's great!

You can buy Gogo Kidz Travelmates at GoGoBabyz.com for $89.99.

—*Lennox McNeary, MD, a mom of a three-year-old son, a specialist in physical medicine and rehabilitation at Carilion Clinic, and a cofounder of the Mommy Doctors Bakery (makers of Milkin' Cookies), in Roanoke, VA*

I started traveling with my oldest son by plane when he was six weeks old because I lived in North Carolina and my relatives lived in California and Minnesota. Traveling with one child was easy once I figured out how to manage all the stuff.

My best advice is: If someone offers to help you get onto or off of the plane, say, "Yes!" Keep your baby and purse and let the other person help you with everything else. There's no prize for being the parent who manages to do it all alone.

On one trip, my son and I had a really long layover at an airport. The bathroom mirror was a lifesaver. My son laughed at himself in the mirror for almost 45 minutes, which was a great break for me.

After my second son was born, when my older son was 26 months old, traveling became a bigger challenge. I still flew alone with them across the country multiple times. I survived, but it wasn't easy.

Packing a bag of new, small toys and books to help to keep their interest while waiting in the airport was a lifesaver. A portable DVD player has also been wonderful.

I started dressing my sons in matching clothes, usually brightly colored shirts that we purchased on a previous trip. This was helpful for several reasons. First, when my sons were dressed alike, it was obvious that they belonged together. Second, it made it much easier to spot them in a crowd. And third, it would have been easy to describe them to someone if need be. Thankfully, I never lost a child, so I never had to test this theory out.

Rather than bringing my kids' car seats on the plane, I found it very handy to rent them from the car rental company once we arrived at our destination. It was one less thing to pack. Plus, I've never seen a rental car company's car seat that wasn't in excellent condition. People request them so infrequently that sometimes they were brand-new with tags still on.

—*Carrie Brown, MD*

My extended family lives in Lebanon and France, and I've taken my children on many overseas trips, some by myself—nine hours on a plane! Because we have worked hard with our children on using good manners at home, they are very well behaved on the plane.

I put together a master packing list for these trips, so that I remember to bring everything we need. Because of the restrictions about liquids on airplanes, I pack chewable or meltaway children's medications. That way, I can bring them in my carry-on bag, and I don't have to check them.

I also bring plenty of things for my children to do on the plane. Digital games can be a lifesaver on long trips. For the younger ones, sticker books are a great distraction. I also bring snacks that take a long time to eat and keep them occupied too, such as gummies and lollipops. I'm careful not to bring snacks that will be messy and might stain.

To help to lighten my load, I bought each of my children their own wheeled carry-on bags. Even my youngest daughter has a Dora the Explorer bag! This way, they can carry their own toys and snacks, and I don't have to lug it all.

—*Aline T. Tanios, MD*

RALLIE'S TIP

With a teenager and two toddlers, my husband and I didn't have the courage to travel very far or very often. It was just too exhausting! When we did travel, we made sure that we were well prepared in advance. One of our first big trips by plane was to Walt Disney World, and I took an extra day of vacation just to pack and plan for the trip. In addition to clothes, shoes, favorite toys, and lovies, I made sure to stock a lightweight travel bag with all of the things that we would need to keep us as healthy as possible while we were traveling, including the following items.

- *A zipper-lock baggie for each person's toothbrush and toothpaste: It's best to have a small tube of toothpaste for each family member. If you don't share toothpaste, you're less likely to share germs.*
- *Small packets of honey from a fast-food restaurant: Honey has antibiotic properties, and it's a great remedy for coughs for toddlers and older children.*
- *A disposable ice bag for bumps and bruises*
- *Children's multivitamin and mineral supplement*
- *Healthy snacks, such as raisins or granola bars in single-serving-size packs*
- *Sugarless chewing gum to ease ear discomfort on the airplane*
- *Tylenol and the dosage cup*
- *Benadryl and the dosage cup*
- *Band-Aids and antibiotic ointment*
- *Sunscreen*

• *Hand sanitizer and wipes to clean the tables and everyone's hands before eating at a restaurant*

Going to an Amusement Park

According to the International Association of Amusement Parks and Attractions, there are more than 400 amusement parks in the United States. Each year, they draw more than 300 million visitors, who enjoy more than 1.7 billion rides. The most visited park? The Magic Kingdom at Walt Disney World in Florida.

My son loves carnivals, and we go to several of them during the spring, summer, and fall. Even though some of the rides are meant for little children, I always watch the ride go through at least one cycle before I let my son ride. I've been surprised by how many of those kiddie rides start and stop abruptly, which can injure a child's neck.

—*Lennox McNeary, MD*

I've taken my daughter to Walt Disney World twice, and we're planning another trip for this year. Before we stepped foot inside the park, I explained to my daughter that there would be many, many people there, and that it would be very, very easy to get lost. I told my daughter that she needed to hold my hand at all times if she wasn't in her stroller. I set that expectation up front so that she wouldn't be surprised, or upset, inside the parks.

—*Christy Valentine, MD, a mom of a six-year-old daughter, a specialist in pediatrics and internal medicine, and the founder of the Valentine Medical Center, in Gretna, LA*

I'm opposed to the harness systems that I see some parents using in airports, amusement parks, and zoos. I can understand that people might feel the harnesses are making their kids safer, but for me, using one would make me feel like I was treating my child like an animal.

—*Carrie Brown, MD*

When my younger kids were toddlers, we wanted to take the older ones to Walt Disney World, so the toddlers came along for the ride. They had a bit of a hard time with all of the flashing things and bright lights.

To keep the toddlers entertained, we made sure to spot Mickey and friends everywhere that we went because even the little ones were familiar with those characters. We also alternated between fast, loud rides for the bigger folk and slower, calmer events for the little ones.

—*Susan Besser, MD, a mom of six grown children, ages 27, 25, 23, 21, 20, and 18, a grandmom of two, a family physician, and the medical director of Doctors Express-Memphis, in Tennessee*

Whenever we went out in public, I always dressed my girls in matching outfits. It was cute, but more importantly, it was always easier for me to spot three similar outfits in a crowd. As my girls got older, this trick was perfect for water parks and pools. Recognizing a bathing suit pattern is so much easier than finding a face that's behind swimming goggles or blowing bubbles in the water.

—*Marra S. Francis, MD*

In the Chicago area, we have a lot of water parks, both indoor and outdoor. They're wonderful parks with water slides, fountains, and lots of great activities for small children. We enjoyed going there to cool off in the summer and also for camaraderie with other kids.

My children learned to swim at early ages, but I still never took my eyes off them in the water parks. One thing I especially worried about was them running, slipping, and falling. I taught my toddlers to walk "lightly" on the wet places of the water park. That way, they didn't run and slip.

—*Teresa Hubka, DO, a mom of a 14-year-old son and an 8-year-old daughter, an ob-gyn and the medical director of Comprehensive Wellness Care in Chicago, and an associate professor of obstetrics and gynecology and the chairman and residency program director of the department of obstetrics and gynecology at the Midwestern University/Chicago College of Osteopathic Medicine, in Downers Grove, Illinois*

Identification tags for kids are a great idea when you're going to be at a place like an amusement park. A product called Who's Shoes IDs attach to a child's shoe, for example, or you could get dog tags for older kids.

When I was a child, my family visited the United States from Pakistan. We went with family to an amusement park, and I got lost. I was terrified! This was before cell phones, and I didn't know my uncle's home phone number for the park employees to call. My family was scheduled to fly out of that city the next day, and I was scared they would leave without me! My family found me after a few very scary minutes spent at the lost-and-found kiosk.

ID tags can be helpful closer to home too. One day, when my triplets were toddlers, one of my sons got out of the house while I was taking a nap and wandered onto the golf course next door. A stranger found my son and waited with him, not sure what to do because he didn't know where my son lived or whom to call for help. If my son had been wearing an ID tag, the man could have called me.

Thank goodness it all worked out okay. I realized my son had gone outside a few minutes later and found him.

—*Sadaf T. Bhutta, MD, a mom of a six-year-old daughter and four-year-old triplets and an assistant professor and the fellowship director of pediatric radiology at the University of Arkansas for Medical Sciences and Arkansas Children's Hospital, both in Little Rock*

RALLIE'S TIP

I learned one of my most important life lessons at King's Island in Mason, Ohio: One adult is no match for four toddlers. My husband and I went to the amusement park with another couple who, like us, had two toddlers. We spent the morning pushing the four boys around the park in their strollers and snapping cute pictures of them on all the kiddie rides.

By noon, the boys had had enough, but my husband and our friends were dying to try out the roller coaster called The Beast. I'd rather have a root canal than ride a roller coaster, especially one named The Beast, so I volunteered to watch the four toddlers while the other adults risked life and limb in their quest for an adrenaline rush. All four boys were sitting angelically around a table eating ice cream cones as we waved good-bye to the grown-ups, but the minute they were out of our sight, my youngest son hopped off his chair and scampered under the table. It took less than a minute for me to lean down and retrieve my son, but as soon as I sat back up, I was horrified to see that my friends' youngest son was no longer sitting in his seat.

I don't think that I've ever experienced such overwhelming fear and panic. I gathered up the three remaining toddlers, which was no easy task, and I started frantically searching the food court and shouting the missing child's name at the top of my lungs. There were dozens of small children around, and I couldn't even remember exactly what the lost boy was wearing. I found a security officer, and I told him that I was a horrible person and that I had managed to lose my friends' child. He quickly cut me off and sprang into action, radioing his fellow officers around the park to be on the lookout. Then he helped me search the food court.

After what felt like an eternity, I spotted the lost toddler next to his stroller, just a few feet away from the table where we had been sitting. I can honestly say that I've never been so happy to see anyone in my entire life. I immediately scooped him up and strapped him and the other three boys snuggly in their strollers and dared them to move a muscle. When I looked at my watch, I was amazed to see that the entire drama had unfolded in less than 15 minutes.

Since then, I've never volunteered to take care of anyone else's children in addition to my own in a crowded environment. Two toddlers are more than most adults can keep up with. I also started dressing my children in shirts that will stand out in a crowd, and I make sure that I remember exactly what they're wearing. I think it's an excellent idea to attach a little luggage tag with your contact information to a child's belt loop or shoelace, and after my experience, I wouldn't think twice about putting a little GPS tracking device in a toddler's pocket.

When my husband and our friends returned from their roller coaster ride, I had to confess what had happened. We were all happy that things turned out so well, but we also learned an important lesson. Toddlers can get away from adults in an instant, and the results could be devastating. After that, we realized that we needed one adult to watch each pair of toddlers. When I count my blessings, I always say a special thanks for the happy ending at King's Island.

Safety While Away

Wanting to keep your toddler safe is part of your job description. That can be challenging enough at home, in your own controlled environment. It can be even more of a challenge when you're on the go.

⌒

I don't have any particular travel safety tips because I never left the kids out of my sight. Although it's a good idea to know the pool policy when traveling. Many hotels and resorts don't have lifeguards on staff.
—*Ann V. Arthur, MD*

⌒

When my family stays in hotels, I do a quick sweep of the room before anyone is free to play in the room and before we unpack. I pick up any small items on the floor that might have been missed by housekeeping, and I move things like pens and notepaper out of reach.

—*Sadaf T. Bhutta, MD*

The first time we stayed in a hotel room with my older daughter, I actually brought outlet covers, corner guards for the desk corners, and a few other little safety items from home to babyproof the room. After that, I had a better idea of what my concerns were and would only bring the few items that I felt were most important for subsequent trips.

—*Jeannette Gonzalez Simon, MD, a mom of three- and one-year-old daughters and a pediatric gastroenterologist in private practice, in Staten Island, NY*

When my boys were toddlers, we stayed in hotels several times even when we visited relatives. This made it easier to keep my boys on their usual sleep schedule and to make the sleeping environment very dark.

When we visited relatives, I would ask them beforehand to help me to borrow a Pack 'n Play for each child so they would have somewhere to sleep in the hotel. My dad did not own one, but when he asked his coworkers at his office, he suddenly had offers for three to borrow.

Sleep is important for both the boys and me. It helps to have separate sleeping areas, even in the same room.

—*Carrie Brown, MD*

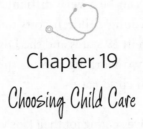

Chapter 19
Choosing Child Care

YOUR TODDLER'S DEVELOPMENT

Choosing child care for your toddler—whether that's a Mommy's helper who comes a few hours a month or all-day, every day care—is one of the most important decisions you'll make for your toddler. No pressure. But you are hiring someone to stand in for you, to care for and love your child in your absence. It might be comforting to know that you have plenty of company. About 70 percent of families place their children in some kind of daily care.

Whether you're continuing with the child care you had when your child was a baby, going back to work and need child care for the first time, or making a change from a baby care to more preschool-like setting, listen to that inner voice that says, "Yes, this feels right."

TAKING CARE OF YOU

After a long day at work, it's tempting to race to the day care or sitter to pick up your child and then race home. Instead, why not build a little time into that process for yourself? After work, give yourself a few minutes to meditate in the car, go for a brief walk outside, or take some time to call a friend to ease the transition before picking up your toddler.

JUSTIFICATION FOR A CELEBRATION

It might be bittersweet, but when your toddler says, "I love school!" and runs to play with his friends is cause for a celebration.

Choosing Care Providers

Choosing child care can be a very difficult and expensive decision. Child care for young children costs more per year than the public-college tuition in 39 states and the District of Columbia. A typical family with two working parents spends up to one-sixth of its gross income on child care.

❧

I see friends with relatives caring for their kids who face the challenge of the family members doing what they want, and not necessarily what the parent wants. That can be an issue with relatives, and you have to give a little.

I found that with paid caregivers, you might still have to make compromises. But it's easier to tell them, "This is what I want you to do."

—*Heather Orman-Lubell, MD, a mom of 11- and 7-year-old sons and a pediatrician in private practice at Yardley Pediatrics of St. Christopher's Hospital for Children, in Pennsylvania*

❧

As a working mother, I had to entrust my children's care to someone else. I was very fortunate to find caregivers who had similar philosophies to mine about the importance of setting limits and establishing simple rules about eating, sleeping, and safety. I think part of this was luck, but also because when I interviewed potential caregivers, I got a sense of how they approached these issues.

When you're looking for a caregiver, think about the qualities that are most important to you. If you don't know what these qualities are ahead of time, how could you hope to find someone who has them?

Talk to mothers whose children are well behaved for their ages. Ask them what they think is important to look for in a caregiver. Remember, those mothers might have older children by the time you speak with them. They've already been through what you are going through now.

—*Cathie Lippman, MD, a mom of 31- and 29-year-old sons and a physician who specializes in environmental and preventive medicine at the Lippman Center for Optimal Health, in Beverly Hills, CA*

While my girls were young, we always had help, either living in or living out. I felt that a lot of the things that my small children needed could be done by someone else, and that person could even do a better job at it than I could. I am not a micromanager. I hired mature women who had raised their own children. I felt that they had good skills, and they did a good job.

One day, I came home from work unexpectedly to find the nanny and my daughter having cookies and café con leche. Can you imagine giving coffee to a two-year-old? I wasn't too happy about the cookies either. But I did appreciate that the nanny loved my daughter and that my daughter was learning a lot of Spanish over her coffee and cookies. I explained to the nanny that I don't drink coffee, and I eat cookies only rarely, and that I think it's important to control what kids eat at this age. I explained, "If you want to have a snack, great. But let's make it a healthy snack." I realize that it's an imperfect world. Even though my daughter was having cookies and coffee for a snack, the world kept spinning.

—*Eva Ritvo, MD, a mom of 21- and 16-year-old daughters, a psychiatrist, and a coauthor of* The Beauty Prescription, *in Miami Beach, FL*

My sons' nanny was with us for nine years! I found her through a friend in my prenatal yoga class. She's my younger son's godmother, and we still see her. Where we live, a lot of the nannies are Spanish speaking, and I appreciated that our nanny spoke Spanish with our kids. She also had a lot of friends who were nannies nearby, and they all got together for playdates and lunches.

Most of all, I appreciated that my nanny did things the way I wanted them done. She was respectful of me, just as I was respectful of her. My husband and I gave her fair raises, and we also gave her and her kids gifts on their birthdays and for Christmas.

—*Lauren Feder, MD, a mom of 18- and 14-year-old sons, a nationally recognized physician who specializes in homeopathic medicine, and the author of* Natural Baby and Childcare *and* The Parents' Concise Guide to Childhood Vaccinations, *in Los Angeles*

When my daughters were toddlers, my parents and my in-laws took turns watching them while I worked. But when my son was born, it was too much for them, and we needed more help.

Our babysitter, Violet, was a member of our family for about eight years. She lived with us during the week, and on weekends she went home. My son became very bonded with her. He was so very well cared for. On weekends, when I'd ask my son to do something like put on his shoes, he'd say, "I can't wait for Violet to come on Monday!" She loved him, and she was very good to him.

I know some moms are jealous when their kids are close to a babysitter or nanny. But I always felt grateful that my kids were so loved. Violet still comes to see us about once a month because we miss her so much, and we love to see her.

—*Siobhan Dolan, MD, MPH, a mom of 16- and 13-year-old daughters and an 11-year-old son, a consultant to the March of Dimes, and an associate professor of obstetrics and gynecology and women's health at Albert Einstein College of Medicine/Montefiore Medical Center, in Bronx, NY*

Making a Change

Change can be hard, but sometimes it's inevitable.

When my kids were toddlers, we had a nanny. I made a point to drop in unannounced to check how she was doing. One day, I caught the nanny napping. I went to wake her.

"Oh no, Mommy, don't wake her up. That makes her mad!" my daughter said.

I woke the nanny right up, and I said, "Poor dear, you must be very tired. Go home, take a nap, and don't come back."

—*Lisa Dado, MD, a mom of 23- and 20-year-old daughters and an 18-year-old son, a pediatric anesthesiologist with Valley Anesthesiology Consultants, and the cofounder and CEO of the nonprofit organization the Center for Humane Living, which teaches life skills with an innovative approach to traditional martial arts training in six centers in and around Phoenix, AZ*

As a working mom during my kids' toddler years, one of the hardest things for me was being on the same page as my caregivers: making sure we were all doing the same things and that our schedule stayed more or less the same, and that they were following our family's same eating habits.

When my older son turned one, we decided we weren't going to use a nanny anymore, but rather try day care. Six months into it, my husband and I went one day to pick our son up. We saw something that upset us so much that we said, "We're done. Tomorrow, we'll figure out what we're going to do next."

When we quit the day care, we were lucky enough to have my mom, a nurse from my office, and a friend to fill the void while we looked for a nanny. It wasn't ideal, but it was the best situation for us at the time.

—*Heather Orman-Lubell, MD*

⌘

If your child is in day care, stop by to visit unannounced. And don't be afraid to take your child home immediately if you don't like what you see.

When our sons were in day care, my husband and I would drop by to visit. One day when my husband stopped by, he saw a little girl outside in the yard in the rain—all by herself. My husband quickly realized that the staff didn't even know she was out there! My husband simply picked up our sons and took them home. Then we talked it over and explained to the day care why we were pulling our kids out of there. We wanted to get our sons out of that situation immediately, and then we wanted to have some time to calmly think it through and decide how to react. Luckily, my husband has a flexible job, so he was able to stay home with our sons for a while until we found a new day care.

—*Carrie Brown, MD, a mom of eight- and six-year-old sons and a general pediatrician who treats medically complex children and specializes in palliative care at Arkansas Children's Hospital, in Little Rock*

⌘

When my son was a toddler, we didn't have so much a child care change as a major life paradigm shift. We lived in Cleveland, far from family and friends, and my husband and I both had demanding jobs. We put our son in day care. It was going fine, at first. Then suddenly, it wasn't working at all.

My son was very unhappy. After several weeks of watching his struggle, the director of his preschool said, "This isn't working for him."

"I don't understand why not. It works for other kids," I remember saying.

"But it does not work for him," the director replied.

After months of trying to tell myself that my son's level of sadness and separation anxiety was age-appropriate and normal, I finally decided that I had made a huge error for him, by relying on day care and other child care providers. My husband and I felt so separated from our family and friends and just had not understood what an amazing blessing it is to have someone to call when you need a hand as a parent. My husband and I decided to move back home. We didn't have jobs waiting for us, but that didn't matter. We packed up and moved.

In time, it all worked out. Our house sold, we got a new one, and we both found new jobs. We rearranged our work hours so that we can be more available to our children, so they can count on us to be there for them.

Today, my son is happy in school. After all of our lessons with our son as our firstborn, we opted for a completely different plan for our daughter. She has a nanny some days, and she attends art class, gymnastics class, and music class because we feel that socialization is important for toddlers. Our daughter is a different child than our son, though, so we learn more about who she is every day. We also realize that while paradigm shifts can be difficult sometimes, things happen for the best. Who knows? Our daughter might be happy as can be if we opt for day care, and we are always open to that possibility.

—*Sigrid Payne DaVeiga, MD, a mom of a six-year-old son and a two-year-old daughter and a pediatric allergist with the Children's Hospital of Philadelphia, in Pennsylvania*

One day when my daughter was 2½, I got a call from a detective at the Seattle police department informing me that one of her day care providers had been arrested for child molestation. The detective wanted to know if my daughter had showed signs of being molested. I told her about one incident when I was strapping her into her car seat when she asked me to play with her pee-pee.

As a child psychiatrist, I was aware toilet talk is extremely common in 2½- to 3-year-olds. However, interest in genital contact is rare unless the child has been sexualized. The detective asked if I wanted my daughter to have an evidentiary interview with anatomically appropriate dolls to find out if anything had happened.

This was an extremely hard decision for me, but I decided not to. Because the staff person had been fired (and arrested), I knew any fondling that might have occurred had stopped. And because my daughter showed no evidence of sleep, emotional, or behavioral disturbances, I thought it was unlikely that any coercion and threats (to harm family members for snitching, for example) had occurred. It's usually the coercion and fear over time that is most troubling to sexually abused children. My main desire was that my daughter would repress the incident, which I felt was less likely if she had to undergo an interview with a strange adult about intimate parts of her body.

I believe I made the right decision in the end. There has been no psychological evidence at any point in her development that my daughter was sexually traumatized.

One might wonder if I changed day cares. No, I didn't. I was really impressed with the way the director handled the situation, and my daughter was strongly attached to both the teachers and the other children.

—*Stuart Jeanne Bramhall, MD, a mom of a 31-year-old daughter and a child and adolescent psychiatrist in New Plymouth, New Zealand*

Finding an Occasional Babysitter or Mommy's Helper

Babysitting has become big business these days with websites such as Care.com and Nanny4Hire.com making it easier than ever to find a babysitter. You can find full- or part-time sitters, even last-minute ones. Often these companies prescreen their sitters and provide references and background checks.

The best babysitters are people that you and your child already know. Ask the director of your child's day care or preschool if any of the teachers babysit on the weekends or weeknights. I found that a few of my children's teachers are usually looking to earn some extra cash.

—Jeannette Gonzalez Simon, MD, a mom of three- and one-year-old daughters and a pediatric gastroenterologist in private practice, in Staten Island, NY

When my triplets were babies, we had a very rapid babysitter turn-over! But thank goodness, the past few years I've had stable, reliable babysitters.

I've found some of our best babysitters through online services such as Care.com and Nannies4Hire.com. These companies charge a fee, but it's worth it for the peace of mind knowing they've done background checks on their sitters.

—Sadaf T. Bhutta, MD, a mom of a six-year-old daughter and four-year-old triplets and an assistant professor and the fellowship director of pediatric radiology at the University of Arkansas for Medical Sciences and Arkansas Children's Hospital, both in Little Rock

I found my most wonderful mommy's helper through a written news-paper ad in which I requested that potential applicants write me a letter about their interest in the job. I discovered that I could tell a lot about a person's reliability, conscientiousness, common sense, and personality through the letters I received in response.

But experience has taught me the crucial importance of getting personal references from previous employers—no matter whether the previous jobs were as a caregiver or in some other capacity alto-gether. You want to hear from prior employers that the person you're

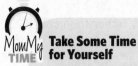

Take Some Time for Yourself

Often when people hire a babysitter, they do so to go out with spouses or friends. But why not hire a babysitter on occasion to carve out a little time for yourself? If you're going to be staying in the house with the sitter and your children, the sitter might not cost as much. Just imagine how much you could get done, or how much relaxing you could do, in just two hours a week, even two hours a month!

considering is rock-solid in terms of honesty and trustworthiness. When you interview the person yourself, you'll be able to judge her warmth, flexibility, and sense of humor directly. But whether people are truly honest and trustworthy is impossible to assess without personal reports from others who have worked with the applicant over a period of time.

—Elizabeth Berger, MD,
a mom of a 29-year-old son
and a 27-year-old daughter,
a child psychiatrist, and the
author of Raising Kids with
Character, *in New York City*

My husband and I have cultivated a good stable of college-age babysitters. When you have four boys, you need a college-age sitter! We live in a college town, and we have some sitters who go to the college and other sitters who live here and come back home on break. So we're covered year-round.

We have a lot of male babysitters, which works out well with our boys. We generally ask them to find their own way here, but we drive them home, certainly after dark. My husband and I go out together once or twice a week.

The University of Pittsburgh's Jewish University Group held a speed-babysitting session for families. It's like speed dating, only you get to meet potential babysitters. We've also placed ads for babysitters in the university's paper.

To test out potential sitters, I have them come over one night at bedtime. This way, I can show them our bedtime routine, and I also get to evaluate how they are with my kids.

To communicate with the babysitters, I text rather than call. I find that they'll respond to a text more quickly than a voicemail.

—*Deborah Gilboa, MD, a mom of nine-, seven-, five-, and three-year-old sons, a parenting speaker whose advice is found at AskDoctorG.com, and a family physician with Squirrel Hill Health Center, in Pittsburgh, PA*

How strange it was hiring someone to love my child. To love in my absence—that was my babysitter's most important function. Arriving on time, housekeeping, feeding, and changing were all secondary.

Ideally, a trusted relative would have babysat my daughter—someone invested in her, and who would have a permanent relationship with her. Unfortunately, that wasn't possible.

So I looked for an older woman who had raised her own children. I knew younger babysitters would leave us for college or other jobs. I didn't want my daughter going through a series of losses like that.

A babysitter needs to be capable of being entrusted with the most valuable thing in the world to you. It's important to keep in mind how vulnerable toddlers are. They're just beginning to talk and to know right from wrong. You can't count on a toddler to report a babysitter's wrongdoing, or to stand up to the sitter.

I wanted a babysitter vouched for through personal connections. I didn't go through an agency, but I asked the nannies of friends. Finally, I found a woman who had raised five daughters. Her grown children were responsibly employed, and they had chosen good husbands. It was obvious from the way she talked about her children that she loved them deeply. Because she was capable of this kind of love, I knew she would also love my daughter.

—*Dora Calott Wang, MD, a mom of a nine-year-old daughter, a psychiatrist and historian at the University of New Mexico School of Medicine, and the author of* The Kitchen Shrink: A Psychiatrist's Reflection on Healing in a Changing World, *in Albuquerque, NM*

Handling Separation Anxiety

Around the first birthday, many kids develop separation anxiety. Knowing this is normal probably doesn't make it easier. Even though your toddler is growing more independent, he can become uncertain and anxious about being separated from you. Whatever pattern your child has developed around his first birthday when you separate from him will probably persist for a while. For example, if he becomes angry or cries when you drop him off at day care, you might have to contend with these challenges for another year or two. Sometimes separation anxiety can be triggered by a change, such as a new caregiver or having a new sibling. In some cases, separation anxiety can last into elementary school.

My girls' father and I started leaving our kids at an early age with relatives and sitters, and they never had separation anxiety, thankfully. Also, because I never made a big deal about leaving my girls, they were not reacting to my anxiety.

—*Marra S. Francis, MD, a mom of eight-, seven-, and five-year-old daughters and a gynecologist, in San Antonio, TX*

I hate leaving my daughter with the nanny when I have to go to work.

"Mommy, do you want to go to work?" my daughter asked me one day.

"No, I'd much rather stay home with you," I answered her quite honestly. I explained to her that going to work for me is like going to school for her. We'd both rather be home. She seemed to really understand that.

—*Lisa Campanella-Coppo, MD, a mom of a three-year-old daughter, an emergency physician, and the emergency department director of academic affairs at Monmouth Medical Center, in New Jersey*

When my son was a toddler and in day care, he had extreme separation anxiety. The hard part about it was that some days were better than others, so I could talk myself through it, like, "it's just a phase" or "he's just getting used to it." I had a lot of trouble dropping my son off at day care and making it to work on time, so I hired a babysitter who would take him in for me in the mornings.

My son would cry and cry, saying, "Don't leave me, Mom. Don't go!" The look on his face was of complete despair while he reached out for me to hold onto him while his babysitter was trying to get him into his car seat. I remember one teacher at his day care saying that watching him made her remember how she felt when her parents left her at college—like he felt a sadness that he didn't have a choice in.

At a certain point, my son's crying and sadness were paralyzing, and he could no longer participate in daily activities at day care. My husband and I had multiple meetings with his teachers and school directors about how to handle it, but we just never found a good solution. It was heartbreaking to think of my warm, intelligent, and loving child spending so many hours of his day struggling like this.

I hoped that in time it would work out and get better, but it never did. Since then, I've heard other moms talk about this feeling, the you-know-when-something-just-doesn't-feel-right feeling. That's what it felt like to me: Something wasn't right, but it was hard to see it and accept it, with all of the competing forces playing in on me as a working parent. One of the day care teachers talked with me about it, which confirmed my feelings. My son just wasn't happy there. He wanted to be home.

One thing that helped a little bit while my son was in that phase was to send in a small photo album of him with separate pages of all of the important people in his life. My son carried it with him at times during the day. He recently found the album and said, "Look at this, Mom. I don't need this anymore, though, because now I'm a big boy."

My husband and I made a major change, sold our house, and moved back home, where we had more family support. I truly feel that the changes we made in our lifestyle for our son have made him such a happy, well-adjusted, confident child. I am so proud of the decisions that we made about our lives to ensure that.

—*Sigrid Payne DaVeiga, MD*

RALLIE'S TIP

Leaving my toddlers at day care the first couple of times was pretty stressful for me, and for them. My youngest son was a mama's boy and a homebody, and I had a feeling that things would go a lot better if I eased him gently into the day care routine. I started out by taking him to his new day care just two days a week, and I left him there for only a couple of hours each time at first. I gradually lengthened the time I left him there until he spent two full mornings each week away from me.

My husband and I always tried to arrange our work schedules so that one of us could stay at home with the children a couple of days each week. That doesn't work for all parents, but we were really lucky to have jobs that allowed us to choose our own schedules to some degree.

I also tried to make sure that I always had plenty of time to get ready on the mornings that my son would be going to day care. I learned from experience that rushing around and feeling stressed made my son anxious, and that always caused him to be a little clingy. On day care days, we'd get up and have a nice breakfast. As we got dressed, I'd tell him that he was going to have a fun day playing with all of his friends. While we were getting ready to leave and enjoying our time together, I'd reassure him that I'd be back to pick him up before lunchtime or right after lunchtime. I wanted him to have a good understanding of how long we'd be apart, because he didn't really understand the concept of "a few hours."

We'd leave the house early so that I would have plenty of time to hang around the day care long enough for my son to get involved with a toy or a playmate. I'd give him his good-bye hug and kiss on the way in, because I didn't want to make a big deal of saying good-bye once we were inside. As soon as we greeted the teacher and my son had relaxed his grip on me and wandered off to focus his attention elsewhere, I'd quietly slip away. I always felt a little guilty leaving this way, but it was a million times better than I felt leaving my son when he was crying and begging me not to go.

Another thing I did to make the handoff a little easier was pack a day care bag with all the essentials: my son's favorite sippy cup and toys and his special blanket that smelled like home. I'll never forget how

happy—and how heartbroken—I was the first time I came to pick up
my son from day care and he told me that he didn't want to go home
with me. He was having too much fun!

Choosing and Starting Preschool

Checking into preschools and filling out applications can feel a bit
like foreshadowing for college someday! Even though many
pre-K programs now accept two-year-olds, holding off for a year
or two can save you thousands of dollars in tuition fees.

⌒◯

My children were with our nanny in the early years, and then we sent
them to preschool at age four. Preschool gave my boys the opportunity to learn to work and play with their peers. It was a good experience for them prior to entering kindergarten.

—*Lauren Feder, MD*

Mommy MD Guides-Recommended Product
Mabel's Labels

Day care centers and preschools ask parents to label everything
their child brings to school, but it's too easy for ink to wash away
when you do laundry, and some items might not have a convenient
place for labeling (winter hats or modern T-shirts without tags, for
example). The perfect solution: Mabel's Labels offers iron-on and
peel-and-stick clothing labels that will stay on even after going
through the washer and dryer.

You can buy packs of 70 peel-and-stick or 40 iron-on labels
with your child's first name for $21 at **MABELSLABELS.COM**. While
you're at the site, you can also browse their bag tags, shoe labels,
allergy alert labels, and sticky labels for cups and lunch boxes that
are dishwasher and microwave safe.

I'm a big believer in preschool, and both of my children started pre-school at age two. I feel very strongly about the importance of early childhood education. I know one-on-one time is critical with your kids, but I feel my kids were so nurtured in preschool. They really enjoyed it, and I saw their language skills and social development improve so dramatically. I think preschool was very beneficial for my kids.

> —*Ann V. Arthur, MD, a mom of a 10-year-old daughter and an 8-year-old son, a pediatric ophthalmologist in private practice at Park Slope Eye Care Associates, and a blogger at WaterWineTravel.com, in New York City*

When my kids started preschool, I found it helpful to go with them the first few times. I wanted to help them to see that preschool was a fun place to be.

I knew there would be tears when I left. It breaks your heart! But I knew that my kids were in good hands. As long as the preschool teachers told me that my kids were fine after I left, I wasn't worried about it. Plus, I peeked in the window a few times to make sure they were okay.

> —*Heather Orman-Lubell, MD*

When my kids were in preschool, they produced incredible amounts of artwork. It seriously could have taken over my house. The preschool had a genius idea: They created a bound book of a selection of my kids' art. I was just looking at my son's portfolio. It was so fun to look back on his finger painting and preschool art!

Even if your child's preschool doesn't do this, it wouldn't be hard to gather up some of his art and bind it into a book.

> —*Siobhan Dolan, MD, MPH*

I'm not big into fear, but at the age when your child will be spending time away from you, such as in day care or preschool, you need to have a talk about private parts and no-touch. Bathtime is a good time to have that discussion.

"Those are private parts," I explained to my daughter. "Only you or Mommy, Daddy, or your doctor can touch them if necessary. Don't let anyone else touch those parts. If anyone tries to, you need to let Mommy know right away."

Keep it short; keep it simple. Don't get into how there are scary people out there who do things to hurt small children!

—*Eva Ritvo, MD*

Adjusting to Work Changes

The only constant in the workplace these days? Change.

I cut my work hours back to five hours a day until my daughter turned four. This made it easier to fit in housekeeping and parenting responsibilities, and it maximized the time I spent with my daughter.

—*Stuart Jeanne Bramhall, MD*

When I went back to work, I changed my schedule so that I worked the evening shift, from 4 pm to 2 am. This way I'm at home for more hours during the day. I sleep until around 8 am, but then I'm home with my kids until around 3:30 pm.

—*Shilpa Amin-Shah, MD, a mom of a two-year-old son and a one-year-old daughter and an emergency physician at Emergency Medical Associates, in Livingston, NJ*

I went back to work soon after each of my babies was born. But I know mothers who didn't. Some of us try to launch our careers and families at the same time, and others stagger them. I don't think any one solution is right for all women. I had a lot of support from my husband and my family, so I launched both at the same time. But every mom has to find her own way.

—*Siobhan Dolan, MD, MPH*

Before my kids gained a sense of independence, it was always challenging to hit the ground running when I got home from work. It was hard to learn to leave everything from the outside world outside when I entered my house, and just focus on my children. Once I made them my priority and resigned myself to the fact that I would work or catch up on household chores only when the kids were sleeping, a lot of frustration was eliminated.

—Mona Gohara, MD, a mom of five- and three-year-old sons, a dermatologist in private practice, an assistant clinical professor in the department of dermatology at Yale University, and a cofounder of K&J Sunprotective Clothing, in Danbury, CT

My father, a medical oncologist, and my mother, a teacher and author of a medical textbook, brought me up to believe that as a girl, I could both have a profession and be a great mother. Many times, I thought this was impossible, but I firmly believe that it's best to show your children what they can do by setting an example. Children learn their work ethic and coping strategies from their parents.

I worked two full days a week and sometimes a half day on Fridays. I kept this up for three years, and then I went to a per-diem schedule, and I went to work when I was called in. When our youngest child went to full-day preschool, I went back to working three days a week and then five days a week because financially we needed to have one parent working full-time. Today, all of my children play sports, so I work part-time and maintain a flexible schedule to accommodate theirs. I try to be at home at 3 pm, and then I work as I'm able all afternoon, around their schedules. Somehow it works.

—Elizabeth Chabner Thompson, MD, MPH, a mom of 13- and 8-year-old daughters and 12- and 10-year-old sons, a radiation oncologist with 21 C. Radiation Oncology, and the inventor of the Mommy Bag, filled with supplies for moms-to-be having C-sections, in Scarsdale, NY

I found my children's toddler years to be a very difficult time. I was in my thirties, just entering the workforce, trying to prove myself and establish my career, and trying to keep up with toddlers at the same time. I found that when my kids were babies, their needs were simpler, but as toddlers, their needs were so much more demanding.

One way I coped was by identifying things that I could delegate without detriment. So, for example, I hired someone to help me with laundry, but I was home in the mornings to get my kids dressed. I hired someone to help me with grocery shopping, but I was home to enjoy meals with my family. I delegated tasks that I thought were less critical for me personally to do, the jobs that didn't matter if I did them or not, so that I had the time to do the things that I felt were important. Some things only *I* can do.

—*Lisa Dado, MD*

I was lucky to have what seemed to me an ideal situation when my children were toddlers. I wanted to work part-time, but I wanted to be home with my offspring during the day. My husband and I worked out a schedule so that he came home from work at dinnertime, and then I would run off to the office to see a few patients in the evening. On weekends, he would spend Saturday mornings with the kids while I saw patients at the office. I felt like a full-time mom, and I kept my hand in my job as a working professional too. This kind of arrangement works smoothly only if both parents' personalities are suited to it and if they both have considerable flexibility in their work schedules.

When our children were old enough for a part-day nursery school, I dropped them off, went to work for two or three hours, and then picked them up again. This requires a fallback plan, in case your child has the flu or some other illness and needs to stay at home. Occasionally, I hired an in-home nurse from an agency to babysit at short notice. At other times, I hired a permanent mother's helper to come to my home daily while I went to work for a few hours.

Each family has to work out its priorities. I wanted to be home with my children primarily and work in the margins and around the edges until my children went to college.

—*Elizabeth Berger, MD*

Both Freud and my Chinese grandmother said that the first years of life determine the rest. I absolutely believe this to be true.

For me, the most challenging aspect of parenting during the

toddler years was simply making time to be there. I received advice from wise psychiatrists, based on research and psychoanalytic theory, to spend only 20 hours per week away from my child. I also looked to Sweden, which has very liberal maternal and paternal leave policies. In Sweden, most children have a parent at home for the first 14 to 16 months of life.

It was a tremendous challenge to keep my career while spending only 20 hours per week away from my child. I cut my work schedule from 10 hours a day to 10 hours a week. Even so, parenting is so consuming that I hired help. Mostly, I sought help with the household. It made no sense to hire a babysitter so that I could clean my house.

I was fortunate that I was able to shift the focus of my career for a few years, from seeing patients toward writing. This was work I could do at home on a flexible schedule, while my daughter slept.

During the toddler years, a lot of a child's personality, level of alertness, and predisposition to anxiety and mood problems are determined. Brain imaging studies show that by age four, the brain is already 90 percent of its adult size. That's not to say that people don't change past age four. But so much is set during the toddler years, depending upon how secure the child feels, and how much attention was paid during those critical early years.

—*Dora Calott Wang, MD*

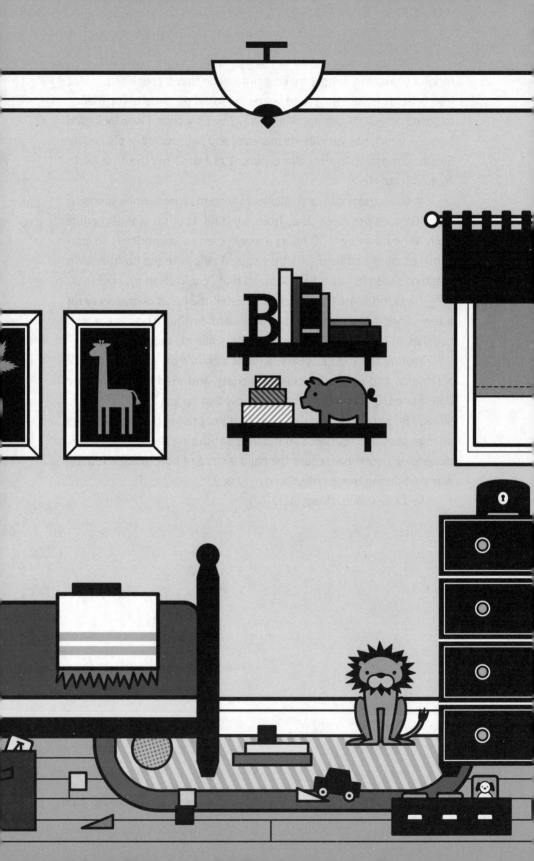

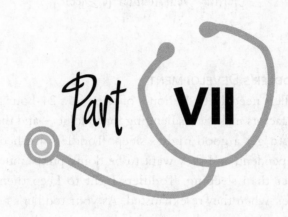

Part VII

SLEEP

Chapter 20
Getting Your Toddler to Sleep

Your Toddler's Development

Most toddlers need 12 to 14 hours of sleep in a 24-hour period. But many factors make it challenging for toddlers—and therefore mothers—to get a good night's sleep. Toddlers are becoming more independent, and they want to be doing pretty much anything other than sleeping. Toddlers fight to keep themselves awake, even when they're exhausted. As your toddler's need for daytime naps decreases, she might be more overtired at night and ironically find it hard to wind down and fall asleep.

To make matters worse, sleep disturbances such as nightmares, night terrors, sleepwalking, and sleeptalking often begin in the toddler years. Toddlers' imaginations kick into overdrive as fear of the dark often begins at this time too. All of these changes conspire to keep your toddler—and you—awake. Good thing Starbucks has a drive-thru.

Taking Care of You

Take a nap. Even after your toddler outgrows naps, it doesn't mean you have to!

Justification for a Celebration

If your toddler still isn't sleeping through the night, you have plenty of company. The first morning that you wake up and realize she slept the entire night—and you did too—will really be a reason to celebrate!

Napping

We are a nation of sleep-deprived caffeine fiends. According to the National Sleep Foundation (NSF), a short nap of 20 to 30 minutes can help to improve mood, alertness, and performance. A study at NASA on sleepy military pilots and astronauts found that a 40-minute nap improved performance by 34 percent and alertness by an incredible 100 percent.

The NSF reports that nappers are in good company: Winston Churchill, John F. Kennedy, Ronald Reagan, Napoleon, Albert Einstein, Thomas Edison, and George W. Bush are known to have valued an afternoon nap. (We find it fascinating that there are no women on their list!)

Naps: They do a toddler good too. A University of Arizona study found that 15-month-olds who napped were able to apply information they'd been given earlier to a new situation. Children who hadn't napped didn't retain the same information.

By the time most babies are a year old, they've dropped to only one nap a day. The average one-year-old naps about two hours. Between two and three years old, most kids nap for about an hour each day. Most children have grown out of naps entirely by age three.

❧

During the toddler years, a lot of children give up naps. Mine did! When your toddler gives up her nap, make sure to adjust her bedtime so that she's still getting enough sleep. Children need to rest as long as they can for proper brain development.

—Eva Ritvo, MD, a mom of 21- and 16-year-old daughters, a psychiatrist, and a coauthor of The Beauty Prescription, in Miami Beach, FL

❧

Most toddlers still need to take naps. As a mother, sometimes it hurts me to deny my daughter something or make her do something she might not want to, such as taking a nap. But I know in the long run she will benefit.

Naps were helpful for me too! I never realized how much

physical and emotional energy I would expend as a parent. There are so many rewards and challenges to parenthood, but I don't really think you appreciate the full extent of what it entails until you actually experience it.

—*Tanya Douglas Holland, MD, a mom of a two-year-old daughter, a women's health advocate, and a consultant in medical affairs to a pharmaceutical company, in Atlanta, GA*

When my older son was about 20 months old, he decided that he didn't need to take naps anymore. My husband and I would go to his room and sit and watch him until he went to sleep, and then we'd sneak back out of the room. We hoped that our son would get back to the point of napping without us in the room. That never happened, so we gave up on his naps when he was three years old.

Our younger son, on the other hand, still takes naps at age six! On weekends, he'll nap for two hours, given the opportunity.

—*Carrie Brown, MD, a mom of eight- and six-year-old sons and a general pediatrician who treats medically complex children and specializes in palliative care at Arkansas Children's Hospital, in Little Rock*

My older son still needs a nap, but he doesn't like taking them. I keep him busy in the morning to wear him out so that he'll hopefully take a nap.

I would love if both of my sons would nap at the same time, but that is an impossible dream. My younger son goes for a nap around 11 or 12 am, and my older son goes around 2 pm. If my older son doesn't get a nap, I have to put him to bed early because he's a miserable child.

—*Sharon Boyce, MD, a mom of three- and one-year-old sons and a family physician at DayOne Family Healthcare Clinic, in Battle Creek, MI*

❧

When my kids were toddlers, I kept afternoon naps short, or they would never sleep well at night. The late afternoon could bleed into evening if I let them nap too long.

My husband and I didn't let our children nap in car seats or on sofas or anywhere but in their beds. I felt doing otherwise was lazy, selfish parenting. Our kids belonged in their beds, if at all possible, not where it was convenient for us.

Many of my friends thought I was crazy to rush home for nap time or say no to invitations when I could not accommodate our kids, but it paid off. Our children are incredibly resilient, and they love to sleep.

—*Elizabeth Chabner Thompson, MD, MPH, a mom of 13- and 8-year-old daughters and 12- and 10-year-old sons, a radiation oncologist with 21 C. Radiation Oncology, and the inventor of the Mommy Bag, filled with supplies for moms-to-be having C-sections, in Scarsdale, NY*

Getting Your Toddler to Sleep

If you had a lot of challenges getting your baby to sleep, you are likely still having plenty of challenges getting your toddler to sleep too. As one pediatric nurse put it, "Some babies are good sleepers; some aren't." If you got a good sleeper, enjoy it! If you didn't get a good sleeper, sleep whenever you can.

My daughter is a very good sleeper. Unless she's very wet, she sleeps 12 hours straight! I would love to think that's because my daughter feels so secure and loved. But really I think how well a child sleeps has to do more with temperament—and a little bit of luck.

—Rachel S. Rohde, MD, a mom of a one-year-old daughter, an assistant professor of orthopaedic surgery at the Oakland University William Beaumont School of Medicine, and an orthopaedic upper-extremity surgeon with Michigan Orthopaedic Institute, P.C., in Southfield, MI

I have one fabulous sleeper and one terrible sleeper. I think the best thing you can do is have a regular bedtime routine so it's the same thing night after night. My husband and I break the rules sometimes, but we try to be consistent. At least my terrible sleeper is a fabulous eater!

—Heather Orman-Lubell, MD, a mom of 11- and 7-year-old sons and a pediatrician in private practice at Yardley Pediatrics of St. Christopher's Hospital for Children, in Pennsylvania

My husband and I have to drive and function in high-stress jobs, whether we get a good night's sleep or not. So I've made choices to help us get our sleep, even if they weren't the "right" parenting decisions. For example, if my daughter will sleep better at night with a pacifier, that means she gets a pacifier at night. There are three of us in this family, and it's important that everyone's mental health is maintained, even if it requires some compromise. Our daughter won't walk down the aisle with her bottle or in diapers, so I'm not worried.

—Lisa Campanella-Coppo, MD, a mom of a three-year-old daughter, an emergency physician, and the emergency department director of academic affairs at Monmouth Medical Center, in New Jersey

Routines are very helpful for toddlers. They can't tell time, after all, so cues about what is happening, and what is going to happen next, help them to understand their world. This is especially helpful at nighttime. My family had a fun nighttime ritual. Each night after bath and books, my husband and I would tuck our kids into bed. Then we'd sing "Twinkle, Twinkle Little Star," but we had made up several versions: a rock version, a lullaby, and a silly version. We'd let our kids pick which version they wanted to hear each night. It was fun, and it helped our kids to wind down for bed.

—*Dana S. Simpler, MD, a mom of 25- and 20-year-old girls and a 23-year-old son and a specialist in internal medicine in private practice, in Baltimore, MD*

My daughter was very hard to get to sleep. She has a very strong, willful personality, which will serve her well, but she can be unrelenting. When my daughter was a toddler, she wouldn't sleep, and I had to sleep train her. She could scream for hours if she didn't want to go to sleep.

How did I cope? I tried different things. Sometimes I'd just go to another room where I couldn't hear her as well. Other times, I'd call a friend who could talk to me and distract me.

—*Dina Strachan, MD, a mom of a six-year-old daughter, a dermatologist and director of Aglow Dermatology, and an assistant clinical professor in the department of dermatology at New York University, in New York City*

One of the biggest challenges when my kids were toddlers was sleep. None of them were good sleepers. The most helpful thing I did was learn how to fall back to sleep quickly after one of them woke me up! I adapted because I had to.

I also read the book *Solve Your Child's Sleep Problems* by Richard Ferber, MD. Each time my children presented me with a new sleep challenge, I followed that book to the letter, and it always helped. It often required letting my toddlers cry it out, which was difficult to do. But it worked.

—*Ann Kulze, MD, a mom of 23- and 17-year-old daughters and 22- and 20-year-old sons; a nationally recognized nutrition expert, motivational speaker, and physician; and the author of the best-selling book* Dr. Ann's Eat Right for Life, *in Charleston, SC*

One of the most common mistakes parents make is rocking, walking, or nursing their babies to sleep. It's so important to teach your toddler to fall asleep by herself in her own bed. This will save you so much time and energy!

Yes, rocking, walking, or nursing your baby to sleep is a very hard habit to break. But if that's the only way your toddler will go to sleep, it's time to make a change. Just imagine what you can do with those 45 minutes each day! Set a bedtime, about the time your toddler usually looks sleepy. Then do your bedtime routine, and put your toddler in bed. Yes, she will cry. Prepare yourself for that! I had to do this during a week that my husband was away on a business trip because he couldn't stand to hear our kids cry.

—*Ayala Laufer-Cahana, MD, a mom of 16- and 14-year-old sons and a 12-year-old daughter, a pediatrician, and the founder of Herbal Water Inc., in Wynnewood, PA*

My son was a colicky baby and a horrible sleeper. When he was about two months old, I breastfed him as much as 15 times a day because it was the *only* thing that calmed him! Finally, after countless sleepless nights, I let him cry it out at five months of age, which worked quite well with him. My then-husband would be the one to stay in the room after I breastfed my son and handed him off. I made sure to leave before lights out, because my son would let his dad leave much more easily than he'd let me.

As my son got older, it became trickier for my ex-husband to leave the room, so he started using different tactics to distract him. He would say, "It's time to go to sleep. Do you want the door to be open or closed? The picture on the wall or off the wall? The night-light on or off?" That way, my son felt like he got a say in "how" he went to sleep, so that he wouldn't resist the act of going to sleep itself!

—*Cheryl Wu, MD, a mom of a four-year-old son, a pediatrician at LaGuardia Place Pediatrics in New York City, and a pediatric emergency physician at the Joseph M. Sanzari Children's Hospital of Hackensack University Medical Center, in New Jersey*

Kids are all about routine, and one special routine I established early on helps to settle my kids for sleep. Each night when I tuck them into bed, I whisper something special into each of their ears.

It could be something supportive like, "You did great on your homework today. I'm so proud of you!" Or it could be a special story about their grandfather, who passed away before they were born. It's nothing long or complicated, something simple like, "Your grandpa had silly ears!"

—Brooke A. Jackson, MD, a mom of 4½-year-old twin girls and a 2½-year-old son, a dermatologist, and the founder and medical director of the Skin Wellness Center of Chicago, in Illinois

My husband and I found it helpful to have special rituals we did each night when we got our daughters ready for bed. These types of events cue a toddler about what is to happen next. They can't tell time, but they know, for example, that after bath comes a story, and then comes bed.

Each night, the last thing my husband did before he said good-night was sing a song. He "composed" it himself.

He'd sing, "Nightie-night, sleepyhead. Close your ears and go to bed." Our girls would giggle, so he'd continue on with the song, "Nightie-night, sleepyhead. Close your nose and go to bed." More giggles, then "Nightie-night, sleepyhead. Close your mouth and go to bed." More giggles, and then finally the comforting end, "Nightie-night, sleepyhead. Close your eyes and go to bed."

"Sleep tight, give me one last kiss goodnight!"

—*Cathy Marshall, MD, a mom of 28-, 14-, and 11-year-old daughters and a pediatrician in private practice, in Encino, CA*

∽

The biggest challenge for me during my twins' toddler years was maintaining a consistent routine and schedule. Yet that's so critical at this age!

Toddlers are developing and changing rapidly, and their personalities are really starting to emerge. With all that change, they need the constant of a predictable schedule.

This was most important for me with sleep. I tried very hard to keep my kids' nap and bedtime schedules the same each day. It was also equally important to me to have a consistent bedtime routine, which included a bath, a story to read, soothing music to listen to, and cuddle time. I didn't want my twins' needs to completely take over my life, but at the same time, it wasn't beneficial to anyone for us to be eating dinner at a restaurant at 9 pm. I tried to structure our life as much as possible around our twins. I think this secure foundation provides the security their developing personalities need that then takes them well into childhood.

—*Ann Contrucci, MD, a mom of 13-year-old boy-girl twins who works as a pediatric emergency physician, in Atlanta, GA*

∽

My husband was often on call at night, so I did the bedtime routine. I'd grab all three of my kids' pajamas and throw them into a big pile on my bed. Then I set up an assembly line. I'd get them all dressed, then I'd comb their heads, then brush their teeth, then have them go to the bathroom. Then I'd tuck one child into bed, then the next, then the last.

I found that each of my kids had very different needs for how they would fall asleep. For example, my younger daughter liked me to sing to her, but my son didn't. One of my daughters liked to be covered up, but my other daughter didn't.

Even when I got that all sorted out, that wasn't the end of it! I'd have to go back to each of them a few times to answer questions, give more kisses, meet needs. It was quite a process, but finally I'd have everyone settled down for the night, and I could go relax.

—Lisa Dado, MD, a mom of 23- and 20-year-old daughters and an 18-year-old son, a pediatric anesthesiologist with Valley Anesthesiology Consultants, and the cofounder and CEO of the nonprofit organization the Center for Humane Living, which teaches life skills with an innovative approach to traditional martial arts training in six centers in and around Phoenix, AZ

I found that a very consistent bedtime routine worked for my family. Each night at very close to the same time, I offered my daughter a drink, we brushed her teeth, read books, sang songs, and then we put her to bed awake and she would fall asleep. She always had her two favorite lovies and her pacifier. The next morning, she woke up happy!

Yes, the strict routine meant I wasn't able to go out as much, but the sacrifice was worth it for us with more sleep and less drama.

My daughter had a favorite lovie and her pacifier (BB). She had a pretty easy temperament, and with our routine, she could self-soothe and slept wonderfully through the night. At about a year, she started throwing things out of the crib and then crying for them, often several times a night. Going in there and handing her a lovie or BB got old—quick. I saw the "crib-tent" online, which is meant to keep pets out and kids from climbing out of the crib, but from the first night when we would zip up the little mesh tent, our problem was solved! She would toss her lovies, and they would simply fall back into the crib where she could reach them, and happily fall back asleep! We used it for about eight months.

—Katja Rowell, MD, a mom of a six-year-old daughter, a family practice physician, and a childhood feeding specialist with TheFeedingDoctor.com, in St. Paul, MN

My son used to be a great sleeper! Then my daughter was born. He was the first grandchild on both sides, and he was used to being the center of attention. When my daughter was born, my son regressed in a lot of areas, especially sleep. He didn't want to sleep in his own room anymore; he wanted to sleep with us. We tried to stick to his old bedtime routine, but it didn't seem to work anymore.

I reduced my son's nap to only one hour a day so that he'll be sleepier at night. Around 6:30, I see he's getting sleepy, so I give him a bath. I let him play for a while to tire him out some more. It still takes him around a half hour to fall asleep. Fortunately, he doesn't cry. He listens to a Baby Einstein lullaby CD. He calls it his "sleepy music." He usually falls asleep with it on.

—*Shilpa Amin-Shah, MD, a mom of a two-year-old son and a one-year-old daughter and an emergency physician at Emergency Medical Associates, in Livingston, NJ*

A challenge with bedtime I first noticed when my twins were toddlers was the delay tactic. When I put my girls to bed, they keep coming up with requests: "Mommy, I need a Band-Aid." "My feet are cold." "I need a drink." "I need this particular stuffed animal I haven't played with in three years."

My best solution for this is to make getting into bed a race. My girls like to have backrubs before they go to sleep. Whoever gets into bed first, and stays there, gets the first backrub.

Even after I've said goodnight, invariably I have to go back up to their room two or three times. After that, I usually say, "Enough is enough!" I allow them to read with a flashlight, but I really do try to keep them in their beds, trying to go to sleep. But sharing a room with your twin means having a slumber party every night.

—*Brooke A. Jackson, MD*

∽◌

I always tried to make my toddlers' bedtime early because I needed a few hours to myself or with my husband. I did not have a lot of patience for a worn-out child at 9 pm. I knew my limitations, and irritable crying was not something I could cope with.

I found that a long bathtime at 6 pm, a warm bottle, and songs or books were a good formula for getting my toddler to sleep. "Bath, bottle, books, bed."

I also never waited until any of our kids was fast asleep to put them in their cribs. I put them in tired and let them soothe themselves to sleep. This leads to a lifetime of good sleeping habits and also the ability to self-soothe. I figured that wherever the kids might be later in life, I could not always be there to pat them or sing to them. They should learn to rely on themselves.

Sure, I spent plenty of nights soothing a crying child, but I never took our kids into our bed or indulged in any nonsense at bedtime. Our children had my attention all day; they did not need it when they were sleeping. Letting a child into our bed (if there was not a really good reason) was no solution in the long run. All of our children learned to be great sleepers.

—*Elizabeth Chabner Thompson, MD, MPH*

Transitioning to a Toddler Bed

Most toddlers are ready to move into a "big-kid" bed around age two. Some children have started to climb out of their cribs long before that, and other toddlers are perfectly comfortable sleeping in their cribs long after. In any event, when you make the switch to the big-kid bed, and your toddler is no longer safely confined to her crib at night, you need to carefully reevaluate your baby-proofing efforts in her room, and beyond.

When my older son was 15 months old, he figured out how to escape from his crib. My husband and I didn't want him falling 3½ feet to the floor, so we transitioned him out of his crib. He didn't have a bed yet, so we simply put his crib mattress on the floor. Now we had a new problem: He could escape from his room.

—*Carrie Brown, MD*

One of my twin daughters was a climber, so I had to transition them both from their cribs to beds when they were two years old.

My son is 2½. He's certainly capable of climbing out of his crib, but he doesn't. My plan is to keep him in that crib as long as I can. I'm not looking forward to him being able to wander around the house at night.

—*Brooke A. Jackson, MD*

My younger son is a climber. A few months ago, we were on a trip, and he climbed out of the hotel's crib. *We'll see how this goes when we get home*, I thought.

Sure enough, my son now climbs out of his crib pretty much right after we put him into it. I know that I have to transition him to a bed. But at least now, we have a few seconds' head start to race out of his room and close the door before my son makes it out of his crib. Once my son is in a bed, we'll lose that advantage!

Of course, I worry that my son will catch his foot on the crib rail, fall, and get hurt. So I think it's time to put him in a bed. At this point, after he climbs out of his crib, he falls asleep on the floor, right inside his door.

—*Rebecca Reamy, MD, a mom of seven- and two-year-old sons and a pediatrician in emergency medicine at Children's Healthcare of Atlanta, in Georgia*

My family moved from a condo to a house when my older son was two years old. He had just started trying to climb out of his crib, so that seemed like the logical time to transition him from his crib to a bed. My younger son was born around that same time, so that made for a lot of changes in a short amount of time for my older son!

I had a really hard time keeping him in his bed. I tried to be as consistent as possible with his bedtime routine and returning him to his bed if he got out. I also tried to make his bed as comfortable as possible, with soft pillows and his favorite stuffed animals.

I also set up a reward system. I told my son that once he stayed in his room for an entire night, I would buy him a present he really wanted. At first, he wanted a kids' guitar. Then a violin. I couldn't deliver on that, so I was able to talk him back to the guitar, which he pretends is a violin.

By about three months after our move and sleeping in his own bed, my son was pretty consistently staying in bed!

—*Deborah Kulick, MD, a mom of two-year-old and eight-month-old sons, a child and adolescent psychiatrist at the Everett Teen Health Center, and an instructor in psychiatry at Harvard Medical School and the Cambridge Health Alliance, in Boston, MA*

Dealing with Nighttime Wakings

According to the National Sleep Foundation, most children spend 40 percent of their childhoods asleep. It might not feel like that, however, when your toddler wakes you from a sound sleep in the middle of the night. A change in routine, such as transitioning to a toddler bed, is a common cause of nighttime wakings.

I found that a hard habit to break is babies and toddlers waking up in the middle of the night for milk. These nighttime rendezvous are hard to stop. Certainly by age three months, babies do not need to eat in the middle of the night. If you continue these nighttime feedings, you're putting yourself farther and farther away from having a good night's sleep.

I've met parents from the Netherlands, where they believe a

healthy newborn baby doesn't need to be fed at night. They actually teach all new parents that. If your toddler wakes up, make sure she's dry and put her back to bed! Yes, you can leave a water bottle where your toddler can get a sip, by herself, but don't let her expect the kitchen to be open at the wee hours. Mommy and Daddy should be off feeding duty at night and sleeping.

—*Ayala Laufer-Cahana, MD*

My son often wakes up at 2 in the morning, runs into our room, and wants to sleep with us. I don't fight it. I know I probably should, but for this year, I'm going to let it slide. I know it won't last forever. He wants to cuddle and be close to me. If that makes him feel more comfortable and secure, that's totally fine with me.

I try to look at the big picture. If letting my son come sleep the rest of the night with me lets him fall asleep, so I can fall back to sleep, we're all getting sleep. That's a good thing.

—*Shilpa Amin-Shah, MD*

It wasn't an issue for me to keep my toddlers in their beds because we slept in a family bed throughout their toddler years. As a working mother, I felt that a family bed gave me more time with my sons. Even sleep is a very important time of communication. No words are said, but there is energy, and also overnight there are thoughts and feelings.

Looking back now, I think my sons would have been fine if I'd weaned them from the family bed sooner, though.

—*Lauren Feder, MD, a mom of 18- and 14-year-old sons, a nationally recognized physician who specializes in homeopathic medicine, and the author of* Natural Baby and Childcare *and* The Parents' Concise Guide to Childhood Vaccinations, *in Los Angeles, CA*

Fortunately, my son didn't wake up often in the night. He really only did so when he was sick, jet-lagged, or teething. However, he went through a period of time where he would scream and thrash about while still sleeping, usually between midnight and 2 am. It turned out that he needed to pee. Even though he was wearing a pull-up diaper, his little brain knew not to pee into it because he was fully potty trained during the day. This stopped when I began restricting fluids at night.

As a very physically active little person, it was hard for my son to physically "turn off" himself at night, even though he was mentally exhausted. I realized he needed to learn how to physically relax his body. So when he was two or three years old, I had to give him very specific "go-to-sleep" instructions at night: 1. Lie down. 2. Close your eyes. 3. Stop moving. 4. Stop talking. 5. Relax! This is all while he was hanging upside down on his bed and yelling, "Mommy, it's so hard to go to sleep!"

I also taught my son how to take deep breaths, and for a while we used the scent of lavender oil to help him relax. I know that the basis behind aromatherapy is that the olfactory center is associated with different emotions, so I hoped that I could condition my son's brain into associating a certain smell with relaxation. It didn't really work (I think it takes a much longer time to condition a brain!), but he did finally learn how to relax his body.

—*Cheryl Wu, MD*

When my children were toddlers, I was a strict schedule mom because I needed my sleep as much as they did. I sleep-trained all three of my girls between four and six months. I used a modified method: When one of my daughters woke up, I would go into her room, but I did not speak or make eye contact with her because both of those are cues for babies to wake up. I gave her a pacifier, a snuggly, and a back rub to soothe her, and then walked out. I would repeat this every 15 to 20 minutes until she stopped crying. It was tough, and it took about three nights before my daughters slept through the night, but it was worth it! I now have the best sleepers.

My pediatrician warned me that it's important for babies to develop healthy sleeping habits by six months because after that, whatever habits they develop, you're stuck with until age five. That was all I needed to hear to suffer through those long nights of sleep training!

Because I started sleep training so early, my girls now have such great sleeping habits that I can recall only a handful of times that they woke up in the middle of the night. When they did, it was always because they were sick.

—*Marra S. Francis, MD, a mom of eight-, seven-, and five-year-old daughters and a gynecologist, in San Antonio, TX*

My kids shared a room when they were toddlers. At first, of course, my son slept in a crib and my daughter slept in a twin bed. Generally, this worked out well, but we did go through a brief period when my daughter wasn't happy to have a little brother, and she'd stick her hand in his crib and tweak him! My husband and I moved her to another room for a while for our son's safety! But otherwise, it worked out very well having them share a room.

My husband and I weren't too strict with the noise. If our kids were laughing and talking, that was fine. As long as they weren't coming out of their room, turning on the lights, or being disruptive, we were happy.

We went through phases where our kids, especially our son, would come into our room to sleep with us. Nine out of 10 times, I was so exhausted that I didn't mind. My husband was a little less enthused about having a third person in bed with us. Up until our son was about 2½, we didn't make a big deal out of it. If he came into our bed at night, that was okay. But as our son got older and more verbal, we became more firm about wanting him to sleep in his own bed. If he came into our room, I'd escort him back to his own bed.

Sometimes I'd stay in my kids' room to help them get back to sleep. I remember one night I woke up totally disconcerted because no one was sleeping where they were supposed to be sleeping! One child was in my bed, and I was on the sofa. I couldn't figure out what had happened overnight!

At that time, it felt like it would never end, and I'd have a 20-year-old sleeping with us. Looking back now, though, I think our kids just wanted to be in a warm bed with their parents. It wasn't a big deal, and they outgrew it. In hindsight, kids really become independent very quickly.

—*Ann V. Arthur, MD, a mom of a 10-year-old daughter and an 8-year-old son, a pediatric ophthalmologist in private practice at Park Slope Eye Care Associates, and a blogger at WaterWineTravel.com, in New York City*

⊛

Regarding sleep, what I tell my patients and what I did are two different things. I'm a big believer in establishing healthy sleep habits early and sleep-training babies when they are young. That's great in theory, but I know that is very hard to do in practice. You have to be very consistent and disciplined. When your child comes into your room, you should return her to her own bed. That's very hard to do when you are sleep deprived and tired or when the parents are on different pages and one can tolerate the child crying but the other can't.

My husband and I ended up having one of our children sleeping on our bedroom floor! He didn't start out there. He crept into our room each night, and we'd find him there in the morning. Our son was still doing that when he was five years old.

One day, one of my colleagues asked me, "What are you doing?" That shamed me into doing the tough love, making my son go back to his own room at night.

—*Victoria McEvoy, MD, a mom who raised four children; a grandmom of six-, four-, and two-year-old grandsons; an assistant professor of pediatrics at Harvard Medical School; the medical director and chief of pediatrics at Mass General West Medical Group; and the author of* 24/7 Baby Doctor, *in Boston, MA*

Coping with Nightmares and Night Terrors

Between 12 and 14 months, children begin actively dreaming. Bad dreams are very common—and very scary—for toddlers because they can't distinguish between imagination and reality. Nightmares are more common when a child is experiencing anxiety or stress. A child who's overtired or sleep deprived is more likely to have disturbed sleep too.

Nightmares occur in the stage of sleep known as rapid eye movement, or REM, sleep, so they usually happen in the second half of the night, when REM sleep is more frequent. Nightmares peak between the ages of three and six years. During those years, about a quarter of children have at least one nightmare a week.

Night terrors, on the other hand, wake a child from non-REM sleep. They usually happen earlier in the night. After a night terror, a child is usually calm and falls back to sleep quickly.

Living in Miami, we have a lot of Latin influence, and people here are more familiar with the concept of the family bed. We didn't actually have a family bed, but in the night if one of my daughters woke from a bad dream and came into bed with me, I didn't mind, and I didn't make the effort to send her back to her own room. I knew she would out-grow it, and she did.

—*Eva Ritvo, MD*

My older daughter had pretty bad nightmares. I found that I couldn't do anything to prevent them. I just had to make sure that my daughter was safe and couldn't hurt herself by falling off the bed. I noticed that my daughter's nightmares lessened when I stopped letting her watch TV before bedtime. After her bath, we would do story time and then go straight to bed.

—*Jeannette Gonzalez Simon, MD, a mom of three- and one-year-old daughters and a pediatric gastroenterologist in private practice, in Staten Island, NY*

Every once in a while, my kids have nightmares. If I hear my kids cry in the night, I run to their room and calm them down.

"I love you," I tell them. "Everything is okay. Mommy and Daddy are here." Then I tuck them back into bed. They're usually very sleepy and go back to sleep easily.

—*Sadaf T. Bhutta, MD, a mom of a six-year-old daughter and four-year-old triplets and an assistant professor and the fellowship director of pediatric radiology at the University of Arkansas for*

Medical Sciences and Arkansas Children's Hospital, both in Little Rock

Most nights, around 2:30, one of my twins comes to visit and climbs in bed with me and my husband. She will not stay in her own bed all night. I think that she might be having bad dreams. I want her to feel that she is safe and that she can come and sleep with us when she's scared.

But another part of me wonders if she does this to have a little time with her parents. I can understand if she's craving some special time to have Mommy and Daddy all to herself.

—*Brooke A. Jackson, MD*

Like many children, my son developed a fear of the dark. (Or maybe just a fear of bedtime.) He became afraid of his room at night, so bedtime was a huge ordeal. Thanks to the suggestion of his teacher, we made a spray bottle of "Monster Spray" and would spray any problem area before going to bed. We also read *Bedtime for Frances*, one of my favorite childhood books, and my son decided that it might help to have his stuffed animals take turns keeping watch just like Frances's

? When to Call Your Doctor

Nightmares, which usually start between age three and five, can feel very real to your toddler and can make her fearful about going back to sleep. Oftentimes comforting her, talking about the nightmare during the day, having a fun bedtime routine, avoiding scary bedtime stories and television shows, sticking with a bedtime schedule, and using your own unique strategies to deal with nightmares will help your child cope.

It's time to call your doctor about your child's nightmares when the bad dreams become worse or start to happen more often, when your child is so afraid that it interferes with activities during the day, when nightmares are extremely distressing to your child, or when a psychological problem might be involved.

animals did. When my son wouldn't sleep without a light on, I hung a strand of Christmas lights on the ceiling as a compromise. I've recently discovered that an even better option is an old wake-up light that I had years ago. I can gradually dim the light while we're reading stories, so he doesn't notice that it's getting darker. It's just enough light to keep him from being scared, but not enough to disrupt his sleep.

—*Lennox McNeary, MD, a mom of a three-year-old son, a specialist in physical medicine and rehabilitation at Carilion Clinic, and a cofounder of the Mommy Doctors Bakery (makers of Milkin' Cookies), in Roanoke, VA*

My husband and I have never been bed sharers. I think it's important for kids to know that Mommy and Daddy need to have a good relationship and time together, and that when Mommy and Daddy are happy, everyone is happy.

When my kids were toddlers and had nightmares, I'd take time to comfort them, but then I'd take them back to their own rooms to go back to sleep. For some reason I've never had much of a problem with this, maybe because we just never let them sleep with us, even as infants. If they get scared, I plug in their night-lights, tuck them back in all cozy, and make sure to put some positive or happy thoughts in their heads so that's the last thing they hear.

—*Antoinette Cheney, DO, a mom of a seven-year-old son and a six-year-old daughter and a family physician with Rocky Vista University College of Osteopathic Medicine, in Parker, CO*

My middle son has terrible nightmares. Several times a week, he wakes up screaming and crying, and it's very difficult to settle him back down.

My husband and I are still trying to figure out what's causing them. We've tried various things, such as calming him down and letting him cry it out to go back to sleep. But nothing seems to make a difference. We're taking my son to his pediatrician to get his advice.

—*Amy Thompson, MD, a mom of five- and three- and two-year-old sons and an ob-gyn at the University of Cincinnati College of Medicine, in Ohio*

RALLIE'S TIP

There's nothing as sweet as a sleepy, cuddly toddler. I loved snuggling with my boys while I read them their favorite bedtime stories. Before tucking them into bed with a goodnight kiss, I'd ask them what they wanted to dream about that night. I'm not sure, but I think it might have helped them to have more sweet dreams and fewer nightmares. Asking them what they wanted to dream about helped focus their minds on positive, happy things as they were drifting off to sleep.

In the morning, I also loved asking my boys what they dreamed about the night before. Listening to your child tell you about his dreams is a great way to learn what's on his mind, good or bad.

Because sweet dreams aren't just for nighttime, I always encouraged my boys to tell me about their dreams for the future—whether it was later in the week or later in life. When my sons were toddlers, we'd sit down with a pile of old magazines and make "dream boards." I'd give them each a big piece of cardboard and some gluesticks, and I'd cut out pictures they found in magazines of things that they wanted to do, have, be, or feel. Sometimes they'd choose pictures of toys they'd like to have, but more often, they'd choose photos of laughing children playing tag, a boy riding a skateboard, a happy family on a picnic, or a fireman in his uniform.

While we were gluing the pictures on the cardboard, we talked about the dreams that they represented—going on a picnic at the playground, learning to ride a skateboard, or growing up to be a fireman.

Even when my boys were toddlers, I began teaching them that it was always within their power to achieve their goals. With enough passion, belief, and hard work, dreams really do come true!

Index

Dolan, Siobhan, 147, 152, 202, 307, 309, 352, 432, 443, 444
Doorknob locks, 147, 150, KidCo Door Knob Locks, <u>150</u>
Door locking, as safety measure, 139, 141, 142, 147, 150, 151, 155
Drawing, 356, 385
Dream boards, 471
Dreaming, 467, 471. *See also* Nightmares
Dressing toddlers, 243, 250–53. *See also* Clothing
Dr. Hana's Nasopure 2 Squirts, <u>185</u>
Driving, avoiding distractions during, 152, 153
Drowning, 157, 160, 161, 163, 231
Dry lips, 201
Dry skin, <u>160, 201</u>
Duralux glasses, 115
DVD player, 392, 413, 419, 421

E

Earaches or ear infections
  allergies and, 184–85
  cause of, 173
  diminished appetite from, 74
  fever with, <u>203, 417</u>
  incidence of, 172
  preventing and treating, 135, 173–76, 221
  from teething, 220–21
  When to Call Your Doctor about, <u>160, 174, 417</u>
Early Intervention support system, 17
Ears, cleaning, 233
Ear tubes, 173, 175, 176
Easter, 352
Eating. *See also* Cooking; Foods
  bottlefeeding for (*see* Bottlefeeding)
  breastfeeding for (*see* Breastfeeding)
  excessive, preventing, 65–69
  at family meals, 52–55
  healthy, encouraging, 57–64
  in high chair, 45–48
  learning to use utensils and dishes for, 80–81

messy
  avoiding, 80
  cleaning up, 48–50
  nighttime, avoiding, 463–64
  picky, 26, 51, 62–63, 69–77
Eating out. *See* Restaurants
Eczema
  allergies and, 40, 44, 109, 200
  in ear, <u>160</u>
  treating, 199–201, <u>201</u>
Education, saving for, 399, 400–401
Eggs
  allergy to, 40, 42–43, 45
  organic, 33
Environment, allergies and, 185
Epiglottitis, 206
Eucerin Cream, 201, <u>201</u>
Exercise
  for children, encouraging, 401, 402–3, 404, 405, 406
  from dog walking, 164
  for moms, 2, 281, 285, 286, 287, <u>318,</u> 402, 404–5, 406
  TV time during, 389
Extinguishing, as discipline technique, 321

F

Facial changes, of toddlers, 3, 8
Failure to thrive, symptoms of, <u>7</u>
Falls
  from climbing (*see* Climbing, accidents from)
  from high chair, 147
  preventing, 140
  treating scrapes from, 409
Family bed, 291, 464, 468
Family meals, 52–55
Family size, poll about, 308–9
Family traditions, 358–60
Feder, Lauren, 91, 283, 291, 326–27, 431, 442, 464
Fertility drugs, 303
Fever
  with colds, <u>179,</u> 181
  with conjunctivitis, <u>208</u>
  determining cause of, 204

tart, sweetening, 60
FunBites, for cutting foods, 29
Furniture, toddler proofing and, 137, 147–48, 149

G

Game night, 358
Games
  car seat, 152
  computer, 377
  iPad, 357, 385
  outdoor, 9, 391, 403
  for trips, 410, 421
Garden, vegetable, 60
Gastroenteritis. *See* Stomach viruses
Gastrointestinal health, probiotics for, 135
Gates, baby, 138–39, 141, 147, 148, 150
Genetically modified foods, 34
Gerber Graduates Grabbers Squeezable Fruit, 367
Germs, minimizing spread of, 177, 255, 396, 408, 414, 415, 422
Gilboa, Deborah, 9–10, 56, 63, 75, 83, 146, 150, 164, 251, 311, 314, 317–18, 322–23, 361–62, 370, 388–89, 395, 409, 437–38
Ginger, for motion sickness, 411
Girls' night out, ideas for, 306
Gluten intolerance, 72
Goggles, for hair washing, 237
Go-Go Kidz Travelmate, 420
Gohara, Mona, 28, 122, 199, 247, 357, 361, 378, 403, 444–45
Gold Bug 2 in 1 Harness Buddy, 424
GoNannies.com, 57
Grocery shopping, with toddlers, 365–66, 368–70
Gross motor skills, 8, 9, 10
Growth, 2, 3–7, 119
  healthy, 67
  slowdown in, 51, 66, 69, 73, 76
  When to Call Your Doctor about, 7, 73
Growth chart, 4, 5, 6, 7, 65, 73
Guilt, of moms, 286, 289
Gums, brushing, 215, 217

H

Haircuts, 238–40
Hairstyle, moms changing, 239
Hair washing and detangling, 236–38
Halloween, 352
Hammock, for MomMy Time, 452
Hand, foot, and mouth disease, 187
Handbags, PonyUP! Kentucky, 243
Hand-eye coordination, 18–21, 25, 79, 377, 404
  When to Call Your Doctor about, 19
Hand sanitizer, 195, 423
Hand washing, 230
  for preventing
    colds, 176–77, 178
    conjunctivitis, 208
    stomach viruses, 195
  during travel, 415
Hanes, Jennifer, 16, 53, 56, 95, 97, 105–6, 114, 132, 153, 168, 173, 179, 207, 216, 223, 226, 237, 239, 247–48, 255, 269, 323, 331, 356, 363, 373, 402
Hanukkah, 354
Harnesses, 423
  CARES Harness, 419
  Gold Bug 2 in 1 Harness Buddy, 424
Head banging, 14, 331, 332
Head circumference, of toddlers, 3, 7
Head injuries, 170–71, 417
Heart disease, from smoking, 136
Heatstroke, When to Call Your Doctor about, 262
Height, of toddlers, 3, 4, 6–7, 63, 67, 68
Helpers. *See also* Babysitters; Child care; Mommy's helpers; Nannies
  finding and hiring, 57, 446, 447
  toddlers as, around the house, 393–97
Hevea's Pond Bath Toys, 235
Highchair Organizer, 46
High chairs, 45–48, 49, 53, 54
  falling from, 147
Hitting, discipline for, 339–41

Hobbies, for moms, 283, 284, 285, 286, 287
Holidays
  celebrating, 351–55, 360
  unique, 348–49
Holland, Tanya Douglas, 4, 18–19, 50, 71, 81, 82, 133, 180, 201, 231, 253, 261, 269, 287, 355, 368–69, 378–79, 394, 402–3, 408, 451–52
Homeaway.com, for finding vacation lodging, 418
Homeopathic remedies
  for behavioral issues, 326–27
  for sore throats, 188
Honey
  for coughs, 179, 422
  for sore throats, 189
  in tea, 183, 189
Hotels, 418, 427–28
Household chores, toddlers helping with, 393–97
Hubka, Teresa, 61, 158–59, 260, 283, 310, 345, 350–51, 363, 374, 379–80, 387, 403–4, 425
Humidifier, 181
Hypothermia, 259

I

Ibuprofen
  accidental ingestion of, 133–34
  for treating
    earaches, 174
    fevers, 132, 202, 203, 203, 204, 205
    pain after shots, 125
    pain from bumps and bruises, 169
    sore throats, 189
    teething pain, 221, 222
Ice packs, 125–26, 132, 168
Identification tags, 425, 427
Illnesses. See also specific illnesses
  When to Call Your Doctor about, 120–21
Immune system, role of, 42, 182, 183, 205

Immunity
  breastfeeding increasing, 85, 86, 88, 115
  probiotics improving, 135, 177
  stress lowering, 300, 414
Immunizations. See Vaccinations
Independence
  development of, 2, 18, 227, 280, 312, 333, 439, 444, 467
  with dressing, 258
  with feeding, 24, 25, 50, 80, 94, 162
  fostering, 299, 328, 387–88
  preventing sleep, 450
  toddlers' craving for, 9, 14, 25, 80, 251, 342, 439
Infections
  diminished appetite from, 74
  ear (see Earaches or ear infections)
  sinus, 74, 135, 181
  urinary tract, 275, 414
Inflate-a-Potty, 274
In-laws, nurturing relationship with, 307, 308
Insect Repellent, Cutter Advanced, 362
Insurance, travel, 416
Internet research, on health concerns, 122
IntraKID liquid multivitamin, 134
iPad, 126, 357, 377, 385
Iron deficiency, 58

J

Jackson, Brooke A., 78, 178, 286, 312, 351, 419–20, 457, 460–61, 462, 469
Jaliman, Debra, 60–61, 108, 111, 164–65, 250, 315–16, 337, 386
Jogging strollers, 403, 406
Journaling, 374, 375
Juice, fruit. See Fruit juice
Juice box, for numbing vaccination site, 125

K

K&J Sunprotective Clothing, 361
Keratosis pilaris, 201

Putting nonfood items into mouth, 18, 21, 36, 222–25
When to Call Your Doctor about, 223, 225
Puzzles, 384–85

Q

Q-tips, 233
Queasy Pop Kids by Three Lollies, 198
Quiet time
for moms, 283
for toddlers, finding fun in, 355–58

R

Rappaport, Nancy, 41, 90, 281
Rash(es)
diaper, 200, 201, 244–45
preventing and treating, 246–48
When to Call Your Doctor about, 200
fever with, 203, 416
viral, 199
Reading. See also Books
before bed, 458, 461, 471
benefits of, 286, 378–81
as hobby for moms, 283, 284, 285
instilling love of, 376, 379
learning, 381, 386
Reamy, Rebecca, 6, 10–11, 20, 27, 81, 138–39, 142, 145, 150, 164, 171, 256, 311, 331, 338, 340, 353, 362–63, 373, 377, 382–83, 390–91, 394, 462
References, about caregivers, 436–37
Refrigerator locks, 141
Safety 1st Refrigerator Door Lock, 144
Regenerative medicine, cord blood used in, 302, 303
Relationships
circle exercise for prioritizing, 280–81
nurturing
with children, 296–301
with friends, 304–6
garden analogy about, 295
with parents, 307–8

with self, 281–89
between siblings, 308–13
with spouse, 290–96
toddlers' formation of, with others, 280, 296
Religion, introducing toddler to, 397–99
Rental equipment, for travel, 415, 421
Restaurants
behavior in, 12
drinking from cup in, 105–6
eating in, 81–83
as family tradition, 359
Rewards, 164, 297, 310, 333, 334, 393, 396, 463. See also M&Ms, as rewards; Stickers, as rewards
Rheumatic fever, 190
Ritvo, Eva, 11, 13, 59, 122–23, 124, 152–53, 155, 161, 265, 317, 324, 327–28, 333–34, 364, 371, 393, 397, 405–6, 431, 443–44, 451, 468
Rohde, Rachel S., 47, 52, 81, 82, 99, 110–11, 113, 119, 127, 142, 148–49, 234, 249, 267, 367, 383, 389, 454
Rosch, Laura M., 61–62, 186–87, 287–88, 299, 357, 365, 369–70, 387–88, 410–11
Rowell, Katja, 26, 44, 46, 49, 54, 67, 71, 95–96, 114–15, 270, 375, 459
Running, 8, 9, 17

S

Safety
bathtub, 140, 143, 231–34
car, 151–54, 164
crib, 137
fireplace, 148–49
kitchen, 78
outdoors, 155–57
around pets, 162–66
pool, 157–62, 262, 427
toddler proofing for (see Toddler proofing)
with toys, 137

travel, 427–28
Safety equipment, for sports, 157
Safety 1st Oven and Refrigerator
       Locks, <u>144</u>
Saline spray or washes
    for allergies, <u>185,</u> 186
    for nasal congestion, 178, 180–81
Scavenger hunts, 356
Scrapes. *See* Cuts and scrapes
Security, fostering feelings of, 300–301
Self-care for moms, 281–89
Self-discipline for toddlers. *See*
       Discipline
Self-esteem, building, 316–19, 371
Separation anxiety, 434, 439–42
Serving sizes, 67
Sexual abuse, 435, 443–44
Shampoos, 233, 236
Shellfish allergy, 40, 43, 45
Shoes
    buying, 255, 256, 257
    ID tag for, 425
    organizing, 256–57, 258
    outgrown, donating, 258–59
    removing at front door, 395
    sandals, 261
    Stride Rite, <u>258</u>
    tying, 243
Shopping, with toddlers, 365–71
Shots, 123–26. *See also* Vaccinations
Siblings
    age gaps between, 301
    encouraging peace between, 308–13
Signing Time, for learning sign
       language, <u>16</u>
Similac SimplySmart bottle, <u>96</u>
Simon, Jeannette Gonzalez, 99, 129,
       193, 213, 242, 257, 296–97,
       342, 344, 428, 436, 468
Simpler, Dana S., 26, 70, 80, 107–8,
       175, 184, 251, 309, 352–53, 355,
       395, 404, 454–55
SimplySmart On-the-Go Powder Cap,
       <u>96</u>
Sinus infections, 181
    antibiotics for, 135
    diminished appetite from, 74

Sippy cups
    for air travel, 412
    cleaning, 112–15
    Foogo, <u>114</u>
    keeping drinks cold in, 113, 115
    preventing tooth decay from, 112–13
    transitioning to, 94, 99, 100, 101,
       103, 104–6
Skin problems. *See also* Dry lips; Dry
       skin; Eczema; Rash(es)
    preventing and treating, 199–201
Sleep
    challenges with, 450, 453–61
    during colds, 178, 180
    dreaming during, 467, 471
    for fevers, 205
    naps for, 450, 451–53
    nightmares and night terrors during,
       467–70
    nighttime wakings from, 463–67
    poor, When to Call Your Doctor
       about, <u>457</u>
    recommended amount of, 450
    routines for (*see* Bedtime routines)
    transitioning to toddler bed for,
       461–63
    during travel, 413, 414, 428
Sleep deprivation, 287, 451, 467
Sleepovers, 365
Sleep training, 455, 465–66, 467
Sleepwear, 137
Sling, as baby carrier, 299
Slippery elm, for nausea and vomiting,
       198
Smoke alarms, 137–38
Smoking
    health risks from, 136
    teaching avoidance of, 405–6
Smoothies, 59, 79, 106, 109, 193
Snacks
    calories in, 69
    nutritious, 63, 70
    preventing overeating of, 66
    for shopping trips, 366, <u>367,</u> 369
    for travel, 422
    unhealthy, for moms, 288–89
Snoring, <u>457</u>

Solomon, Hana R., 15, 27, 50, 79, 185–86, <u>185,</u> 305, 372
Solve Your Child's Sleep Problems, 455
Sore throats. *See also* Strep throat
    fever with, <u>203</u>
    preventing and treating, 177, 179, 187–90
    When to Call Your Doctor about, <u>188,</u> <u>417</u>
Soy allergy, 40, 41, 45
Soy milk, 106, 107, 109
Spanking, 321, 322, 326, 329, 330
Spa treatments, for moms, 230, 283
Speech delays
    evaluating, 14, 15–17
    When to Call Your Doctor about, <u>13,</u> <u>384</u>
Speech development, 3, 11–17
Speedo Kid's UV Neoprene Swim Vest, <u>159</u>
Sports, safety equipment for, 157
Spouse, nurturing relationship with, 290–96
Stair climbing, 8, 10, 148
Stem cells, in umbilical cord blood, 302, <u>302</u>
Stickers, as rewards, 123, 152, 268, 269, 272, <u>333</u>
Stomach upset. *See* Bellyaches; Nausea; Stomach viruses; Vomiting
Stomach viruses, 194–95, 196
Stove safety, 141
    Prince LionHeart Stove Guard for, <u>146</u>
    Safety 1st Oven Door Lock for, <u>144</u>
Strachan, Dina, 8, 28–29, 34, 58–59, 138, 181, 249, 297, 336–37, 455
Strawberries, allergy to, 41, 43
Straws, for drinking from cup, 99, 104, 106, 114
    cleaning, 113–14
Strep throat, 187, <u>188,</u> 189, 190, 204
Stress, lowering immunity, 300, 414
Stride Rite Shoes, <u>258</u>
Strollers
    jogging, 403, 406
    for shopping with toddlers, 366–67
    for trips, 409, 412, 415
Stroller Strides classes, 406
Suffocation hazards, 137, 140, 148
Summer, keeping cool in, 261–62
Summer Infant Dr. Mom Nail Clipper Set, <u>242</u>
Sun protection, 261–62
Sunscreen, 155–56, 361, 422
Sunshine Kids Radian 65 car seat, 152
Sunsweet Essence Orange-Flavored Prunes, <u>194</u>
Supplements, 132. *See also* Calcium supplements; Vitamins
Suppositories, FeverAll, <u>207</u>
Sweetener, agave nectar as, 60
Swimmer's ear, When to Call Your Doctor about, <u>160</u>
Swimming lessons, 157, 158–59, 160–61, 389
Swimming safety. *See* Pool safety
Swim Vest, Speedo Kid's UV Neoprene, <u>159</u>
Symptoms, When to Call Your Doctor about, <u>120–21</u>

T

Take & Toss cups, 105
Talking, 8, 11–17
Tanios, Aline T., 37, 104, 126, 160, 184, 224, 231, 235, 274, 309, 314, 322, 396–97, 408–9, 421–22
Tantrums. *See* Temper tantrums
Tea
    for colds, 183
    peppermint, for bellyaches, 199
    for relaxation, 287
Teeth. *See also* Dental care; Dentist
    baby
        age at losing, 209
        number of, 209
        premature loss of, <u>216</u>
    brushing, 215–19
        biting during, 340
    decayed (*see* Tooth decay)
    pacifier or thumb-sucking affecting, 225, 227

Teething, biting during, 340
Teething pain, 220–22
    When to Call Your Dentist about,
        221
Teething rings, 221–22, 221
Television. *See* TV
Temper tantrums, 153, 320, 324, 331,
        332–38, 342, 366
Temple, taking toddler to, 397, 398
Tent
    crib, 459
    for indoor play, 357
Thermometer, rectal, 204
Thompson, Amy, 178, 196–97, 199–
        200, 206, 238, 244, 257, 259–
        60, 314–15, 322, 470
Thompson, Elizabeth Chabner, 48–49,
        55, 62–63, 101, 290, 297, 318,
        335, 365, 392, 404–5, 445, 453,
        461
Thumb-sucking, weaning from, 225,
        226, 227
Time-out place, for moms, 320–21
Time-outs, for discipline, 314, 320,
        321, 324, 325–26, 333
Toddler bed, transitioning to, 461–63
Toddler proofing, 18, 136. *See also*
        Safety
    bathrooms and kitchen, 139–47
    hotel rooms, 428
    living areas, 147–51
    nursery, 137–39
    after transitioning to toddler bed,
        462
Toenails, trimming, 241–42
Toilet locks, 140, 142
    KidCo Toilet Lid Lock, 143
Tom's of Maine Toothpaste, 217
Tooth decay
    causes of
        bottlefeeding, 98, 100, 102, 104
        fruit juice, 111, 112
        nursing to sleep, 91
        sippy cups, 112–13
    preventing, 112–13, 209, 215–20
    problems from, 209, 216
Toothpaste, 218, 219

Tom's of Maine Toothpaste,
        217
Towel, Avon Toddler Hooded,
        232
Toys
    bath
        cleaning, 234–36
        Hevea's Pond Bath Toys, 235
    caring for, 372–73, 394
    gender-balanced, 373–74
    pet, safety with, 163
    recycling, 352–53, 373
    safety with, 137
    time-outs for, 326
    for travel, 409, 412, 413, 419, 419,
        421, 422
Traditions, family, 358–60
Training pants, cloth, 271
Train travel, 413
Trauma shears, for haircuts, 239
Travel
    to amusement parks, 423–27
    without children, 291, 293
    day trips, 408–12
    planning downtime after, 407
    safety during, 427–28
    sickness during, When to Call Your
        Doctor about, 416–17
    toys for, 409, 412, 413, 419, 419, 421,
        422
    vacations, 407, 412–23
Travel bag, packing, 387, 408–9, 413,
        415, 419, 421–23
Travel insurance, 416
Travelmate, Go-Go Kidz, 420
Tree nut allergy, 40, 44, 45, 106
Triple Paste, for diaper rash, 247
Triplets. *See also* Twins
    development of, 8–9
    transitioning to sippy cup, 100
Trips. *See* Travel
T-shirts, sun-protective, 361
Tulenko, Kate, 17, 41, 57, 67–68, 107,
        128, 157, 161, 173, 177, 195, 285,
        291, 315, 318, 357–58, 364,
        366, 373–74, 385–86, 392, 400,
        402, 409–10, 413

TV
    for moms, <u>390</u>
    for toddlers
        bedtime and, 468, <u>469</u>
        monitoring, 389–93
Twins. *See also* Triplets
    appetites of, 66
    bedtime routines for, 458, 460–61
    breastfeeding, 86
    competition between, 312
    doctor visits for, 127–28
    dressing, 249, 250
    growth of, 5
    hiring help for, 287–88
    messy eating and, 49–50
    potty training, 266, 274–75
    shopping with, 366, 369
    spending time away from, 289
    whole milk for, 108
Tylenol. *See* Acetaminophen
Tylenol Children's Meltaways, 133

U

Umbilical cord blood banking, 301–3,
        <u>302,</u> 304
Underweight, <u>73</u>
Upset stomach. *See* Bellyaches;
        Nausea; Stomach viruses;
        Vomiting
Urinary incontinence, in women, 263
Urinary tract infection (UTI)
    from travel, 414
    When to Call Your Doctor about, <u>275</u>
U.S. Savings Bonds, 401
Utensils
    learning to use, 80–81
    for restaurant meals, 82
UTI. *See* Urinary tract infection

V

Vacations, 407, 412–23. *See also* Travel
    sickness during, When to Call Your
        Doctor about, <u>416–17</u>
Vaccinations
    for children, 123–26, 173, 184
        fever after, <u>203</u>
    for pets, 163

Valentine, Christy, 59, 226, 264–65,
        298, 305–6, 324, 339, 350, 352,
        353, 391, 399, 423, <u>424</u>
Values, teaching, 314, 315, 358, 405–6
Vaseline, for skin care, 201, 247
Vegetables
    encouraging eating of, 64
    homegrown, 60
    new, trying or introducing, 26, 111
    in nutritious meals, 56, 58, 59, 61
    organic, 33, 34
    pesticides and, 32–33
    for preventing
        colds, 178
        constipation, <u>192,</u> 193
        overeating, 66
    with restaurant meals, 83
Vegetarianism, 28–29, 61, 83
Viruses
    exposure to, during travel, 414
    stomach, 194–95, 196
Vitamin C
    for preventing colds, 177
    for sore throats, 188
Vitamin D
    deficiency of, 58
    sources of, 106, 107
    supplements, 109, 134
Vitamins. *See also specific vitamins*
    multivitamin and mineral, 110, 134,
        422
    safe storage of, 140, 142
Vomiting
    from motion sickness, 411–12
    preventing and treating, 194–99
    When to Call Your Doctor about,
        <u>196, 416</u>

W

Walking, 2–3, 8–9, 10, 17
    problems with, When to Call Your
        Doctor about, <u>10</u>
Walt Disney World, 422, 423, 424,
        <u>424</u>
Wang, Dora Calott, 34–35, 56–57,
        299–300, 328–29, 331, 334,
        438, 446–47

About the Authors

RALLIE MCALLISTER, MD, MPH, MSEH

Dr. McAllister is a family physician and nationally known health expert. She is also a cofounder of Momosa Publishing LLC, publisher of MommyMDGuides.com and DaddyMD Guides.com and the Mommy MD Guides book series. She is a coauthor of *The Mommy MD Guide to Pregnancy and Birth* and *The Mommy MD Guide to Your Baby's First Year*.

Dr. McAllister's nationally syndicated newspaper column, Your Health, appeared in more than 30 newspapers in the United States and Canada, and it was read by more than a million people each week.

A nationally recognized physician, Dr. McAllister has been the featured medical expert on more than 100 radio and television shows, including *Good Morning America Health* and *FoxNews*. She's the former host of *Rallie on Health*, a weekly regional health magazine on WJHL News Channel 11 with more than one million viewers in a five-state area, and *No Bones about It*, a weekly radio talk show. A dynamic public speaker, Dr. McAllister educates and entertains audiences from coast to coast with her upbeat, down-to-earth delivery of the latest health news.

Dr. McAllister's healthy-eating tips and interviews have been featured in dozens of popular publications, including *USA Today*, *Women's Day*, *Better Homes and Gardens*, *Redbook*, *Family Circle*, *Parenting*, *Prevention*, *Men's Health*, *Women's World*, *Cosmo*, *Glamour*, *Health Magazine*, *Energy Times*, *Arthritis Today*, and dozens of other newspapers.

Dr. McAllister has authored hundreds of health articles, with millions of additional readers, on dozens of health-related websites, including WebMD.com, LifetimeTV.com, iVillage.com, ParentsMagazine.com, MSN.com, ParentingBookmark.com, FamilyResources.com, ChristianMommies.com, WomenOf.com, and BabyCenter.com.